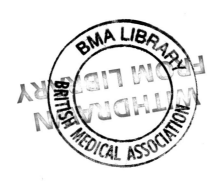
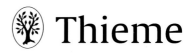

This book is dedicated to the task of advancing our understanding of the earliest manifestations of breast cancer, when the disease is an entirely different clinical entity from its more advanced stages.

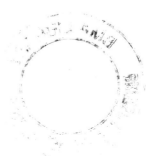

Breast Cancer

Early Detection with Mammography

Crushed Stone–like Calcifications:
The Most Frequent Malignant Type

László Tabár, MD, FACR (Hon)
Professor of Radiology
University of Uppsala School of Medicine
Uppsala, Sweden
Medical Director
Department of Mammography
Central Hospital
Falun, Sweden

Tibor Tot, MD, PhD
Associate Professor of Pathology
University of Uppsala School of Medicine
Uppsala, Sweden
Chairman
Department of Pathology and Clinical Cytology
Central Hospital
Falun, Sweden

Peter B. Dean, MD
Professor
Department of Diagnostic Radiology
University of Turku
Turku, Finland
Formerly Visiting Professor
Brigham and Women's Hospital
Harvard Medical School
Boston, MA, USA

With contributions by
Tony Hsiu-Hsi Chen, DDS, PhD; Stephen W. Duffy, MSc; Amy Ming-Fang Yen, PhD;
Sherry Yueh-Hsia Chiu, PhD

1022 illustrations

Thieme
Stuttgart · New York

Library of Congress Cataloging-in-Publication Data is available from the publisher.

Important note: Medicine is an ever-changing science undergoing continual development. Research and clinical experience are continually expanding our knowledge, in particular our knowledge of proper treatment and drug therapy. Insofar as this book mentions any dosage or application, readers may rest assured that the authors, editors, and publishers have made every effort to ensure that such references are in accordance with **the state of knowledge at the time of production of the book.**

Nevertheless, this does not involve, imply, or express any guarantee or responsibility on the part of the publishers in respect to any dosage instructions and forms of applications stated in the book. **Every user is requested to examine carefully** the manufacturers' leaflets accompanying each drug and to check, if necessary in consultation with a physician or specialist, whether the dosage schedules mentioned therein or the contraindications stated by the manufacturers differ from the statements made in the present book. Such examination is particularly important with drugs that are either rarely used or have been newly released on the market. Every dosage schedule or every form of application used is entirely at the user's own risk and responsibility. The authors and publishers request every user to report to the publishers any discrepancies or inaccuracies noticed. If errors in this work are found after publication, errata will be posted at www.thieme.com on the product description page.

Some of the product names, patents, and registered designs referred to in this book are in fact registered trademarks or proprietary names even though specific reference to this fact is not always made in the text. Therefore, the appearance of a name without designation as proprietary is not to be construed as a representation by the publisher that it is in the public domain.

© 2008 Georg Thieme Verlag,
Rüdigerstrasse 14, 70469 Stuttgart, Germany
http://www.thieme.de
Thieme New York, 333 Seventh Avenue,
New York, NY 10001, USA
http://www.thieme.com

Cover design: Thieme Publishing Group
Typesetting by primustype Hurler GmbH, Notzingen, Germany
Printed in Germany by Druckerei Grammlich, Pliezhausen

ISBN 978-3-13-148531-1

1 2 3 4 5 6

Preface

This book is the second volume of our series *Breast Cancer: Early Detection with Mammography*. The series describes the paradigm shift that early detection of breast cancer can accomplish. In each volume the approach used emphasizes the importance of familiarity with the subgross anatomy of the breast, the pathogenesis of different disease processes, and the capabilities and limitations of the imaging methods in order to be able to understand the nature of the imaging findings. The long-term follow-up of patients diagnosed with the earliest detectable phases of breast cancer completes the circle. Our goal is to inform both the medical community and the women at risk that the development of technology capable of revealing breast cancer at an ever earlier stage has opened the door into a new era in the diagnosis and treatment of breast cancer.

It is important to emphasize the enormous difference between the advanced, palpable breast cancers and the mammographically detected in situ or 1–9 mm invasive carcinomas in every respect, particularly in terms of outcome and treatment requirements. The mammographic tumor features, upon which this series of volumes is based, provide a reliable and reproducible tool for prognostic classification. A characteristic mammographic image of each particular prognostic feature is attached to the corresponding, specific long-term survival curves published in these books. These provide a reliable tool to assist in planning custom-tailored treatment.

Our previous volume *Casting Type Calcifications: Sign of a Subtype with Deceptive Features* singled out one well-defined subgroup of breast cancer having a surprisingly poor prognosis despite its being currently classified as belonging to the size range of small, 1–14 mm tumors. In contrast, this volume deals with a subgroup having a far better prognosis. These books demonstrate how the mammographic prognostic features are capable of distinguishing the breast cancer subtypes originating within the TDLUs (crushed stone–like calcifications) from those subtypes originating within the ducts (casting type calcifications). This important distinction helps describe the precise origin and location of the breast cancer subtypes with distinctly different outcomes. For these reasons we have attempted to clarify the terminology, based on a thorough analysis of the subgross, 3D histological features and the long-term disease outcome. In particular, we point out that the accumulation of malignant cells confined to the TDLUs should not be called "ductal" carcinoma in situ. Also, the growth of cancer cells within the ducts is often associated with an unexpectedly poor outcome, which brings into question whether the term ductal carcinoma "in situ" correctly describes the actual process. Combining these separate disease entities under a common term "ductal carcinoma in situ" (DCIS) leads to confusion in communication and potentially impairs custom-tailored management.

László Tabár
Tibor Tot
Peter B. Dean

List of contributors

The authors are particularly indebted to the principal bio-statisticians in the Two-County Research Team for their long-term commitment to the task of increasing our knowledge of breast cancer in its earliest detectable phase.

Tony Hsiu-Hsi Chen, DDS; Amy Ming-Fang Yen, PhD; and Sherry Yueh-Hsia Chiu, PhD
Institute of Preventive Medicine
Division of Biostatistics
Centre of Biostatistics Consultation
College of Public Health
National Taiwan University
Taiwan

Stephen W. Duffy, MSc
Professor of Cancer Screening
Cancer Research Centre for Epidemiology,
Mathematics and Statistics
Wolfson Institute of Preventive Medicine
London, UK

Acknowledgments

The authors wish to express their sincere appreciation to the following:

Nadja Lindhe, MD and Mats Ingvarsson, MD, Department of Mammography, Central Hospital, Falun, Sweden, for their professional standards and for our excellent teamwork;

Ms. Britt-Marie Ericsson and Ms. Elisabeth Klockare, Department of Clinical Pathology and Cytology, Central Hospital, Falun, Sweden, for carefully preparing the exquisite sub-gross, 3D histology specimens;

Marla Lander, MD, Breast Health Center, Indio, CA, USA, for kindly reviewing the manuscript.

Contents

Chapter 1 The Diagnostic Approach to Malignant Type Calcifications on the Mammogram

Calcifications on the mammogram are relatively easy to perceive, regardless of the mammographic parenchymal pattern. The main difficulty lies in differentiating the malignant type calcifications from the benign type. This poses a considerable challenge, and we must often resort to interventional procedures for a histological diagnosis. Effective mammographic analysis requires an understanding of the underlying pathophysiological processes leading to the various types of calcifications. A careful analysis combined with a selective use of larger-bore needle biopsy will help us reach the correct diagnosis and optimize treatment planning.

The first step in analyzing the calcifications is to **determine their site of origin**:

- **Within the ducts:** Casting type and secretory disease type calcifications, the subject of the previous volume in this series.[1]
- **Within the terminal ductal lobular units** (TDLUs):
  - Crushed stone–like calcifications: the subject of this volume.
  - Powdery/cotton ball–like calcifications: the subject of the next volume in this series.
- **Outside the glandular tissue** (miscellaneous types): calcifications in the walls of blood vessels, in sebaceous glands in the skin, or in sclerotic stroma are usually characteristic for benign processes and seldom cause differential diagnostic problems.

Each of the **three groups of malignant type calcifications**—the casting type, the crushed stone–like and the powdery—has its own unique characteristics from the viewpoint of histology, imaging (see Table **1.1**), and outcome.

(A) Casting type calcifications are easy to perceive and diagnose radiologically and histologically, but there is a considerable discrepancy between their tumor characteristics and their surprisingly poor outcome.[1] The underlying malignant process is often diagnosed as in situ carcinoma or as Grade 3 in situ carcinoma occurring over a large area associated with microinvasion and/or small (1–9 mm, 10–14 mm) invasive tumor foci, but the outcome may correspond to that of an advanced carcinoma. This important breast cancer subgroup requires a concerted interdisciplinary effort if we are to succeed in improving the currently poor prognosis of patients presenting with extensive casting type calcifications on the mammogram.

(B) At the other extreme, **powdery calcifications** may be barely perceptible on the mammogram. Unlike the casting type calcifications that represent a clearly defined disease subgroup, powdery calcifications—corresponding to psammoma body type calcifications on histology—may represent a number of benign breast lesions (sclerosing adenosis with or without atypia, blunt duct adenosis, lactational change) in addition to Grade 1 in situ carcinoma. The mammographic appearance of these different diseases may be identical, making a definitive radiological diagnosis impossible. While surgical excision of casting type calcifications will result in a malignant histological diagnosis in more than 95 % of the cases, even if there is no associated tumor mass (Figs. **1.1**-4 & 5), the corresponding figure is about 50 % when only powdery calcifications are seen on the mammogram (Figs. **1.1**-8). Also, preoperative vacuum-assisted biopsy is strongly recommended in cases with casting type calcifications, since the malignant cells and their product, the amorphous calcifications, are in close proximity. In powdery calcification cases, the psammoma body like calcifications may be located in a benign process, at a site remote from an incidental malignant process, or they may be associated with the Grade 1 in situ carcinoma itself. For this reason, the effectiveness and reliability of preoperative vacuum-assisted biopsy is limited. Excisional biopsy is the method of choice for the definitive diagnosis of powdery calcifications.

(C) Crushed stone–like calcifications are those most frequently encountered in mammography screening and also require the most extensive preoperative work-up. This is because their benign differential diagnostic counterparts—fibrocystic change, fibroadenoma, and papilloma—are far more frequent than breast cancer and can be managed satisfactorily with the use of large-bore percutaneous needle biopsy procedures. The differential diagnosis is a challenge, because Grade 2 in situ carcinoma, fibrocystic change, and fibroadenoma all originate from the TDLU. Therefore, when both the malignant and benign processes have associated crushed stone–like calcifications, the result will be a cluster or multiple clusters of similar calcifications. Subgross, 3D histology is of considerable help for understanding the underlying pathophysiological processes producing these diseases and learning the capabilities and limitations of radiological differential diagnosis.

Table **1.1**   General characteristics of the three histologically verified malignant type calcifications

	Casting Type	**Crushed Stone–like**	**Powdery**
Relative frequency	**29 %** (158/553)	**49 %** (272/553)	**22 %** (123/553)
Perceptibility	**Easily perceived**	**Usually easy to perceive**	**May be barely perceptible**
Reliability of the mammographic diagnosis	Likelihood of malignancy: **96 %**	Likelihood of malignancy: **66 %**	Likelihood of malignancy: **47 %**
Value of preoperative vacuum-assisted biopsy	**Highly valuable**; should be performed in every case	**Highly valuable**; essential for differential diagnosis; should be performed in every case	**Limited effectiveness** and reliability since the malignant process may be at some distance from the calcifications. Surgery is necessary

Overview of the Diagnostic and Management Problems Encountered When Malignant Type Calcifications Are Detected on the Mammogram

The relative frequencies of the casting type, crushed stone-like and powdery calcifications in malignant and benign breast diseases, with and without an associated tumor mass, are given in the following pie charts. The data originate from a prospective, consecutive series of patients referred to open surgical biopsy during a 12-year period at the Department of Mammography, Falun Central Hospital, Sweden.

Crushed stone–like calcifications account for about half of all calcification cases referred to open surgical biopsy, regardless of whether we consider the malignant type calcifications alone or in combination with the histologically verified benign cases (Figs. **1.1**-1 & 3). The relative frequency

of the three types of histologically proven malignant type calcifications remains virtually unchanged regardless of whether they are associated with a tumor mass or not (Figs. **1.1**-2 & 3). The value of casting type calcifications in predicting malignancy is 96 % without and 99 % with an associated tumor mass (Figs. **1.1**-4 & 5). This is not the case with crushed stone–like or powdery calcifications. As Figs. **1.1**-4 to 9 demonstrate, crushed stone–like and powdery calcifications are less predictive of malignancy without an associated tumor mass. This uncertainty may cause considerable differential diagnostic problems.

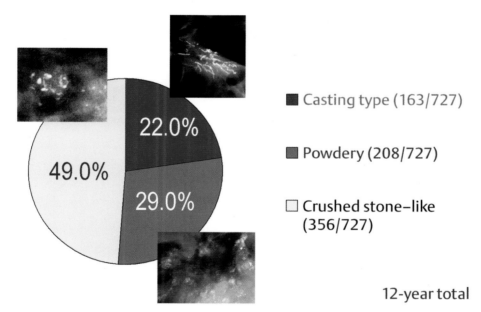

- Casting type (163/727)
- Powdery (208/727)
- Crushed stone–like (356/727)

12-year total   1.1-1

Fig. **1.1**-1   Relative frequency of occurrence of malignant type calcifications among **all surgically removed calcification cases** in women with or without an associated tumor mass. Women of all ages.

■ Relative Frequency of Calcification Occurrence

Distribution of All Histologically Verified Malignant Type Calcifications

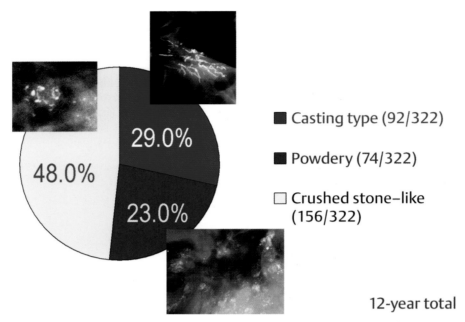

■ Casting type (92/322)

■ Powdery (74/322)

□ Crushed stone–like (156/322)

12-year total

1.1-2

Fig. **1.1**-2 Relative frequency of occurrence of **verified malignant type calcifications** among women **without** an associated tumor mass.

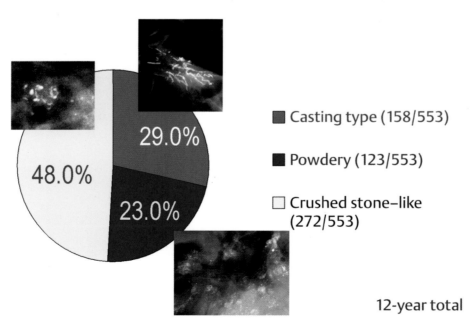

■ Casting type (158/553)

■ Powdery (123/553)

□ Crushed stone–like (272/553)

12-year total

1.1-3

Fig. **1.1**-3 Relative frequency of occurrence of **verified malignant type calcifications** among women **with and without** an associated tumor mass.

Malignancy Ratio of Casting Type Calcification Cases

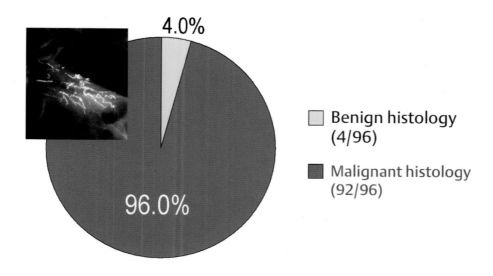

4.0%

96.0%

☐ Benign histology
(4/96)

■ Malignant histology
(92/96)

12-year total · · · · · · · · · · · · 1.1-4

Fig. **1.1**-4 Even in the absence of an associated tumor mass, casting type calcifications are still highly predictive of malignancy.

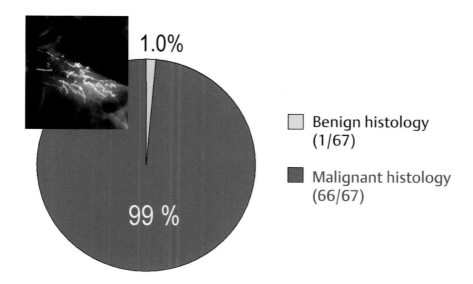

1.0%

99 %

☐ Benign histology
(1/67)

■ Malignant histology
(66/67)

12-year total · · · · · · · · · · · · 1.1-5

Fig. **1.1**-5 Casting type calcifications associated with a tumor mass are the most reliable mammographic sign of malignancy.

Malignancy Ratio of Crushed Stone–like / Pleomorphic Calcification Cases

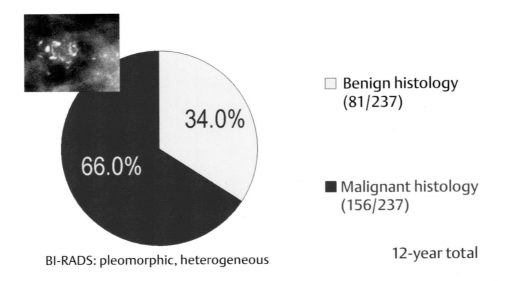

☐ Benign histology
(81/237)

34.0%

66.0%

■ Malignant histology
(156/237)

1.1-6   BI-RADS: pleomorphic, heterogeneous   12-year total

Fig. **1.1**-6   In the absence of an associated tumor mass, crushed stone–like calcifications are less predictive of malignancy and cause considerable differential diagnostic problems.

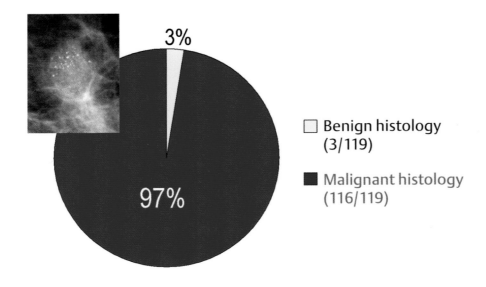

3%

☐ Benign histology
(3/119)

■ Malignant histology
(116/119)

97%

1.1-7   BI-RADS: pleomorphic, heterogeneous   12-year total

Fig. **1.1**-7   Crushed stone–like calcifications associated with a tumor mass are highly predictive of malignancy.

Malignancy Ratio of Powdery Calcification Cases

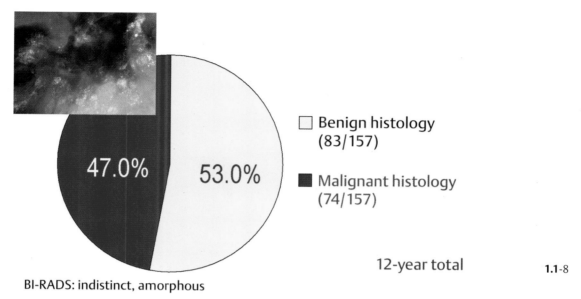

47.0%   53.0%

☐ Benign histology
(83/157)

■ Malignant histology
(74/157)

12-year total   1.1-8

BI-RADS: indistinct, amorphous

Fig. **1.1**-8   Nearly half of all consecutive powdery calcification cases without an associated tumor mass had breast cancer at histological examination.

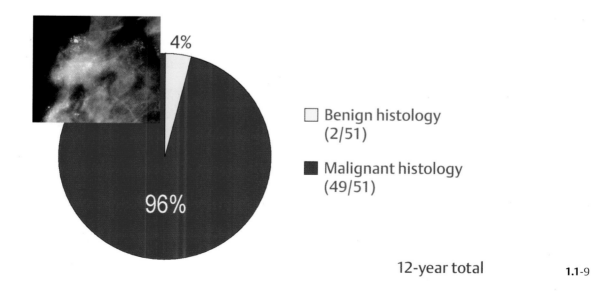

4%

96%

☐ Benign histology
(2/51)

■ Malignant histology
(49/51)

12-year total   1.1-9

Fig. **1.1**-9   Powdery calcifications associated with a tumor mass are highly predictive of malignancy.

Crushed Stone–like and Powdery / Cotton Ball–like Calcifications on the Mammogram

The TDLU (Figs. **1.2**-1 to 4) is the origin of many heterogeneous pathological processes, including in situ carcinoma of different grades. However, most abnormalities arising within the TDLUs are benign hyperplastic breast changes. These diseases may produce proliferating cells and/or an excessive amount of fluid, either of which will distend and distort the TDLUs by increasing the intraluminal pressure. In either case calcifications may be produced within and confined to preexisting TDLUs and may be detectable on the mammogram as single or multiple clusters. These resulting calcifications can be classified into two different categories:

1. The individual calcifications are discernible, resembling crushed stones (Figs. **1.3**-1 & 2); a thorough analysis of their distribution, shape, size and density will assist in determining the underlying benign or malignant pathophysiological process.
2. The individual calcifications are indiscernible, powdery, dusty, resembling cotton balls. The limited resolution of mammography does not reveal the individual calcification particles in powdery calcifications (Figs. **1.3**-3 & 4).

Crushed stone–like and powdery calcifications seen at mammography can each represent both benign and malignant breast diseases. For both types of calcifications, benign and malignant processes may produce an identical appearance on the mammogram (Figs. **1.3**-1 to 4).

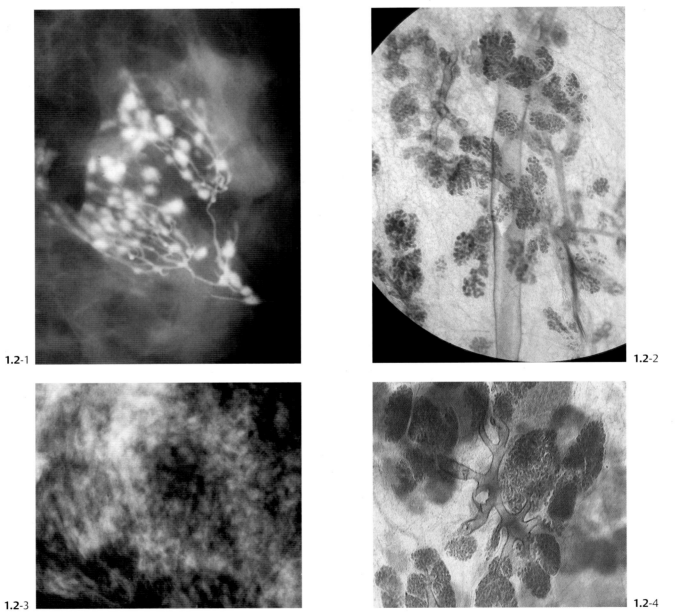

1.2-1

1.2-2

1.2-3

1.2-4

Figs. **1.2**-1 to 4   The normal distribution of the individual TDLUs is demonstrated using galactography (1), subgross/3D histology (2 & 4) and mammography (3).

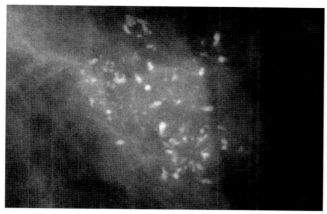

1.3-1

Fig. **1.3**-1   Specimen radiograph showing a cluster of crushed stone–like calcifications caused by Grade 2 carcinoma in situ.

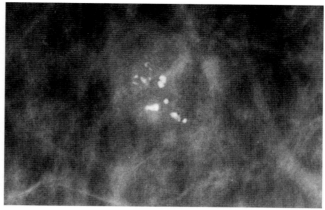

1.3-2

Fig. **1.3**-2   A cluster of crushed stone–like calcifications in a histologically proven fibroadenoma.

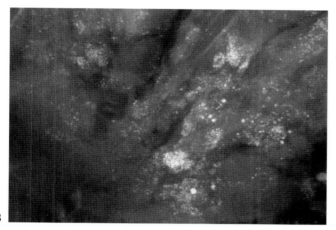

.3-3

Fig. **1.3**-3   Specimen radiograph. Multiple clusters of powdery, cotton ball–like calcifications in sclerosing adenosis.

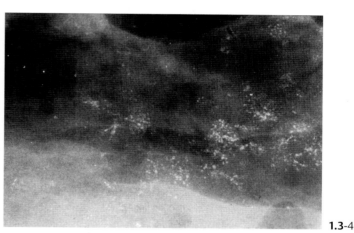

1.3-4

Fig. **1.3**-4   Specimen radiograph. Multiple clusters of powdery, cotton ball–like calcifications in Grade 1 in situ carcinoma.

Comment

The use of large-format subgross/thick-section histology technique is an instructive way to visualize how the morphology of the TDLU is altered by the gradual accumulation of fluid or cell proliferation/necrosis/calcifications. Comparison of subgross, 3D histological, and mammographic images is a most effective way to gain an understanding of the underlying breast diseases and their mammographic presentation. Examination of the subgross, thick-section 3D histological images presented in this book will demonstrate many cases in which the malignant cells are confined to the terminal ductal lobular unit (TDLU) with no ductal involvement. Use of the term "ductal" when describing these cases, although widely practiced, provides a misleading description of the location of the disease. For these cases we have used the terminology of Grade 1 or 2 or 3 in situ carcinoma. The grading system applied considers nuclear grade and presence or absence of central necrosis.[1, 2] The term in situ carcinoma used in this book should be considered identical to DCIS of the same grade according to the currently used terminology.

In situ carcinoma, Grade 1: low nuclear grade without central necrosis.

In situ carcinoma, Grade 2: either malignant cells with low nuclear grade and central necrosis or malignant cells with intermediate nuclear grade, with or without central necrosis.

In situ carcinoma, Grade 3: malignant cells with high nuclear grade with or without central necrosis. Cases with the cellular features of **LCIS** are not graded.

A thorough mammographic work-up with proper analysis in combination with the frequent use of larger-bore percutaneous needle biopsy will help in planning proper management when the finding is **crushed stone–like calcifications**. This is possible because the calcifications and the pathological processes producing them are in close proximity to each other, regardless of whether the crushed stone–like calcifications have been produced by hyperplastic change (calcified fibroadenoma, papilloma, or fibrocystic change) or by in situ carcinoma localized within the TDLUs. A different approach must be taken for the work-up of **powdery calcifications**. Because the same type of calcification, the so-called psammoma body type, may occur both in benign processes (such as sclerosing adenosis, blunt duct adenosis, etc.) and in Grade 1 in situ carcinoma, mammographic analysis cannot distinguish between the two. In addition, larger-bore needle biopsy will not provide a definitive diagnosis in all cases of powdery calcifications, because it frequently happens that these calcifications are produced by a benign process, while a low-grade malignancy not containing calcifications may be elsewhere in the same lobe. For these reasons, surgical excision of the region with powdery calcifications is recommended.

Example 1.1 demonstrates clustered calcifications localized within adjacent TDLUs that have been distended by a malignant process of two different grades. The result is two different types of calcifications within TDLUs that have been distended to various sizes. This case also demonstrates that both the crushed stone–like and powdery calcifications may remain unchanged for several years, making short-term follow up an unreliable means of management.

Example 1.1

A 58-year-old asymptomatic woman, screening examination. A cluster of crushed stone–like calcifications was perceived at screening and the patient was called back for further evaluation.

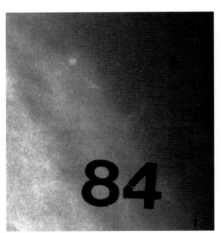

Ex. **1.1**-1

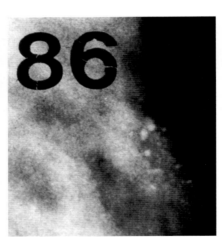

Ex. **1.1**-2

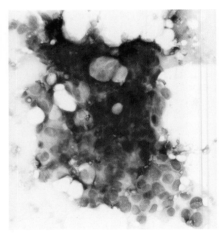

Ex. **1.1**-3

Ex. **1.1**-1   Previous screening mammogram from 1984, detail of the left MLO projection. Non-specific calcifications are visible without a tumor mass.

Ex. **1.1**-2   Microfocus magnification of the solitary cluster at the time of its detection in 1986: the crushed stone–like calcifications are closely spaced and irregular in size and shape, mammographically suspicious for malignancy.

Ex. **1.1**-3   Fine-needle aspiration biopsy performed under stereotactic guidance: cribriform group of malignant cells.

Example 1.1 continued

Surgical excision was recommended. Although the patient was fully informed of the nature of her disease, she declined surgical intervention. She returned for follow-up examinations at irregular intervals, but continued to decline surgery until 8 years after cytological diagnosis.

Ex. **1.1**-4 & 5   The cluster 1 and 2 years after cytological examination: 1987 and 1988, respectively.

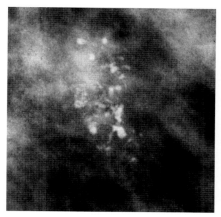

Ex. **1.1**-4

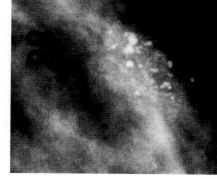

Ex. **1.1**-5

Ex. **1.1**-4 to 7 The size of the calcification cluster remained unchanged over the first 5 years after biopsy. 6 & 7 Images of the cluster from 1989 and 1992.

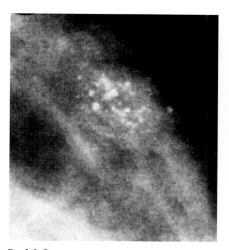

Ex. **1.1**-6

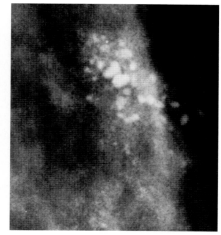

Ex. **1.1**-7

Comment

A careful analysis of the images of this microscopically proven carcinoma demonstrates some of the pitfalls encountered when patients with clusters of crushed stone–like calcifications are placed on follow-up:

1. Lack of change does not rule out the presence of cancer, even over a period of years.
2. The ongoing process of necrosis adds further deposits to the individual calcification particles, reducing the variations in shape and density, variations that are so helpful in differential diagnosis. The individual, previously irregular calcifications having variable size and density gradually become rounded and smoothly contoured.
3. Consequently, important differential diagnostic features can be lost during follow-up.

Example 1.1 continued

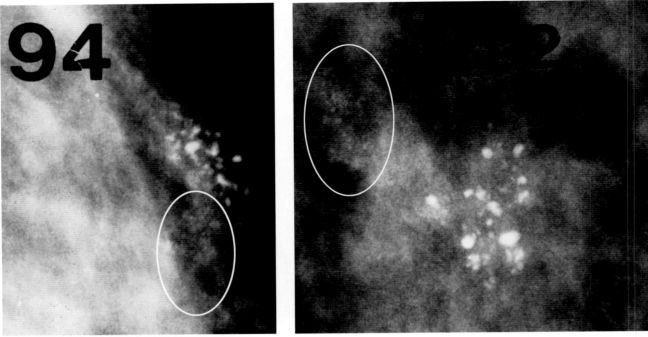

Ex. **1.1**-8

Ex.
1.1-

Ex. **1.1**-8 & 9 Detail of the MLO and microfocus magnification image in the CC projection. Eight years after documentation of her malignancy, small clusters of powdery calcifications have become evident. This new finding helped convince the patient to undergo surgical biopsy.

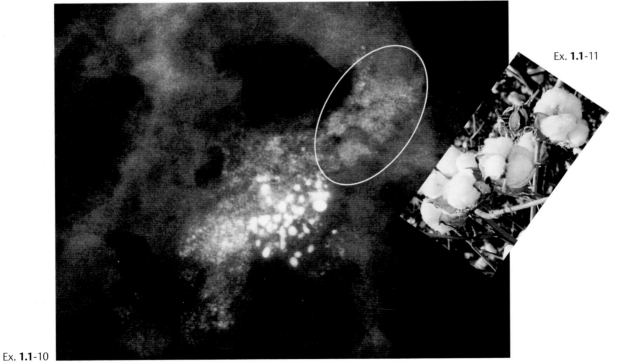

Ex. **1.1**-11

Ex. **1.1**-10

Ex. **1.1**-10 Specimen radiograph. Two types of calcifications are present, each in clusters. The large central cluster contains crushed stone–like, individually discernible particles. Surrounding this cluster are numerous smaller clusters containing powdery calcifications (several are encircled), resembling cotton balls.

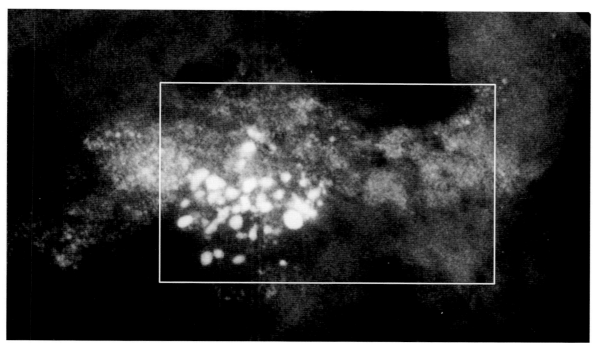

Ex. **1.1**-12   Specimen radiograph for direct comparison with subgross, thick-section histology.

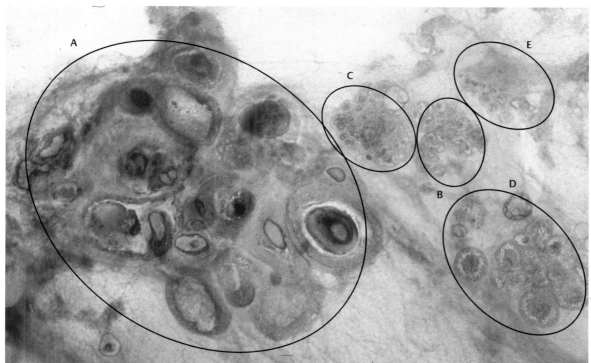

Ex. **1.1**-13   Subgross, 3D histological image of the area within the rectangle in Ex. **1.1**-12, showing several neighboring TDLUs, all containing in situ carcinoma. The largest TDLU (A) is grossly distended by Grade 2 in situ carcinoma and the associated **amorphous calcifications** contained within the individual acini (see comment on p. 17). These discernible calcifications **correspond to the crushed stone–like calcifications** on the specimen radiograph. The adjacent TDLUs (B to E) are distended to a lesser degree by Grade 1 in situ carcinoma associated with **psammoma body type calcifications,** and correspond to the **multiple cluster powdery calcifications** on the specimen radiograph (Ex. **1.1**-12).

Example 1.1 continued

Detailed comparison of the mammographic, subgross/3D histological and conventional histological images of the TDLU containing the **crushed stone–like calcifications** is shown in Ex. **1.1**-14 to 22.

Calcifications localized within the TDLUs are either the result of tissue necrosis or are associated with a secretory process.

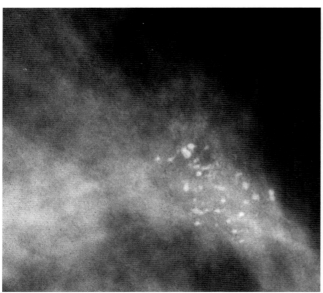

Ex. **1.1**-14

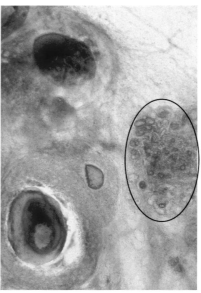

Ex. **1.1**-15

Ex. **1.1**-14   Detail of a microfocus magnification mammogram in the MLO projection. The crushed stone–like calcifications form a cluster, are individually discernible, vary in size and shape, and are in close proximity to each other.

Ex. **1.1**-15   Detail of the subgross histological image showing the discrepancy in size between the large, amorphous calcifications in Grade 2 in situ carcinoma as compared to the psammoma body type calcifications caused by Grade 1 in situ carcinoma in the adjacent TDLU (encircled).

Cluster Calcifications in Necrotic Malignant Tissue

The distorted TDLUs will measure only a few millimeters in size, as reflected by the size of the calcification cluster. The amorphous, necrotic debris may contain microcalcifications large enough to be individually discernible. Since most of

these calcifications appear within the distended lumens of the acini, they will be in **close proximity** to each other, an important differential diagnostic feature. When analyzing the **shape and density** of the individual calcification particles associated with a malignant process, we will find a considerable variation, resembling the random appearance of crushed stones. BI-RADS® classifies these as pleomorphic, heterogeneous.[4]

3D Image

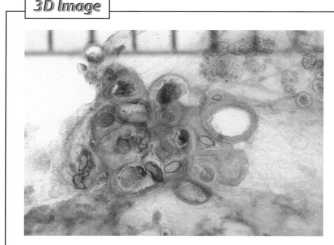

Ex. **1.1**-16

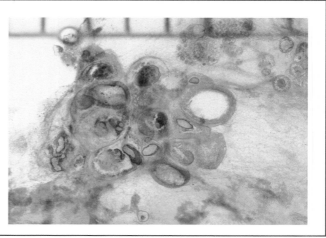

Ex. **1.1**-

Ex. **1.1**-16 & 17   Stereoscopic subgross histological image of the crushed stone–like calcifications within the greatly distended acini of a single TDLU containing the Grade 2 in situ carcinoma. Note that the largest calcification seen on Ex. **1.1**-12 has fallen out during specimen handling. Millimeter scale along the upper edge. A smaller TDLU containing psammoma body–like calcifications is in the foreground at the top of the image just to the right of midline.

3D Image

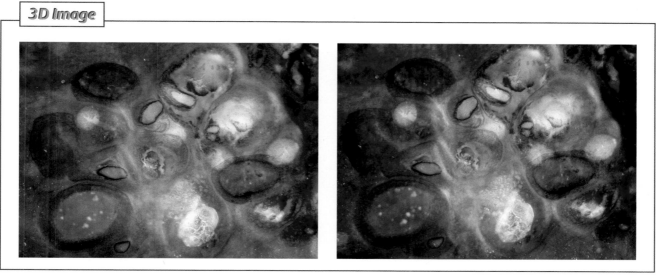

Ex. **1.1**-18 & 19 Stereoscopic subgross histological image showing the amorphous calcifications using indirect illumination.

Ex. **1.1**-20 Medium-power histological image showing the amorphous calcifications illuminated with polarized light.

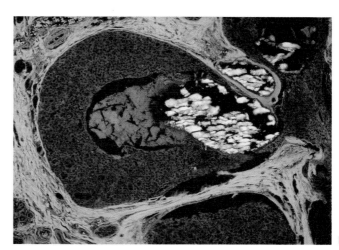

Ex. **1.1**-20

3D Image

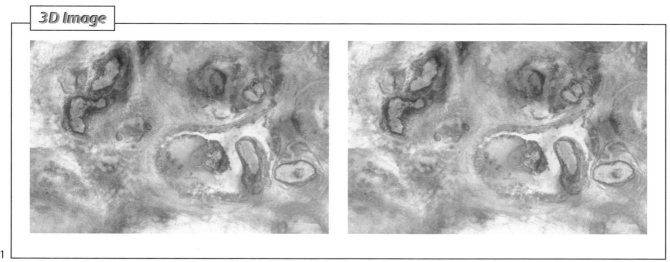

Ex. **1.1**-21 & 22 Comparison of stereoscopic, subgross images with conventional histological image (Ex. **1.1**–20). The amorphous calcifications are within the acini which have been distended by malignant cells, necrosis, and calcifications.

Example 1.1 continued

Detailed comparison of the mammographic, subgross/3D histological and conventional histological images of the TDLUs containing the **psammoma body type calcifications** is shown in Ex. **1.1**-23 to 31.

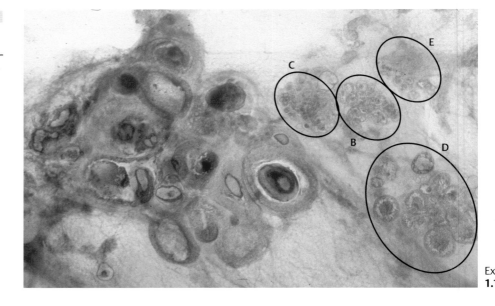

Ex. **1.1**

Ex. **1.1**-23   The psammoma body type calcifications are within the TDLUs containing the Grade 1 insitu carcinoma.

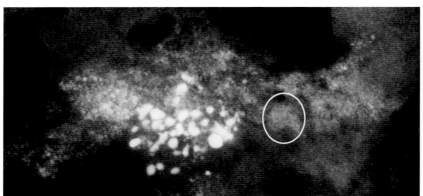

Ex. **1.1**-24

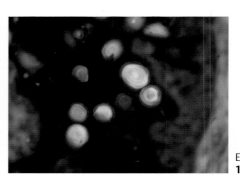

Ex. **1.1**

Ex. **1.1**-24   The psammoma body type calcifications within the TDLUs containing the Grade 1 in situ carcinoma cannot be individually perceived. The summation image of many calcium particles within the TDLUs is reminiscent of cotton balls (Ex. **1.1**–11).

Ex. **1.1**-25   Histological image of the laminated, psammoma body–like calcifications illuminated with polarized light.

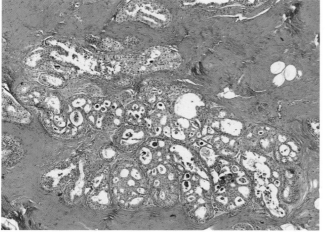

Ex. **1.1**-26

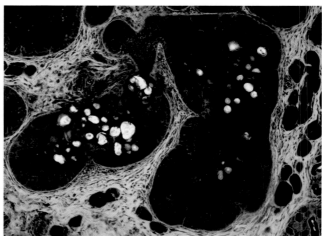

Ex. **1.1**

Ex. **1.1**-26 & 27   Low-power histological image of one lobule with Grade 1 in situ carcinoma and associated psammoma body type calcifications; H&E staining (26) and illuminated with polarized light (27).

3D Image

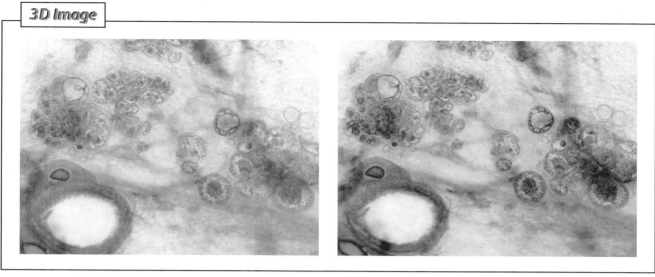

Ex. **1.1**-28 & 29   Stereoscopic view of the TDLUs containing the Grade 1 in situ carcinoma and the psammoma body type calcifications.

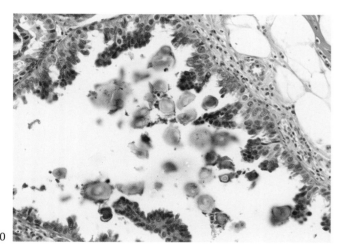
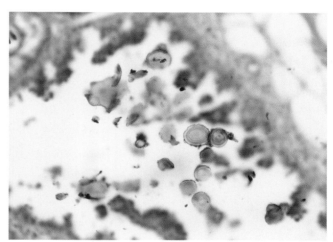

Ex. **1.1**-30 & 31   Medium-power histological image pair; on one of them (30) the cellular details are in focus (Grade 1 carcinoma in situ) while on the other (31) the psammoma body–like calcifications are in focus.

Comment

This case demonstrates the importance of using imaging terminology which correctly describes the pathological findings and which is consistent with the terminology already in use by other medical specialties. In this case the "crushed stone–like calcifications" (correctly described by BI-RADS® as "pleomorphic") correspond to amorphous calcifications arising within necrotic debris. The pathologists' established terminology for these calcifications is "amorphous calcifications." The psammoma body–like calcifications demonstrated above in images Ex. **1.1**-23 to 29 are regularly shaped crystalline structures arising in fluid produced by the malignant cells. Unfortunately, the BI-RADS® terminology for this type of calcifications is "amorphous," which is not only an incorrect description but also has the potential of confusing communication between radiologists and pathologists. Due to the small size of the individual psammoma body–like calcifications, only aggregates of many such calcifications localized within TDLUs can be seen at mammogra-

phy. Clusters of such TDLUs resemble cotton balls (Ex. **1.1**-24), and this terminology is used in the series of *Breast Cancer. Early Detection with Mammography*, along with the term "powdery" calcifications.

Whenever there is a mammographic finding, regardless of whether it is calcifications, a tumor mass, architectural distortion, or some combination of these findings, the challenge is to differentiate between malignant and benign breast lesions, especially those that have been collectively termed "**A**berrations of **N**ormal **D**evelopment and **I**nvolution (ANDI)" by Hughes in 1987.[5] These include different types of adenosis (simple, sclerosing, microcystic, blunt duct), simple cysts and fibrocystic change, fibroadenomas, radial scars, PASH (pseudoangiomatous stromal hyperplasia), papillomas, ductectasia, etc. This book deals with those hyperplastic breast changes and the in-situ carcinomas that are associated with crushed stone–like calcifications.

Classification of Crushed Stone–like Calcifications Produced by Malignant Processes

Correlation of subgross, 3D histological and mammographic images provides a basis for the following classification of crushed stone–like calcifications produced by malignant processes.

■ Group 1

Mammograms showing **one or two clusters of crushed stone–like calcifications** that represent:

Group 1A.　The main morphological finding. In these cases there is **concordance** between mammography and the underlying histology. The temporal changes may be deceptively gradual. The outcome is excellent, even when invasion develops, provided the tumor is surgically removed when it is still in the 1–14 mm size range. The role of MRI in detecting these cases has yet to be defined.

Group 1B.　The subtle mammographic finding may represent only the "tip of the iceberg." In these cases the true extent of the disease is seriously **underestimated** by mammography, although it may be adequately outlined by functional imaging methods such as MRI, since the disease involves numerous TDLUs, ducts and neoducts with little or no intervening normal tissue. The unexpectedly large tumor burden may result in a poor outcome, which can only become worse when underestimation of the disease leads to delayed or inadequate therapy.

Figs. **1.4**-1 & 2　Mammographic–thick-section histological demonstration of a typical Group 1A case.

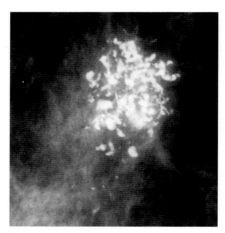

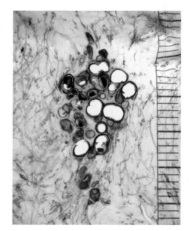

1.4-1

1.4-2

Figs. **1.5**-1 & 2. Mammographic–MRI demonstration of a typical Group 1B case.

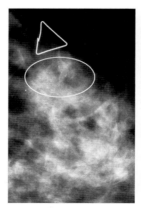

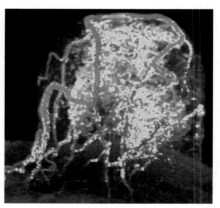

1.5-1

1.5-2

■ Group 2

Mammograms showing **multiple clusters** (or rarely a single cluster) of crushed stone–like calcifications that represent only a portion of the underlying disease, which may be only in situ carcinoma, but histology occasionally reveal associated invasive carcinoma as well. **Correlating the mammographic findings with large-section histological examination combined with subgross, thick-section histology distinguishes the following two groups:**

Group 2A. The in situ process is primarily **confined to TDLUs that are separated from each other by normal tissue**, although histology may reveal a few involved ducts. In these cases there is reasonable concordance between the mammographic and histological findings.

Also, the crushed stone–like calcifications may be associated with powdery calcifications, seen in close proximity on the mammograms, representing Grade 2 and Grade 1 in situ carcinoma side by side.

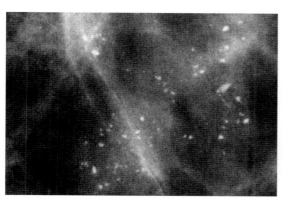
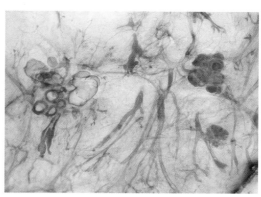

.6-1   1.6-2

Figs. **1.6**-1 & 2   Mammographic–thick-section histological demonstration of a typical Group 2A case.

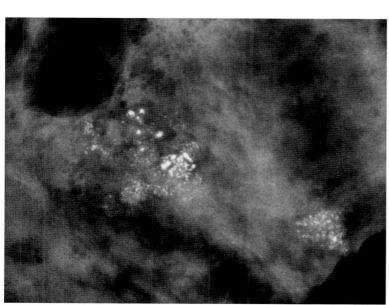
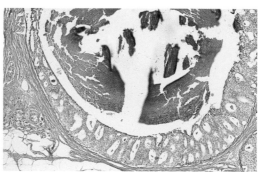
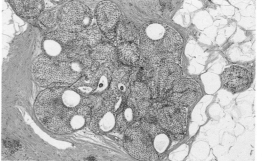

7-1   1.7-2   1.7-3

Figs. **1.7**-1 to 3   Mammographic–histological illustration of another type of Group 2A case in which both crushed stone–like and powdery calcifications are found in the same tumor bed.

Group 2B. Although the mammographic image may show multiple clusters which appear similar to those in Group 2A, large-section histological examination demonstrates tightly packed cancerous TDLUs and ducts covering a larger area than that indicated by the calcifications detected at mammography. MRI of the breast plays an important role in revealing the true extent and confluent nature of the underlying disease. In some extreme cases very large numbers of clusters of crushed stone–like calcifications are visible on the mammogram, often associated with some casting type calcifications. The larger the number of clusters, the more difficult it is to discern the individual clusters. Correlation with large-section and subgross, 3D histology shows a high density of tightly packed cancerous TDLUs and ducts with little, if any, normal tissue in between. Histological signs of neoductgenesis and lymph vessel invasion are often present and may account for the occasional poor outcome.

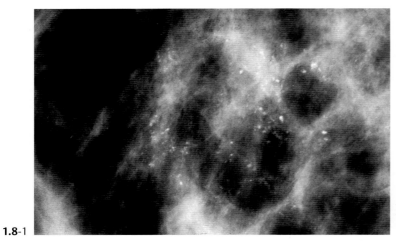 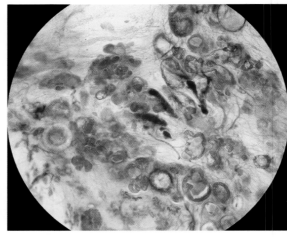

1.8-1   1.8-

Figs. **1.8**-1 & 2   Mammographic–thick-section histological demonstration of a typical Group 2B case.

Chapter 2 Group 1: One or Two Clusters of Crushed Stone-like Calcifications on the Mammogram Produced by Malignant Processes

Mammograms showing **one or two clusters of crushed stone–like calcifications** can be subdivided into the following two subgroups:

Group 1A. The mammographic finding represents the main morphological finding. In these cases there is **concordance** between mammography and the underlying histology. The temporal changes may be deceptively gradual. The outcome is excellent, even when invasion develops, provided the tumor is surgically removed when it is still in the 1–14 mm size range. The role of MRI in detecting these cases has yet to be defined.

Group 1B. The subtle mammographic finding may represent only the "tip of the iceberg." In these cases the true extent of the disease is seriously **underestimated** by mammography, although it may be adequately outlined by functional imaging methods such as MRI, since the disease involves numerous TDLUs, ducts, and neoducts with little or no intervening normal tissue. The unexpectedly large tumor burden may result in a poor outcome, which can only become worse when underestimation of the disease leads to delayed or inadequate therapy.

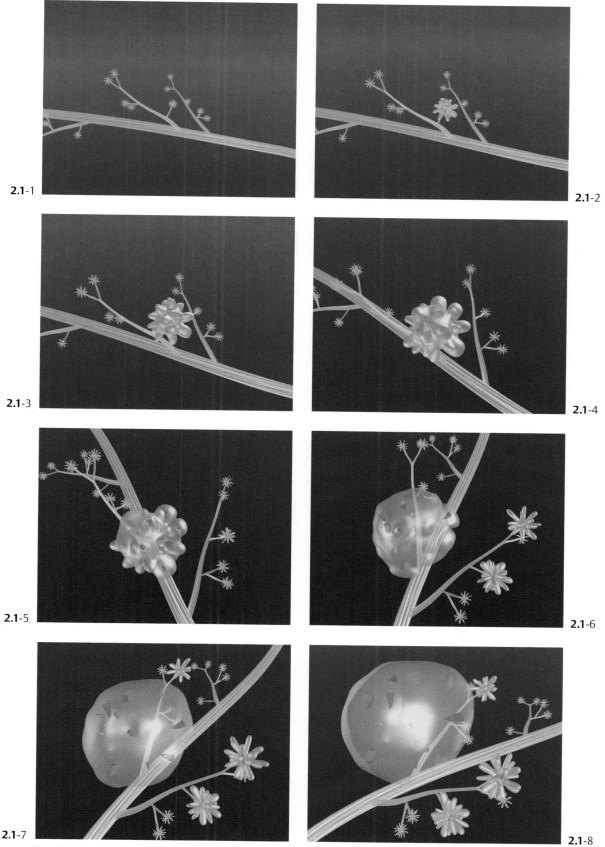

Figs. **2.1**-1 to 8   Computer simulation images of the development of Grade 2 in situ carcinoma within a TDLU. The lobule becomes gradually distended and deformed. Calcifications are formed within the necrotic debris and are seen on the mammogram as **crushed stone–like calcifications**.

Group 1A: The Mammographic Finding Represents the Main Histological Finding

Example 2.1

A 57-year-old asymptomatic woman, screening examination. Called back to the assessment center for further examination of the small cluster of calcifications in her left breast detected at screening.

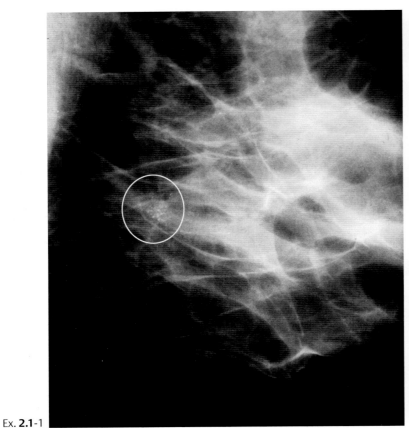

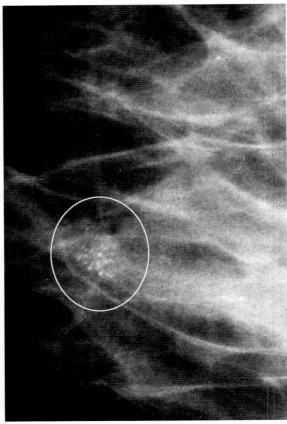

Ex. 2.1-1

Ex. 2

Ex. **2.1**-1 & 2   Mediolateral oblique (MLO) projection and detail of the MLO view of the left breast. A small cluster of calcifications is seen without an associated tumor mass.

Ex. **2.1**-3   Craniocaudal (CC) projection of the left breast. The small cluster of calcifications is located in the retroglandular clear space.

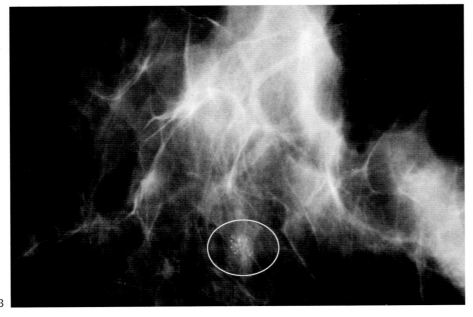

Ex. 2.1-3

Ex. **2.1**-4 Microfocus magnification in the CC projection. The individual calcifications are closely spaced and vary in size and density, and their shape resembles crushed stones. These are of the mammographically malignant type.

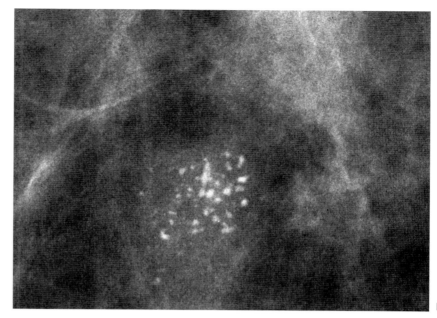

Ex. **2.1**-4

3D Image

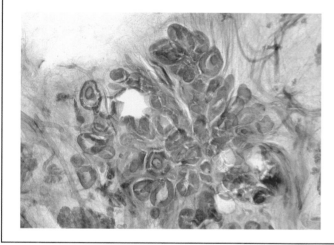 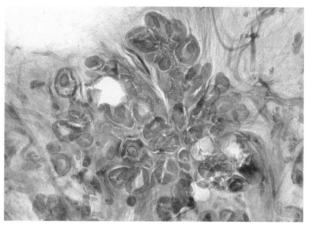

2.1-5

Ex. **2.1**-6

Ex. **2.1**-5 & 6 Stereoscopic image pair of a 1 mm-thick slice of the TDLU containing the crushed stone–like calcifications seen on the specimen radiograph. It is apparent from these images that the in situ carcinoma is confined to the acini of the distended TDLU and is not within ducts. Although such cancers are still termed "ductal" carcinoma in situ, 3D histological images show that this is not the case. There were no other malignant foci in the specimen, but several types of hyperplastic changes were found adjacent to the malignant focus (see Figs. **2.1**-12 to 17).

Example 2.1 continued

Ex. **2.1**-7   Specimen radiograph showing the malignant type calcifications removed with a good margin (15 mm at histological examination).

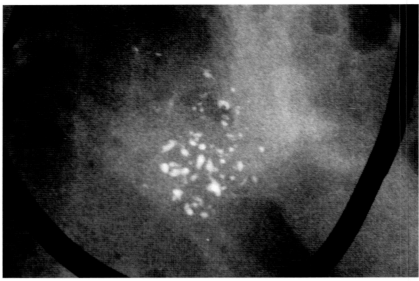

Ex. 1

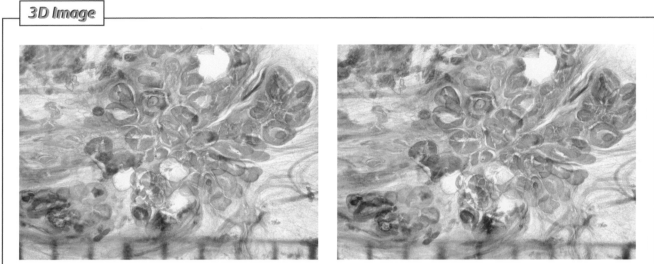

3D Image

Ex. **2.1**-8

Ex. 2

Ex. **2.1**-8 & 9   Stereoscopic images of the TDLUs containing the in situ carcinoma. The individual acini are markedly distended by the combination of malignant cellular growth, central necrosis, and intraluminal amorphous calcification. The TDLUs measure 6 and 3 mm in diameter, with each individual acinus being larger than a normal-sized TDLU.

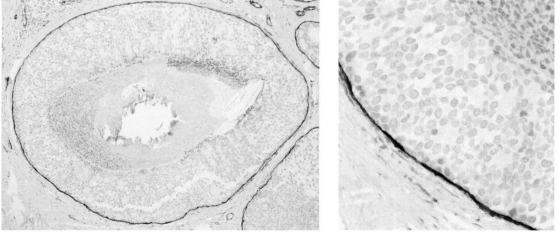

Ex. **2.1**-10

Ex. **2.1**-11

Ex. **2.1**-10 & 11   Medium- and high-power magnification histological images, with α-smooth-muscle actin immunostaining demonstrating a preserved myoepithelial cell layer that outlines a single acinus distended by many layers of Grade 2 in situ carcinoma, central necrosis, and amorphous calcification.

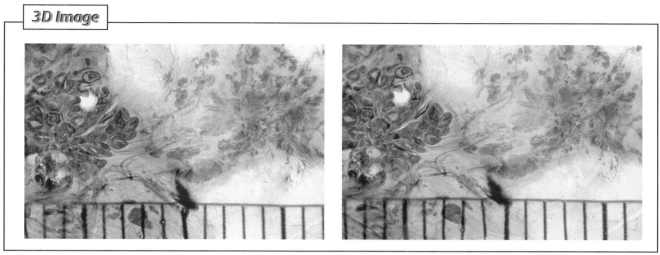

Ex. **2.1**-12 & 13   Comparison of two adjacent TDLUs. The one on the left is altered by in situ carcinoma and the one on the right is deformed by sclerosing adenosis.

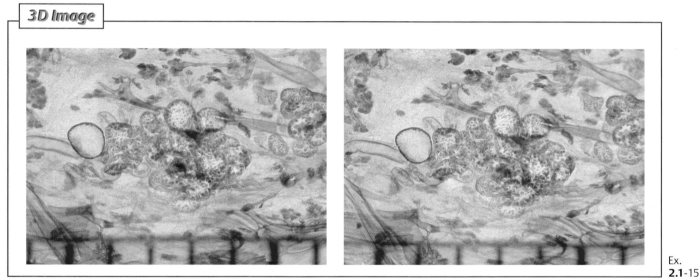

Ex. **2.1**-14 & 15   Stereoscopic images of TDLUs distended by fluid. The underlying hyperplastic breast change is apocrine metaplasia (seen as micropapillary growths within the cystically dilated acini).

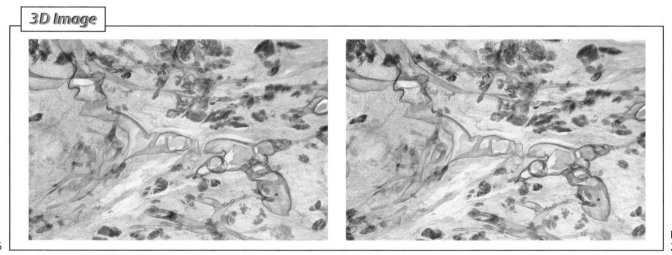

Ex. **2.1**-16 & 17   The fluid produced by the apocrine metaplasia has distended several ducts and their branches. Normal TDLUs surround the dilated ducts.

Treatment and follow-up: Wide surgical excision with no adjuvant therapy. The patient was free of disease at the most recent follow-up 13 years following surgery.

Example 2.2

A 70-year-old asymptomatic woman, screening examination. The faint cluster of crushed stone–like calcifications was not perceived. At her next screening examination 18 months later she was still asymptomatic and was called back for further assessment of the cluster of calcifications.

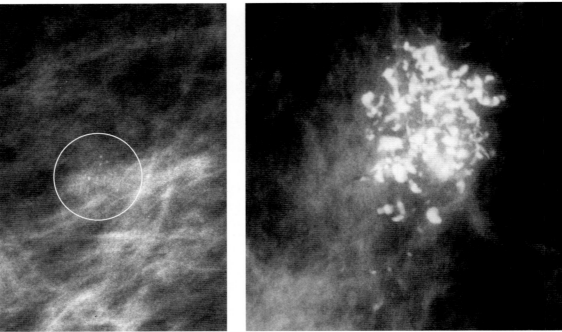

Ex. **2.2**-1

Ex. **2.2**-2

Ex. **2.2**-1 & 2   Detail of the MLO projection in two consecutive screenings with an interval of 18 months. The barely perceptible cluster of discernible, crushed stone–like calcifications (within the circle) has evolved to a mixture of crushed stone–like and casting type calcifications, occupying a much larger volume.

3D Image

Ex. **2.2**-3

Ex. 2

Ex. **2.2**-3 & 4   Stereoscopic images of one extremely distended TDLU (22 mm in diameter!). There are a few atrophic TDLUs in the surrounding tissue for comparison of size. The individual cancerous acini measure up to 2–3 mm in diameter, much larger than one entire normal sized TDLU. The central necrotic contents and the intraluminal calcification of some of the acini have fallen out during specimen preparation.

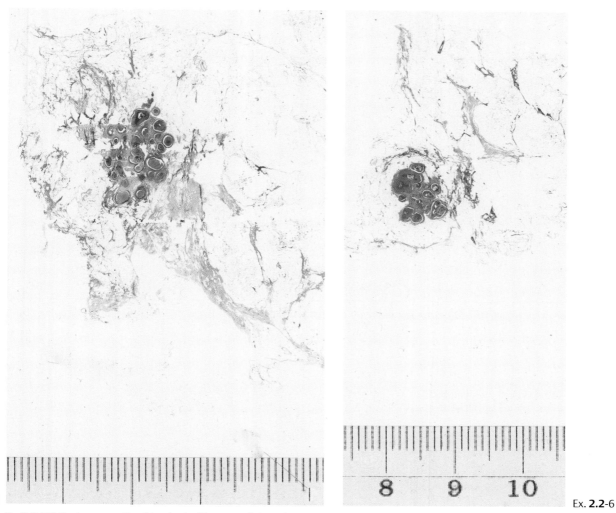

2.2-5

Ex. **2.2**-6

Ex. **2.2**-5 & 6 Large-section histological images of the solitary TDLU at two different slice levels. The TDLU is extremely distended by in situ carcinoma, central necrosis, and amorphous calcifications.

Histological diagnosis: 18 mm × 11 mm × 8 mm Grade 3 in-situ carcinoma with solid and cribriform cell architecture, containing multiple foci of microinvasion.

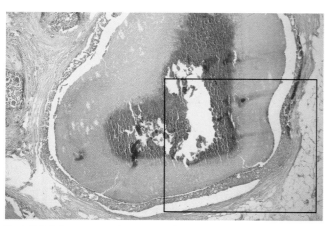
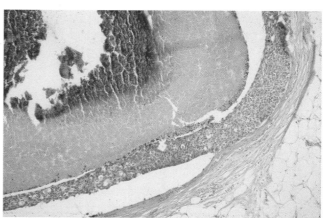

.2-7

Ex. **2.2**-8

Ex. **2.2**-7 & 8 Intermediate magnification of the extremely distended acini containing solid cell proliferation, extensive central necrosis, and large intraluminal, amorphous calcifications.

Example 2.2 continued

3D Image

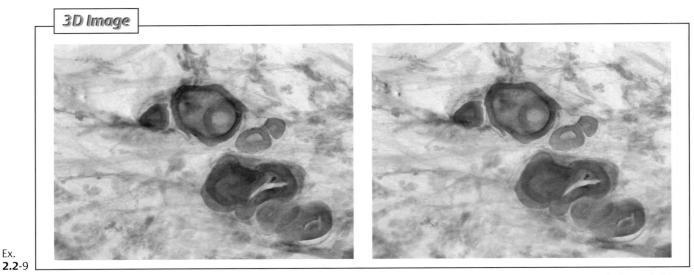

Ex.
2.2-9

Ex.
2.2-

Ex. **2.2**-9 & 10   Stereoscopic images of atrophic breast tissue for comparison with the individual acini, which are greatly distended by in situ carcinoma.

Ex. **2.2**-11   Medium-power histological image (H&E) of an acinus with solid cell proliferation, central necrosis, and amorphous calcification.

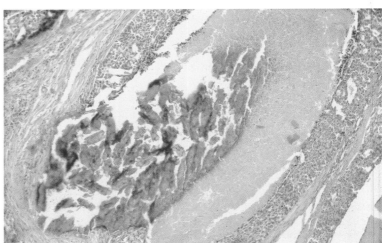

Ex.
2.2-

3D Image

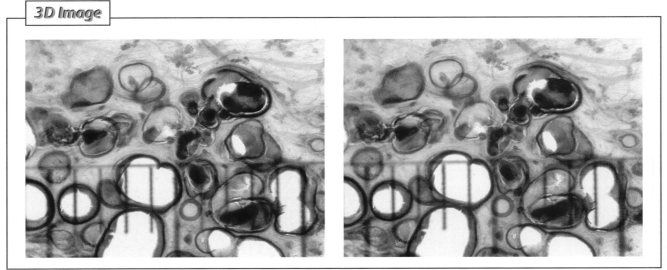

Ex.
2.2-12

Ex.
2.2-

Ex. **2.2**-12 & 13   Higher-magnification **stereoscopic subgross, thick-section (3D) images** of the acini that have been greatly distended by the in situ carcinoma, necrosis, and amorphous calcifications. Some of the acini measure 2–3 mm, which is two to three times larger than an entire normal TDLU.

Ex. **2.2**-14   Medium-power histological image (illumination with polarized light) of one acinus distended by solid cell proliferation (**1**), central necrosis (**2**), and amorphous calcification (**3**).

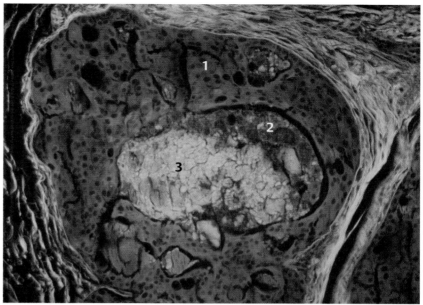

Ex. **2.2**-14

3D Image

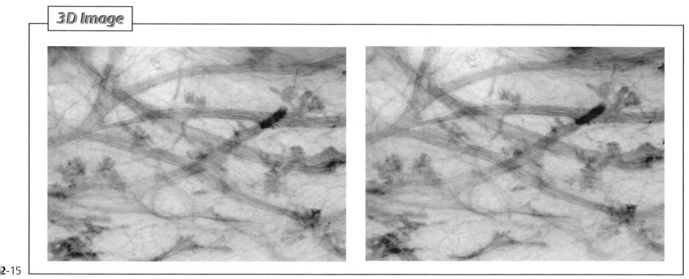

2-15

Ex. **2.2**-16

Ex. **2.2**-15 & 16   Stereoscopic image pair of the surrounding normal breast tissue with pleated ducts and atrophic TDLUs.

Treatment and follow-up: Sector resection was performed. No postoperative radiotherapy or other adjuvant treatment was given. The patient had no evidence of breast cancer at the most recent follow-up, 12 years after operation.

Comment
The large-section histological image and the subgross 3D images clearly show that the disease was limited to a single, extremely distended TDLU. The malignant cells were confined to the acini of the lobule and no ductal involvement was found. These observations are at odds with the conventional term "ductal" carcinoma in situ. Sefton R. Wellings and his co-workers pointed out that pathologists, viewing traditional, small histological sections, might have mistaken the extremely distended acini for ducts.[1] The fact that the disease is restricted to a single, isolated TDLU should be a justification for less radical treatment, such as surgical excision alone without adjunctive therapy.

Example 2.3

A 64-year-old asymptomatic woman, screening examination.

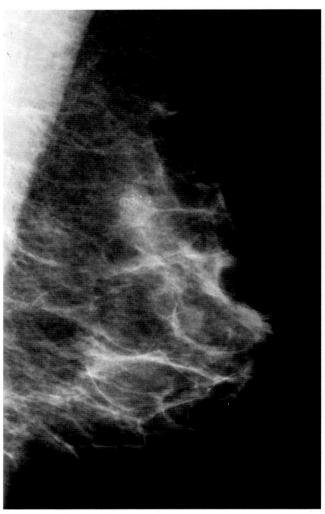

Ex. **2.3**-1

Ex. **2.3**-1   Left breast, MLO projection. A tiny group of calcifications is seen in the upper portion of the breast.

Ex. **2.3**-2   Microfocus magnification image in the MLO projection. The calcifications are tightly packed within a solitary cluster and vary in size and density. Mammographically malignant type calcifications.

Ex. 2

Ex. **2.3**-3   Microfocus magnification image in the CC projection. The solitary group of crushed stone–like calcifications is surrounded by an ill-defined density.

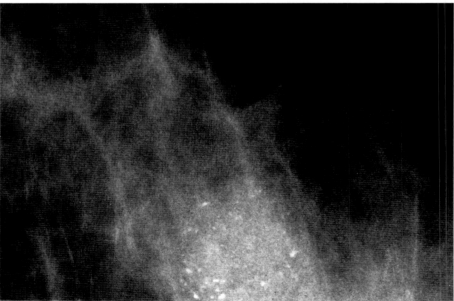

Ex. 2

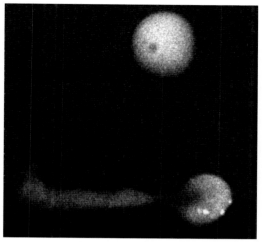

3-4

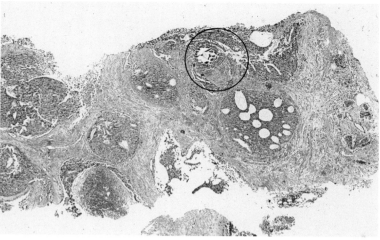

Ex. **2.3**-5

Ex. **2.3**-4   Microfocus magnification image of the vacuum biopsy specimen.

Ex. **2.3**-5 & 6   Histology (H&E) of the vacuum biopsy specimen shows in situ carcinoma with necrosis and amorphous calcifications (encircled).

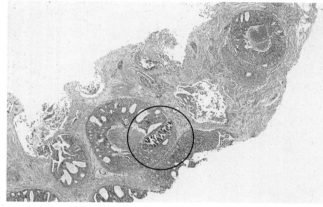

3-6

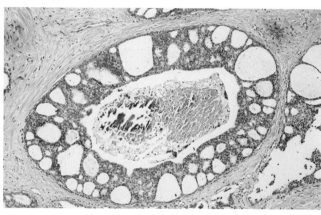

Ex. **2.3**-7

Ex. **2.3**-6   See above.

Ex. **2.3**-7   Low-power histological image: Grade 2 in situ carcinoma with cribriform cell architecture, central necrosis, and amorphous calcification

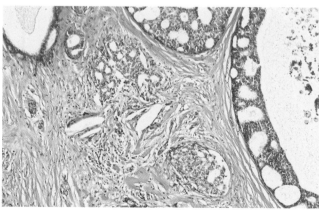

3-8

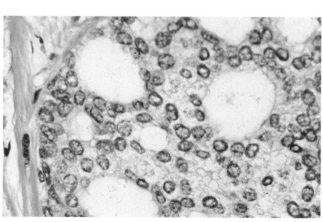

Ex. **2.3**-9

Ex. **2.3**-8 & 9   Histological images of this cribriform in situ carcinoma with increasing magnification.

Treatment and outcome: Sector resection and postoperative irradiation. The patient had no evidence of recurrence at the most recent follow-up 9 years after treatment.

Example 2.4

A 58-year-old asymptomatic woman, screening examination.

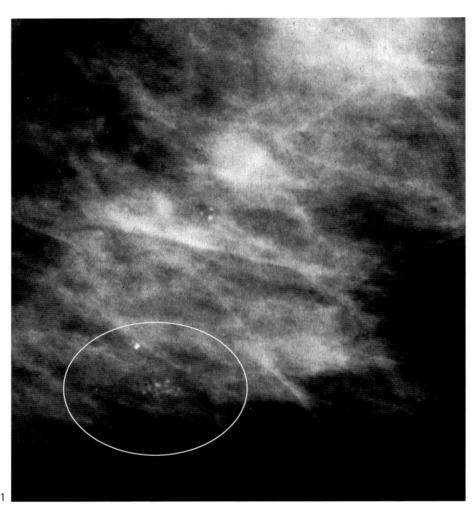

Ex. **2.4**-1

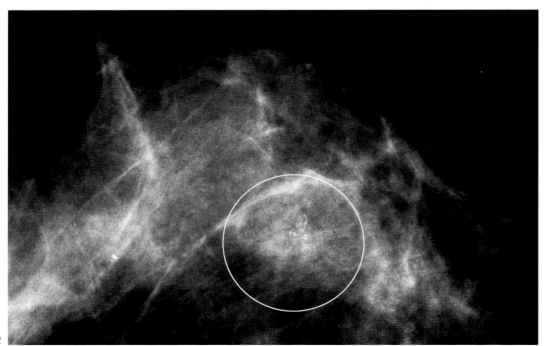

Ex. **2.4**-2

Ex. **2.4**-1 & 2   Detail of the MLO and CC projections. There is a tiny cluster of calcifications in the lower-outer quadrant of the breast with no associated tumor mass.

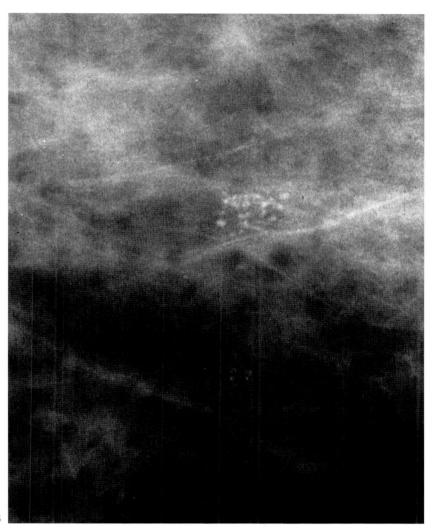

Ex. **2.4**-3 & 4   Microfocus magnification images, MLO (3) and CC (4) projections. The crushed stone–like calcifications within the single cluster are in close proximity to each other, and they vary in size, shape, and density. These are mammographically malignant type calcifications.

4-3

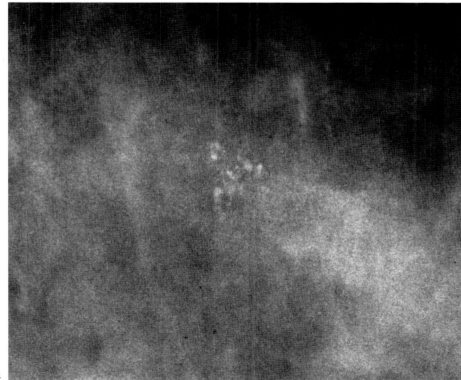

4-4

Example 2.4 continued

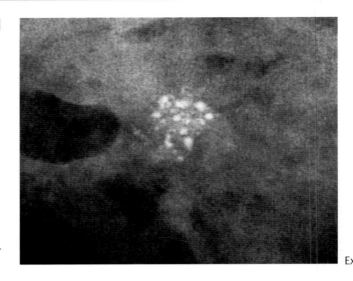

Ex. **2.4**-5 Specimen radiograph. The calcifications have been removed with good margins.

Ex.

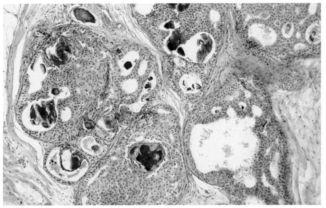

Ex. 2.4-6

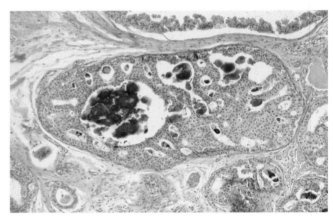

Ex.

Ex. **2.4**-6 & 7 Histology (H&E) images show of a distended TDLU containing Grade 2 in situ carcinoma with a cribriform pattern. The associated calcifications are a mixture of the amorphous and psammoma body–like.

Ex. **2.4**-8 Immunochemical demonstration of estrogen receptor expression in the tumor cells.

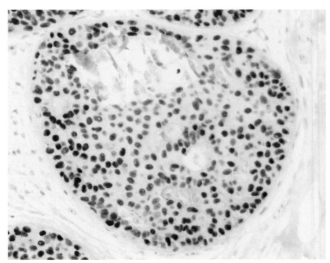

Ex.

Ex. **2.4**-9   Radiograph of the paraffin block.

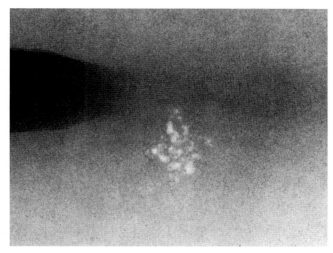

Ex. **2.4**-9

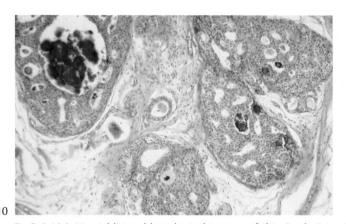

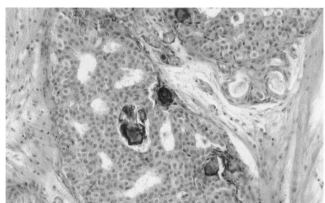

Ex.
2.4-11

10

Ex. **2.4**-10 & 11   Additional histological images of this Grade 2 in situ carcinoma.

Treatment and outcome: Sector resection and postoperative irradiation. The patient was disease-free at the most recent follow-up examination, 14 years after treatment.

Example 2.5

A 52-year-old asymptomatic woman, first screening examination.

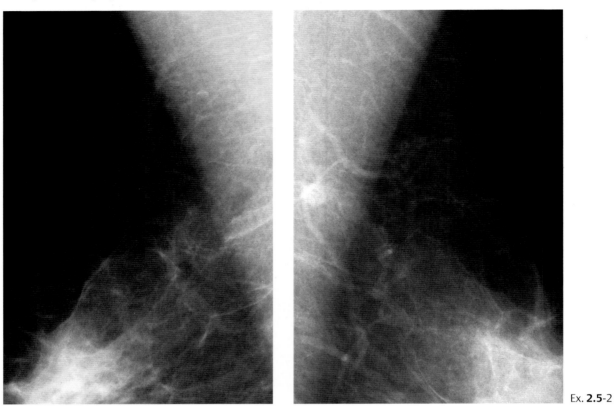

Ex. **2.5**-1   Ex. **2.5**-2

Ex. **2.5**-1 & 2   Right and left breasts, detail of the MLO projections. There is no demonstrable mammographic abnormality on the mammograms.

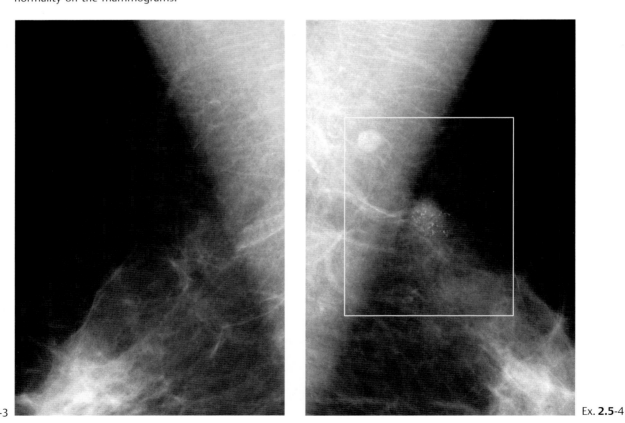

Ex. **2.5**-3   Ex. **2.5**-4

Ex. **2.5**-3 & 4   Next screening examination 2 years later. She is still asymptomatic and is now 54 years old. A group of microcalcifications surrounded by an ill-defined density has developed in the axillary tail of the left breast (rectangle).

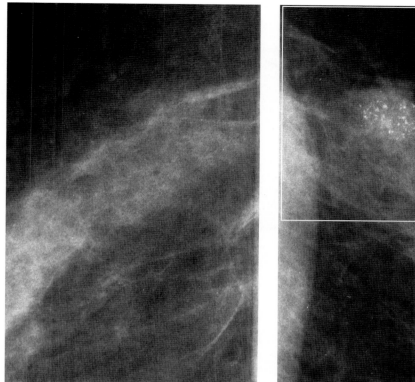

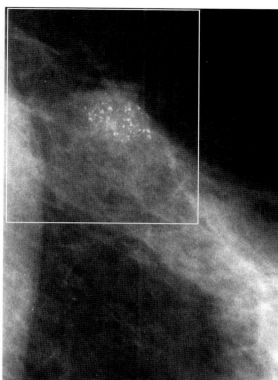

Ex. **2.5**-5 & 6   Detail of the left and right CC projections. The small, solitary group of calcifications is in the upper-outer quadrant of the left breast.

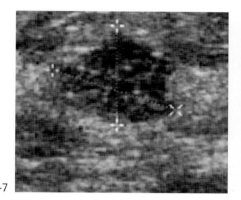

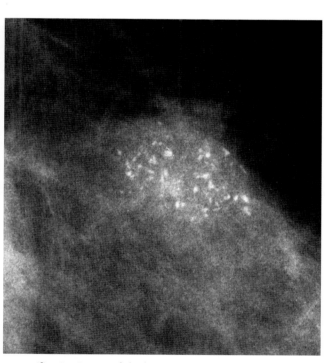

Ex. **2.5**-7 & 8   Breast ultrasound and microfocus magnification image of the lesion containing the crushed stone–like, mammographically malignant type calcifications.

Example 2.5 continued

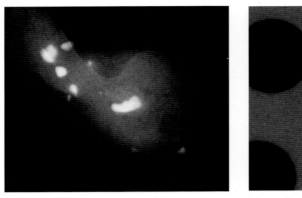

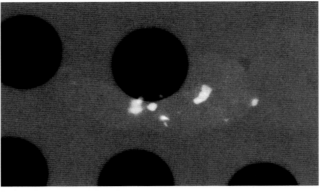

Ex. **2.5**-9

Ex. **2.5**-10

Ex. **2.5**-9 & 10   Radiographs of the vacuum-assisted needle biopsy specimen.

Ex. **2.5**-11 to 13   Histology (H&E) of the vacuum-assisted needle biopsy specimen: Grade 2 in situ carcinoma at increasing magnifications.

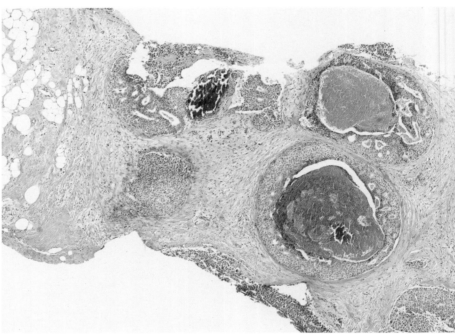

Ex. **2.5**

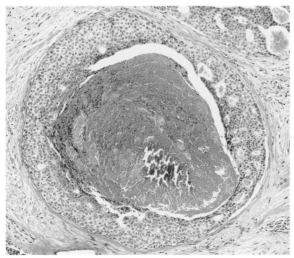

Ex. **2.5**-12

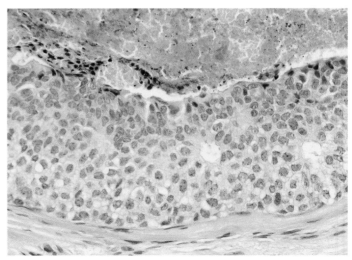

Ex. **2.5**

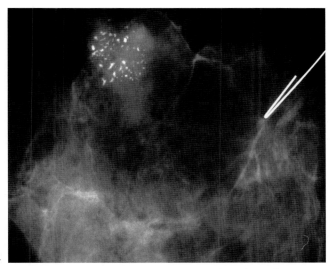

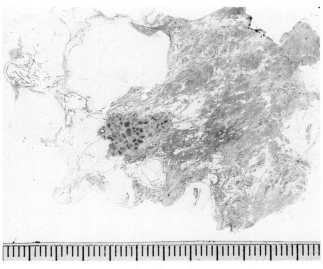

Ex. **2.5**-14   Specimen radiograph shows that the calcifications and the "tumor mass" around them have been removed in their entirety.

Ex. **2.5**-15   Large-section histological image. The cancerous TDLU measures 15 mm × 15 mm. The acini are extremely distended by the malignant cells, intraluminal necrosis and calcifications. There is no sign of invasion.

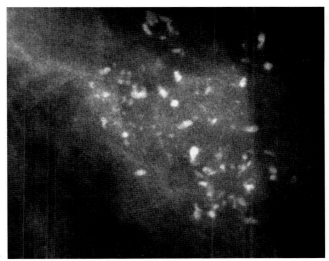

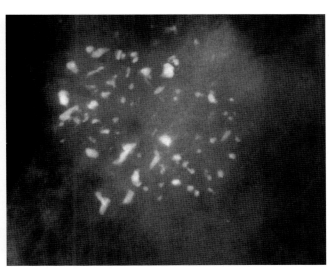

Ex. **2.5**-16   Radiograph of the operative specimen slice demonstrating the characteristic features of malignant type, crushed stone–like calcifications: the individual calcifications are in close proximity to each other and exhibit considerable variation in shape, density, and size.

Ex. **2.5**-17   Microfocus magnification of the specimen. The microcalcifications are in close proximity to each other. The size, shape, and density of the individual calcifications vary considerably. These features are characteristic of a malignant process.

Treatment and outcome. Sector resection and postoperative irradiation. The patient had no sign of recurrence at the most recent follow-up examination 2 years after operation.

■ The Long-term Outcome of Cases in Group 1A

Regular mammographic screening offers us the opportunity of documenting the progression of the underlying disease in those occasional cases where the calcifications have been missed or misinterpreted as benign type and placed on follow-up, or where surgery has been delayed for other reasons. Consecutive mammographic examinations can document temporal changes in the appearance of the crushed stone–like calcifications (increasing or decreasing). These changes over time can help us learn more about the natural history of those breast cancer subtypes that develop within the TDLUs.

Two or more sequential mammographic examinations of Group 1A cases may reflect disease progression as follows:

1. The mammographic image of crushed stone–like calcifications may show **little apparent change** at one or more follow-up examinations. In these cases short-term follow-up does not reliably exclude malignancy (see Example 1.1 on page 11).

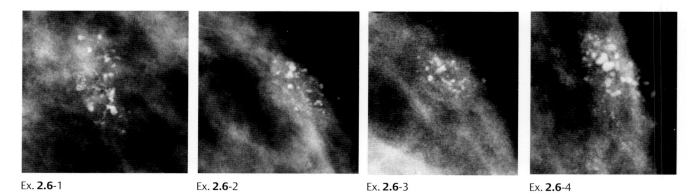

Ex. **2.6**-1   Ex. **2.6**-2   Ex. **2.6**-3   Ex. **2.6**-4

Ex. **2.6**-1 to 4   Images from four consecutive examinations spanning a period of 5 years (figures from Example 1.1, Ex. **1.1**-4 to 7).

2. The crushed stone–like calcifications **may disappear or decrease considerably in number**, concurrent with the development of an invasive tumor (Examples **2.7 & 2.8**). See also Figures 6.51 and 6.52 in *Breast Cancer. The Art and Science of Early Detection with Mammography*[2], pp. 214–215 and Example 2.11 in *Breast Cancer. Early Detection with Mammography. Casting Type Calcifications: Sign of a Subtype with Deceptive Features*[3], p. 124.

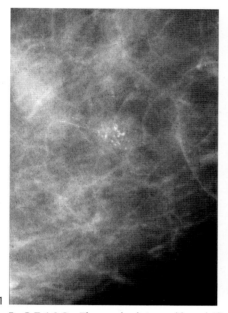 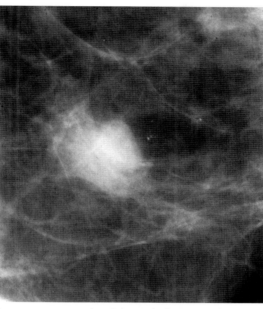

.7-1   Ex. **2.7**-2

Ex. **2.7**-1 & 2   The crushed stone–like calcifications were perceived and correctly diagnosed, but treatment was delayed by one year due to a competing disease. The in situ carcinoma has become invasive and the stromelysin-3 enzyme acts to dissolve the amorphous calcifications.

Another example where the crushed stone–like calcifications disappear concurrently with the development of an invasive tumor.

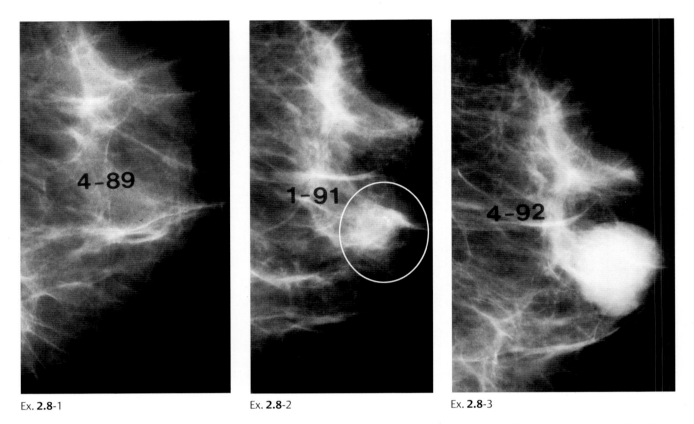

Ex. **2.8**-1   Ex. **2.8**-2   Ex. **2.8**-3

Ex. **2.8**-1 to 3   Three consecutive mammograms of the left breast, retroareolar region. No abnormality can be seen in the first study, but 21 months later there is a tiny group of crushed stone–like calcifications with an associated density. Fifteen months later a mammographically malignant tumor mass has developed, while at the same time the calcifications have been dissolved.

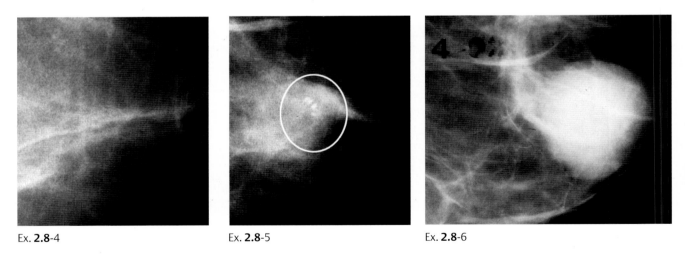

Ex. **2.8**-4   Ex. **2.8**-5   Ex. **2.8**-6

Ex. **2.8**-4 to 6   Photographic magnification of the above three images showing the retroareolar region.

Can breast MRI demonstrate a solitary TDLU containing in situ carcinoma that is seen on the mammogram as a single cluster of crushed stone–like calcifications?
This question has yet to be answered by a prospective study including a sufficient number of cases that fulfills the following criteria:
1. The mammographic finding consists of a solitary cluster of crushed stone–like calcifications (Examples **2.1** to **2.5** in this book, pp. 24–41).
2. Breast MRI is performed **prior to** needle biopsy.
3. Large-section and subgross, 3D histology determine that the disease is confined to a solitary TDLU or to a few adjacent TDLUs.

One of the following two outcomes can be expected:
1. Mammography and histology **demonstrate** the presence of in situ carcinoma within the TDLU, but breast MRI **fails** to demonstrate the presence of any malignant process.
2. MRI **demonstrates** the lesion and accurately estimates its localized nature.

The results of such a study would have considerable practical implications, since if MRI were able to distinguish those in situ carcinomas that are localized to one or a few adjacent TDLUs, a limited surgical resection would be sufficient treatment.

The cases in Groups 1 A & B have a **similar mammographic appearance, but vastly different underlying pathology.** The next section deals with the **Group 1 B** calcification cases, where the mammograms show one or two clusters of crushed stone–like calcifications, which **seriously underestimate** the true extent of the disease. Functional imaging methods such as MRI may more accurately outline the full extent of the malignant process. Large-section histological examination and subgross, thick-section histology will demonstrate cancerous TDLUs and ducts with little intervening normal tissue. Underestimation of the tumor burden may lead to delayed or inadequate therapy, resulting in a poor outcome.

Group 1B: Contiguous and Extensive Disease on Histology

Example 2.9

This 78-year-old woman underwent right mastectomy for breast cancer 43 years earlier. At routine follow-up mammography, a tiny cluster of calcifications was detected. She was asymptomatic and clinical breast examination was unremarkable.

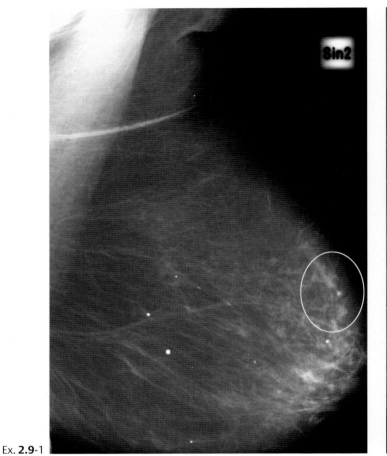

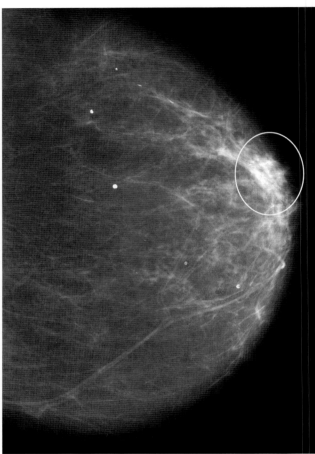

Ex. **2.9**-1

Ex. 2

Ex. **2.9**-1 & 2   Left breast MLO and CC projections. A tiny group of calcifications is encircled.

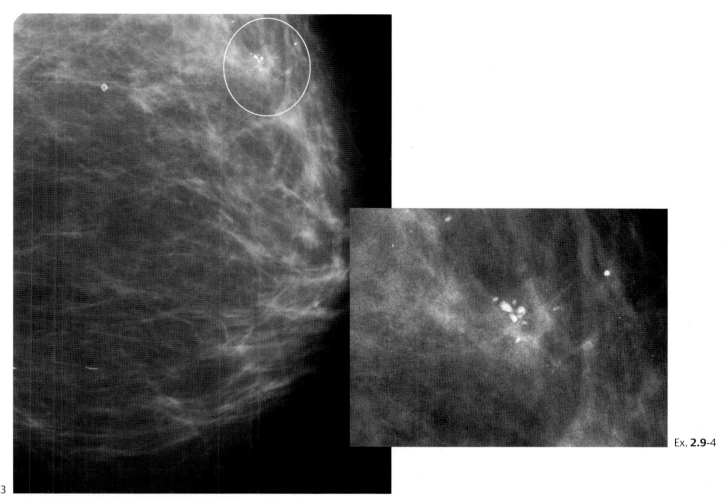

Ex. **2.9**-3

Ex. **2.9**-3   Left breast lateromedial horizontal projection.

Ex. **2.9**-4

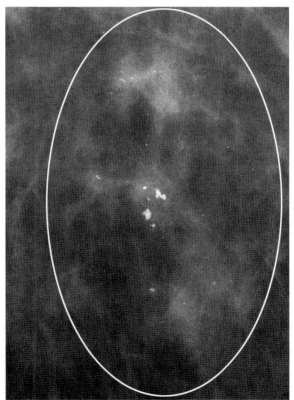

Ex. **2.9**-4 & 5   These microfocus magnification images show a cluster of crushed stone–like calcifications, faint densities, and additional tiny calcifications (encircled).

Ex. **2.9**-5

Example 2.9 continued

Ex. **2.9**-6 to 8 Vacuum-assisted percutaneous stereotactic biopsy specimen radiographs.

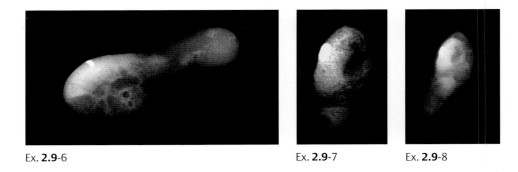

Ex. **2.9**-6   Ex. **2.9**-7   Ex. **2.9**-8

Ex. **2.9**-9 & 10 Histology: Grade 3 in situ carcinoma with necrosis and calcification.

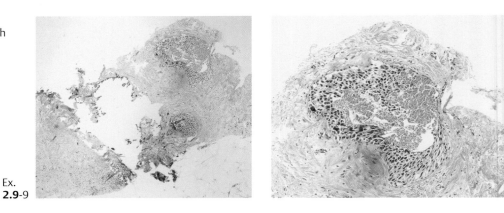

Ex. **2.9**-9   Ex. **2.9**

Ex. **2.9**-11 Radiograph of the operative specimen.

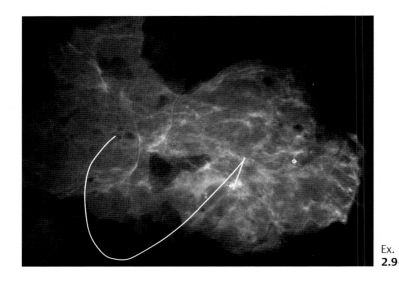

Ex. **2.9**

Ex. **2.9**-12 & 13 Mammographic–histological comparison of the area with the microcalcifications. Pleomorphic cancer cells and necrosis surround the amorphous calcification (a portion of the calcification has been lost at histological preparation).

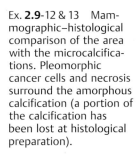 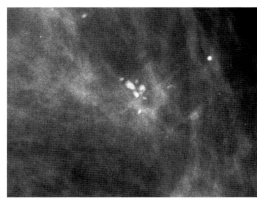 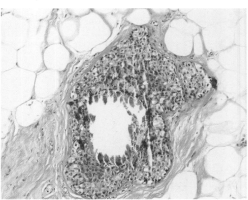

Ex. **2.9**-12   Ex. **2.9**

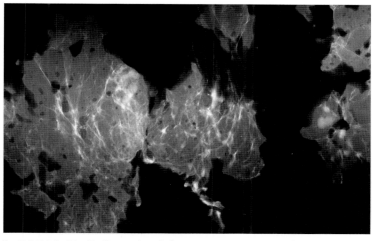

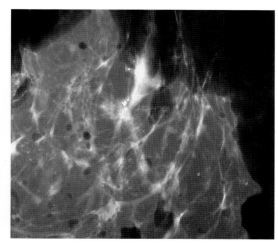

Ex. **2.9**-14 & 15   Radiographs of the operative specimen slices.

Ex. **2.9**-15

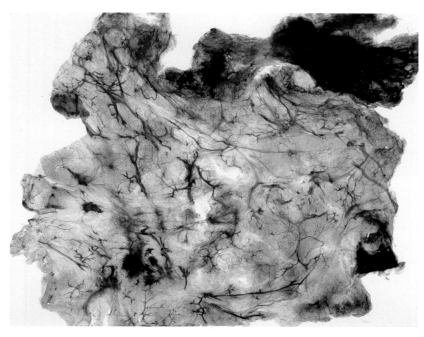

Ex. **2.9**-16

3D Image

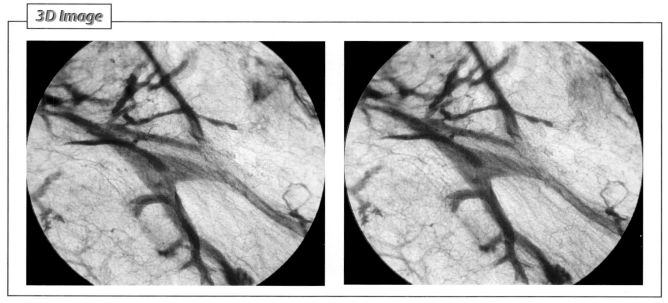

Ex. **2.9**-18

Ex. **2.9**-14 to 18   Mammographic–histological correlation of this **60 mm Grade 3 in situ carcinoma**. The subgross, large-section histological images (16–18) show the contiguous duct system distended by malignant cells.

Example 2.9 continued

Ex. **2.9**-19   Radiographic magnification of one of the operative specimen slices. The involved duct system is outlined.

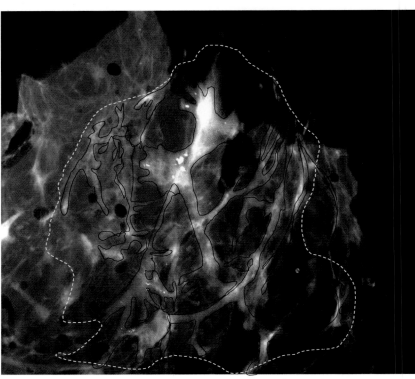

Ex. **2.9**-

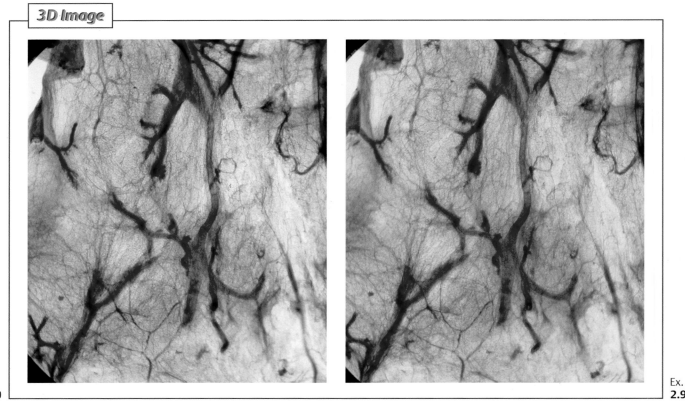

Ex. **2.9**-20

Ex. **2.9**

Ex. **2.9**-20 & 21   Stereoscopic subgross, thick-section (3D) histological images demonstrate the cancerous ducts and their branches. No TDLUs are seen.

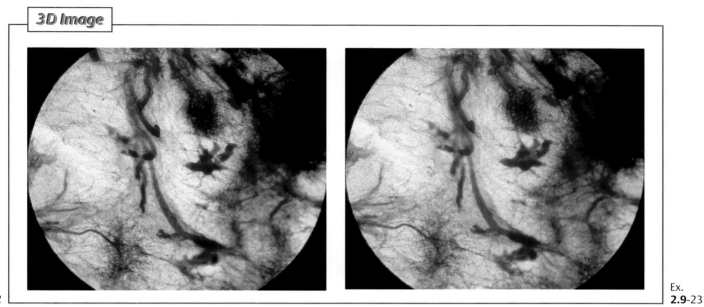

Ex. **2.9**-22 & 23   Stereoscopic subgross, thick-section (3D) histological images of several ducts distended by cancer cells, branching unnaturally in seemingly haphazard directions. The dark-brown areas on the right side of the image are post-biopsy hematoma.

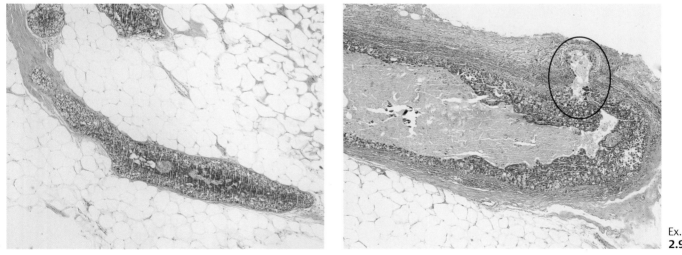

Ex. **2.9**-24 & 25   Histological images of unusually long subsegmental ducts filled with poorly differentiated cancer cells. There are no associated TDLUs. The thick periductal desmoplastic reaction, lymphocytic infiltration and the protruding new duct lined with cancer cells (encircled) suggest the process of neoductgenesis (25).

Example 2.9 continued

3D Image

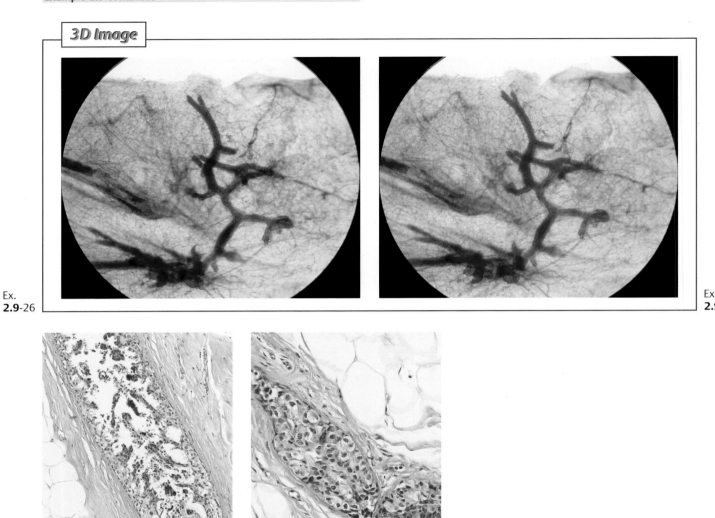

Ex.
2.9-26

Ex.
2.9-

Ex.
2.9-28

Ex.
2.9-29

3D Image

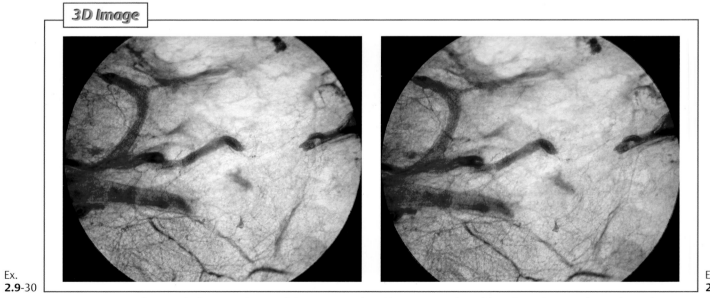

Ex.
2.9-30

Ex.
2.9-

Ex. **2.9**-26 to 31   Subgross, thick-section (1.5 mm) (26, 27, 30, 31) and large-section (4 μm) histological images (28, 29). Grade 3 in situ carcinoma distends a large number of ducts and their branches over a 60 mm × 44 mm area at histological examination, with a combination of micropapillary (28) and solid (29) cell architecture.

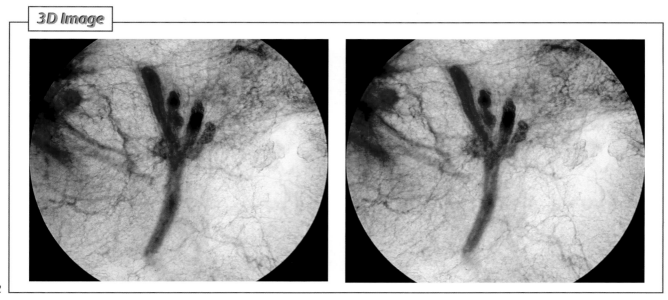

Ex. **2.9**-32 & 33   Stereoscopic subgross, thick-section (3D) histological images of unnaturally branching, irregular cancerous ducts with no associated TDLUs.

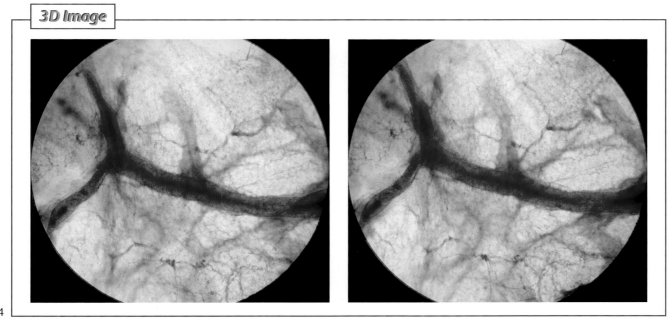

Ex. **2.9**-34 & 35   Thick-section (3D) histological images of an unusually long duct distended by cancer cells.

Example 2.9 continued

3D Image

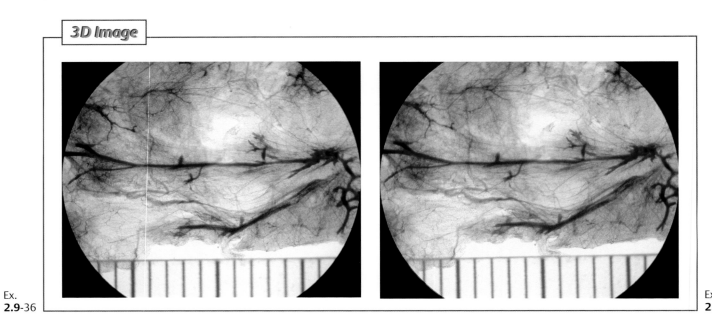

Ex.
2.9-36

Ex.
2.9

Ex.
2.9-38

3D Image

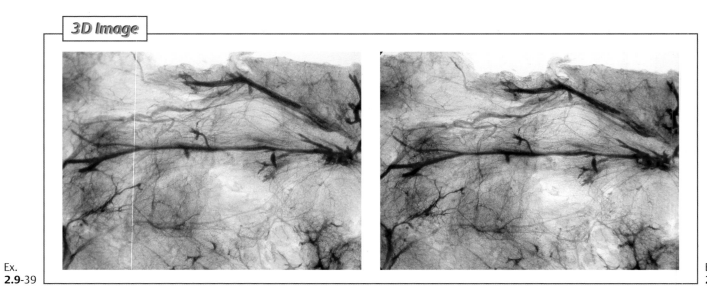

Ex.
2.9-39

Ex.
2.9

Ex. **2.9**-36 to 40   Subgross, thick-section (3D) (large thick-section) (36, 37, 39, 40) and large thin-section (4 μm) (38) histological images of the unnaturally long ducts containing poorly differentiated cancer cells. There are no associated TDLUs. Also, the short side-branches suggest neoductgenesis.

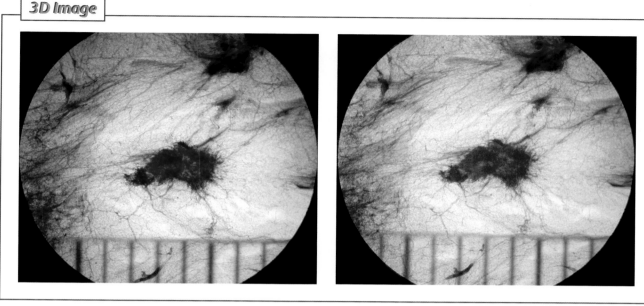

Ex. **2.9**-41 & 42   Subgross, thick-section (3D) histological image of the largest Grade 2 invasive focus.

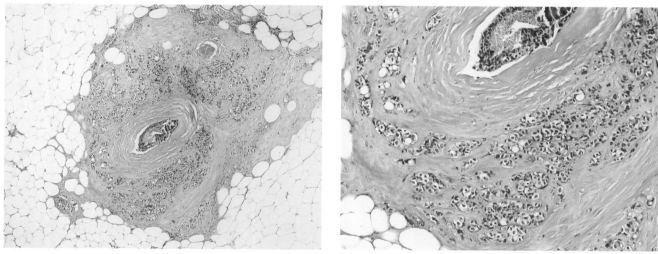

Ex. **2.9**-43 & 44   Several foci of microinvasion were found throughout the specimen. The invasive component is histological Grade 2, while the surrounding in situ carcinoma is Grade 3. The largest invasive component measured 3 mm.

Comment

The screening mammograms showed only the "tip of the iceberg"—a tiny cluster of crushed stone–like calcifications with no associated tumor mass. In this case the disease involved an entire lobe with multiple microinvasive foci. Treatment could have been more appropriately planned if the full extent of the disease could have been assessed preoperatively. Breast MRI offers such an opportunity (see Examples 2.10 and 2.11).

Treatment and outcome: Mastectomy. There was no evidence of recurrence 5 years after surgery.

Example 2.10

[Case courtesy of Bruce A. Porter, M.D., FACR, First Hill Diagnostic Imaging, Seattle, WA, USA.]

A 48-year-old woman presented with diffuse thickening and firmness in the left upper-outer quadrant at clinical breast examination. In addition, there was left nipple discharge. Palpation-guided core biopsy: solid and cribriform in situ carcinoma. The patient was referred to MRI examination of the breasts to assess the extent of the disease. Color Doppler: diffusely increased flow.

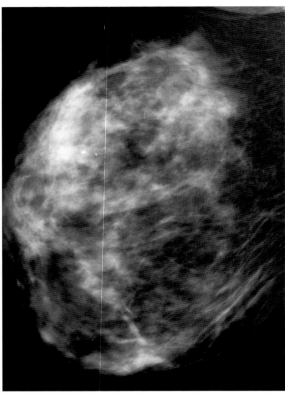

Ex. **2.10**-1

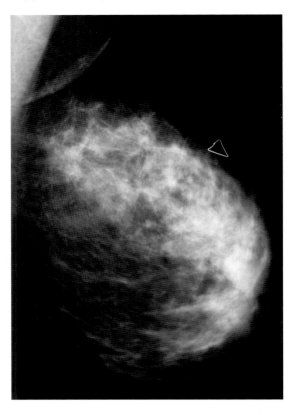

Ex. **2.10**-2

Ex. **2.10**-1 to 3   Right and left breasts, MLO projection. There is a tiny group of nonspecific calcifications in the upper-outer quadrant of the left breast with no associated tumor mass (best seen encircled on the CC magnification image [3]).

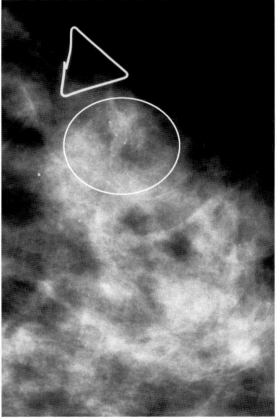

Ex. **2.10**-3

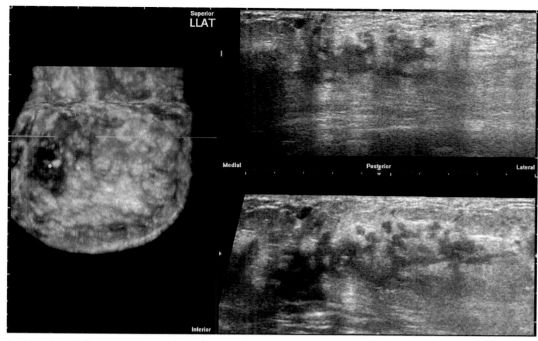

Ex. **2.10**-4

Ex. **2.10**-4 Left breast, automated 3D ultrasound examination in three orthogonal planes: 2 mm thick reconstructed coronal section (left), transverse (upper right), and sagittal (lower right) sections. The malignant process distends the ducts, which have become elongated and tortuous.

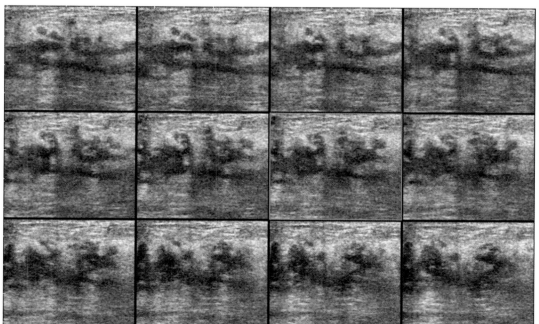

Ex. **2.10**-5

Ex. **2.10**-5 Sequential thin ultrasound slices ("Multislice") through the cancerous, tortuous ducts in the left breast in the axial projection.

Example 2.10 continued

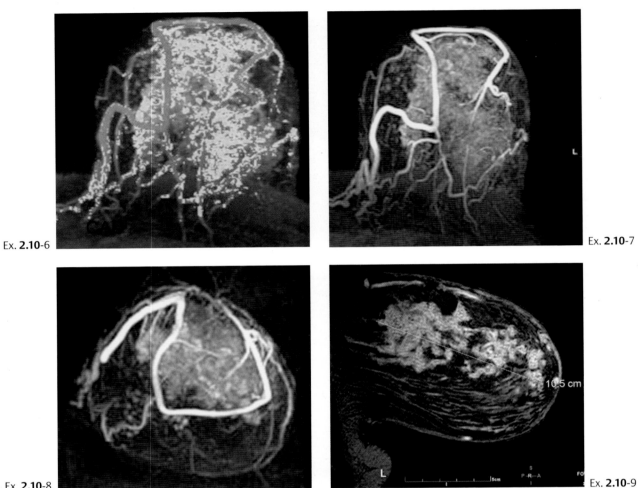

Ex. **2.10**-6

Ex. **2.10**-7

Ex. **2.10**-8

Ex. **2.10**-9

Ex. **2.10**-6 to 10   Contrast-enhanced MR images demonstrating intense enhancement, which measures more than 10 cm, throughout the major portion of the left breast. There was no corresponding uptake in the right breast.

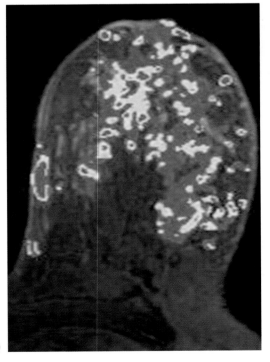

Ex. **2.10**-10

Comment

This case and Examples 2.7 and 2.9 from *Breast Cancer: Early Detection with Mammography. Casting Type Calcifications: Sign of a Subtype with Deceptive Features*[3] demonstrate the potential of breast MRI to visualize the full extent of breast cancer which is seen on the mammogram only as a cluster or multiple clusters of either nonspecific or crushed stone–like calcifications without an apparent tumor mass.

Example 2.11

[Case courtesy of Michael Vendrell, M.D., First Hill Diagnostic Imaging, Seattle, WA, USA.]

A 52-year-old asymptomatic woman, screening examination.

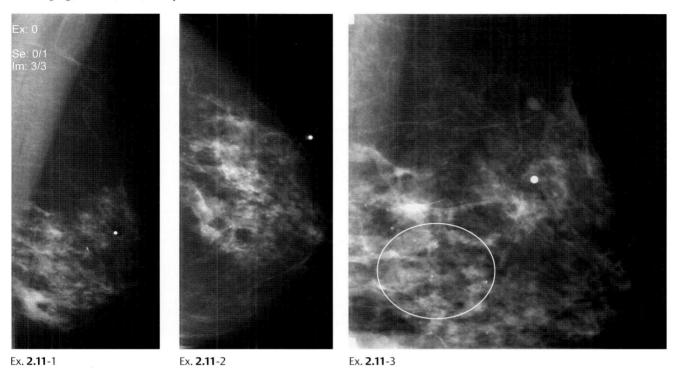

Ex. **2.11**-1   Ex. **2.11**-2   Ex. **2.11**-3

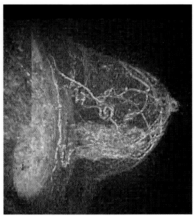

Ex. **2.11**-1 to 3   Left breast, MLO (1) and CC (2) projections and microfocus magnification (3). There are a few clusters of nonspecific discernible calcifications without an associated tumor mass.

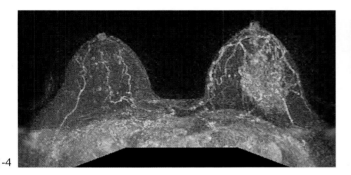

-4

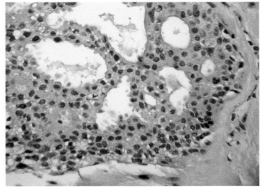

Ex. **2.11**-4 & 5   The MR images demonstrate contrast enhancement of a single large lobe in the left breast, suggesting extensive malignant involvement.

Ex.
2.11-5

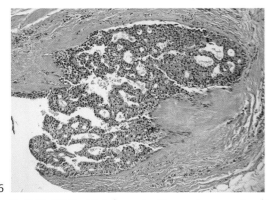

-6

Ex.
2.11-7

Ex. **2.11**-6 & 7   **Histology:** in situ carcinoma extending to the nipple.

Example 2.12

A 63-year-old asymptomatic woman, screening examination. Called back for evaluation of the microcalcifications detected in her left breast.

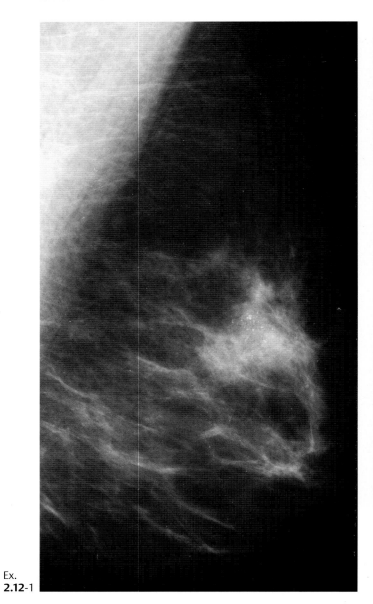

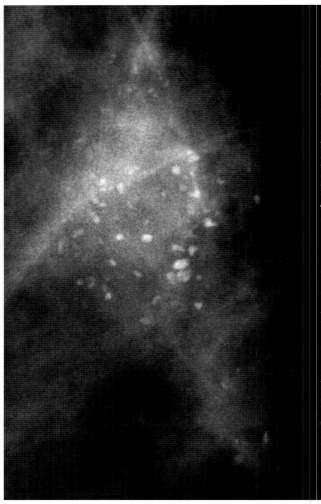

Ex.
2.12-1

Ex.
2.1

Ex. **2.12**-1 & 2   Left breast, MLO projection (1) and microfocus magnification (2). There is a large group of crushed stone–like, mammographically malignant calcifications surrounded by a non-specific soft-tissue density in the upper portion of the breast.

Ex. **2.12**-3   Breast Doppler ultrasound: hypoechoic malignant tumor with increased vascularity.

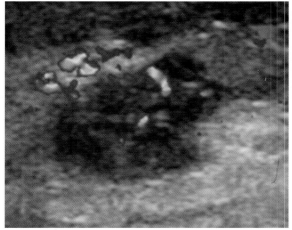

Ex.
2.1

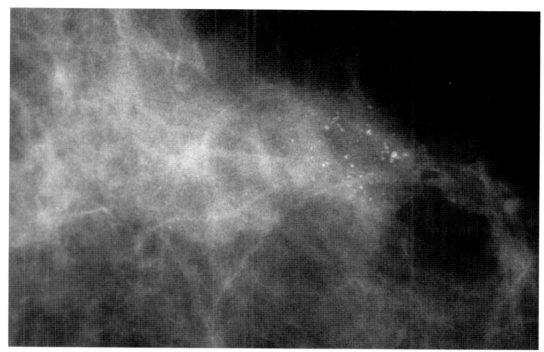

Ex. **2.12**-4

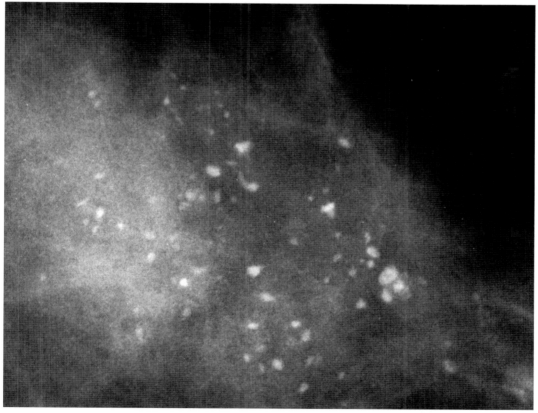

Ex. **2.12**-5

Ex. **2.12**-4 & 5   Detail of the left CC projection (4) and microfocus magnification (5). These are typical crushed stone–like, mammographically malignant type calcifications.

Example 2.12 continued

Ex. **2.12**-6   Medium-power histological image of the tightly packed cancerous structures and an associated desmoplastic reaction.

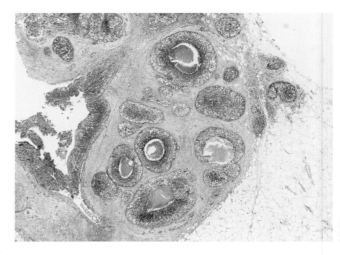

Ex.
2.1

Ex. **2.12**-7   Operative specimen radiograph.

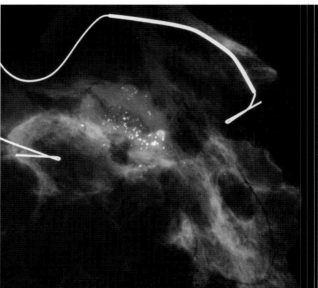

Ex.
2.1

Ex. **2.12**-8   Microfocus magnification radiograph of the sliced operative specimen.

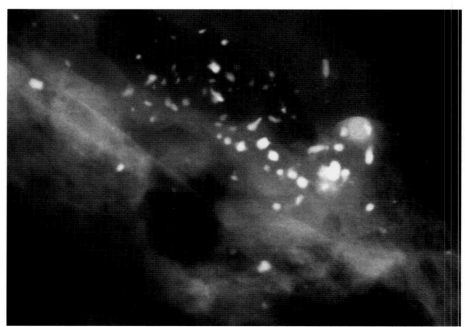

Ex.
2.1

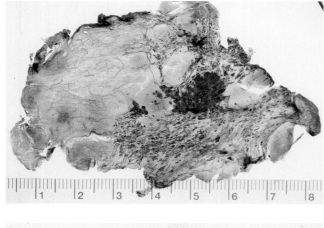

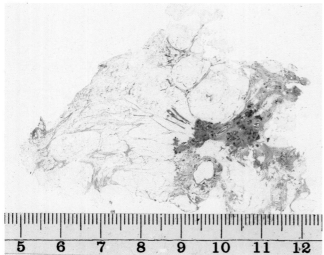

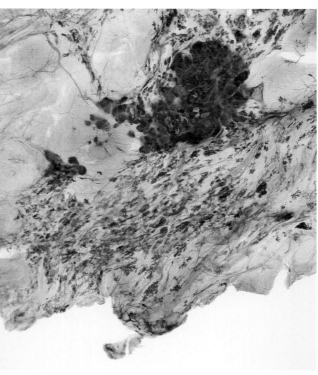

Ex. **2.12**-9 a & 9 b   Large subgross (9 a) and large thin-section (9 b) histological images demonstrating the malignant tumor and the surrounding tissue.

Ex. **2.12**-10   Detailed image of the subgross, 3D histology showing the multifocal tumor surrounded by normal breast tissue.

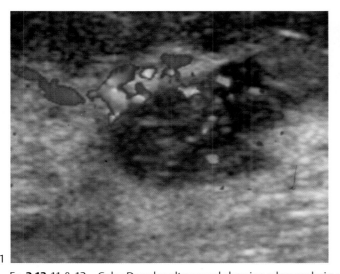

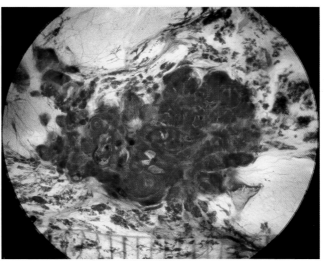

Ex. **2.12**-11 & 12   Color Doppler ultrasound showing a hypoechoic, well-vascularized tumor (11). Corresponding to the ultrasound finding and the soft-tissue mass on mammography and specimen radiography, there is an unnatural concentration of cancer-filled ductlike structures surrounded by a desmoplastic reaction (12). The disparity between the cancer-filled ductlike structures and the surrounding normal TDLUs is striking.

Example 2.12 continued

Histology: 30 mm × 15 mm Grade 3 in situ carcinoma associated with three invasive ductal carcinoma foci measuring 5 mm × 5 m, 3 mm × 3 m and 1 mm × 1 m. The four sentinel nodes removed were free from metastases.

Ex. **2.12**-13   Tenascin staining. The ductlike structures are closely spaced and show tenascin overexpression, suggesting neoductgenesis.

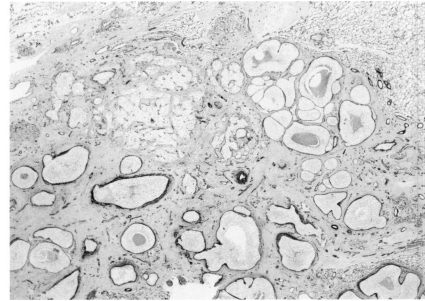

Ex. **2.12**

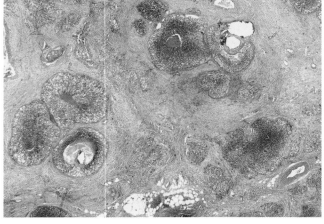

Ex. **2.12**-14

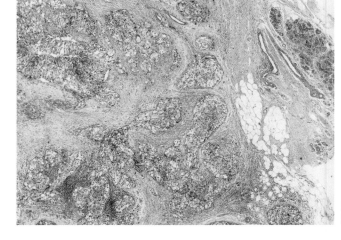

Ex. **2.12**

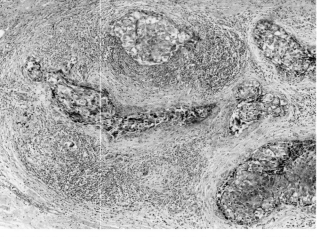

Ex. **2.12**-16

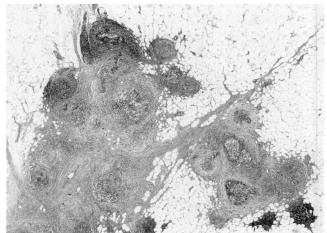

Ex. **2.1**

Ex. **2.12**-14 to 17   The conventional histology images (H&E, 14 to 16) show that the unnaturally concentrated ductlike structures are surrounded by an extensive desmoplastic reaction and lymphocytic infiltration, as often seen in cases with neoductgenesis. Ex. **2.12**-17 shows one of the three microinvasive foci.

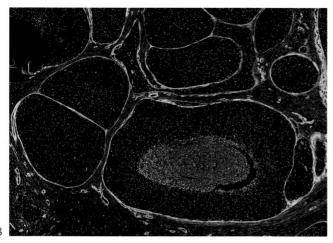

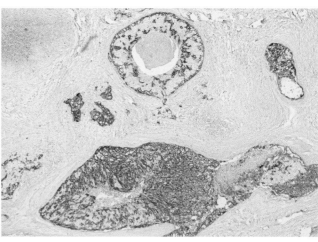

Ex. **2.12**-18

Ex. **2.12**-19

Ex. **2.12**-18   The basement membrane surrounding the ductlike structures is intact (laminin 4 immunostaining). Inverted image.

Ex. **2.12**-19   Immunohistochemical staining for c-erbB-2/Her-2-neu is positive.

Ex. **2.12**-20   Specimen slice radiograph showing calcifications and an ill defined "tumor mass."

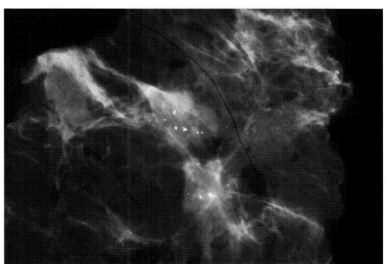

Ex. **2.12**-20

3D Image

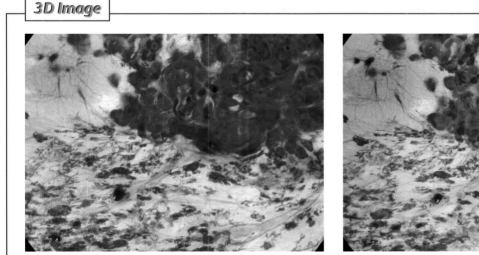

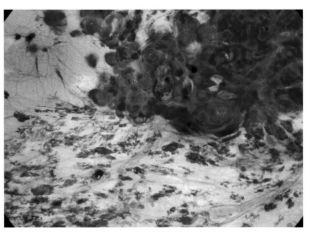

Ex. **2.12**-21

Ex. **2.12**-22

Ex. **2.12**-21 & 22   Subgross, thick-section (3D) histological images reveal that the "tumor mass" consists of a conglomerate of ductlike structures, conventionally termed "ductal carcinoma in situ" or "tumor forming DCIS." In reality, these are cancer-filled neoducts that often act as an invasive cancer does.[3] Note the adjacent entirely normal TDLUs and ducts.

Treatment and outcome: Sector resection and postoperative irradiation. This is a very recent case with only 1 year of follow-up.

Example 2.13

A 36-year-old woman who recently felt a small hard lump in the upper-outer quadrant of her left breast. Clinical breast examination confirms a freely mobile, 1 cm hard tumor. There are no skin changes or discharge.

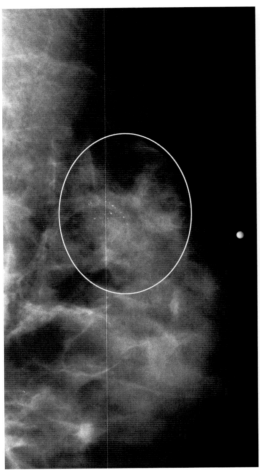

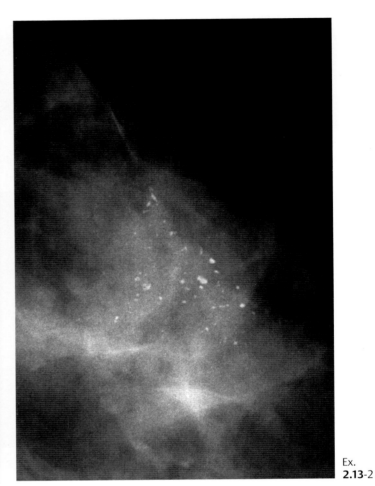

Ex.
2.13-1

Ex.
2.13-2

Ex. **2.13**-1 to 3   Left breast, detail of the MLO projection (1) and microfocus magnification images (2 & 3) of the region with the palpable lesion. The microcalcifications in the 12 mm × 10 mm cluster vary considerably in size and density. These crushed stone–like, broken needle tip–like pleomorphic calcifications are of the mammographically malignant type.

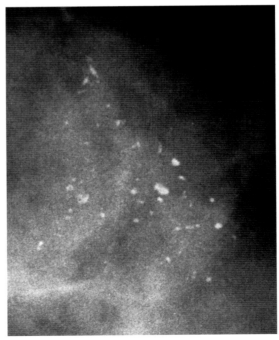

Ex.
2.13-3

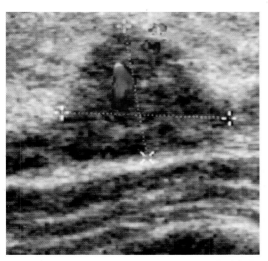
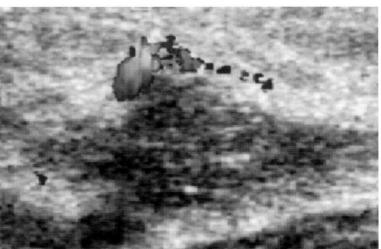

3-4

Ex.
2.13-5

Ex. **2.13**-4 & 5   Breast ultrasound of the palpable lesion.

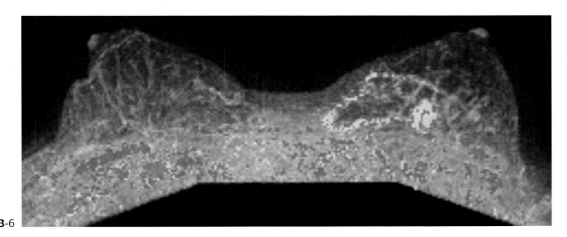

3-6

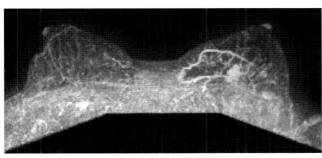

3-7

Ex. **2.13**-6 & 7   Breast MRI: There is a contrast enhancement corresponding to the palpable and mammo-graphic findings, suggesting malignancy.

Example 2.13 continued

Ex. **2.13**-8   Ultrasound image of the tumor with calcifications.

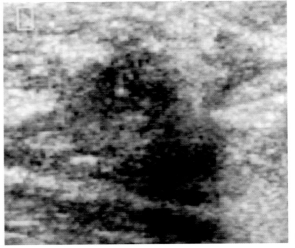

Ex. **2.13**-8

Ex. **2.13**-9   Ultrasound-guided 14-gauge core biopsy.

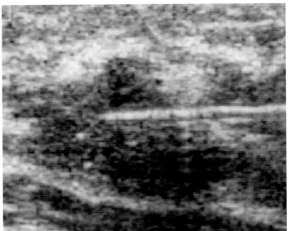

Ex. **2.13**-9

Ex. **2.13**-10 & 11   Histology of the core biopsy specimen: areas of in situ carcinoma.

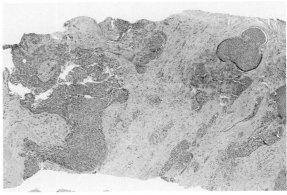

Ex. **2.13**-10

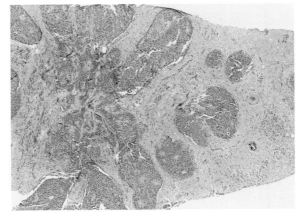

Ex. **2.13**-11

Ex. **2.13**-12   Detail of the left MLO projection.

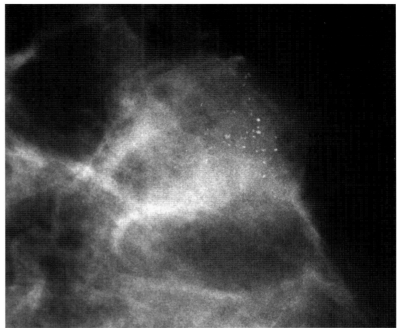

Ex. **2.13**-12

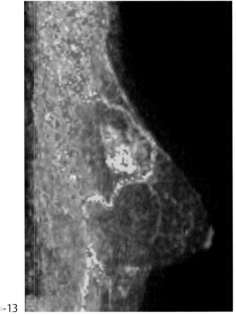

-13

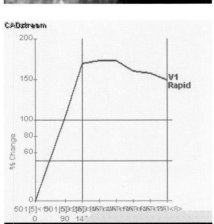

CADstream

3A

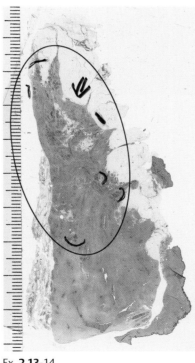

Ex. **2.13**-14

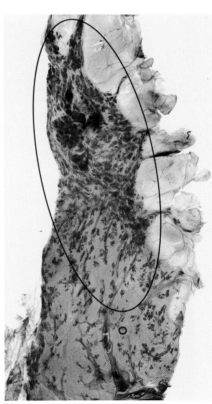

Ex. **2.13**-15

Ex. **2.13**-12 to 15   Comparison of the mammogram (12), breast MRI (13), large thin-section histology (14) and subgross, large thick-section slide (15). The enhancement curve (13A) shows the pattern typical for a malignant tumor. The histological examination revealed Grade 2 & 3 in situ carcinoma over an area measuring 50 mm × 20 mm. In addition, three foci (5, 3, and 1 mm) of Grade 2 invasive carcinoma were found within the same region.

Example 2.13 continued

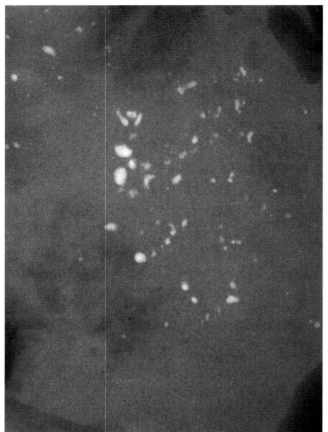

Ex.
2.13-16

Ex. **2.13**-16   Microfocus magnification of one of the surgical specimen slices that contain the calcifications.

Ex. **2.13**-17   Detail of the large-section histology slide demonstrating the area corresponding to the calcifications seen in Ex. **2.13**-16.

Ex.
2.1

3D Image

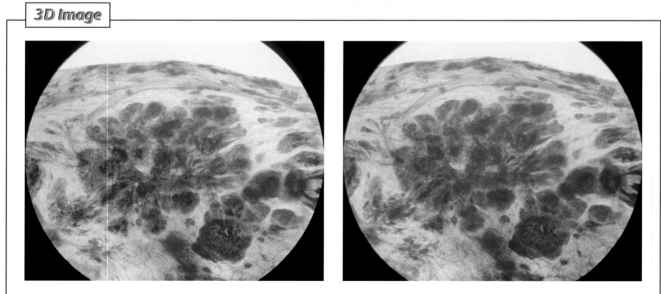

Ex.
2.13-18

Ex.
2.1

Ex. **2.13**-18 & 19   Subgross, thick-section histological image pair of a TDLU distended and distorted by cancer cells. Cellular details are shown at increasing magnification in Ex. **2.13**-20 to 25.

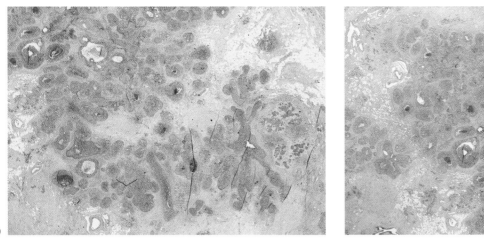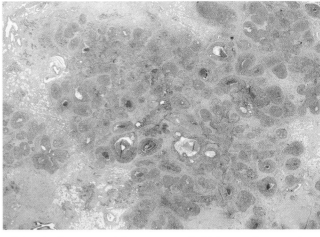

Ex. **2.13**-20

Ex. **2.13**-20 & 21   Medium-power histological images of cancer-filled acini and subsegmental ducts, many of which contain amorphous calcifications.

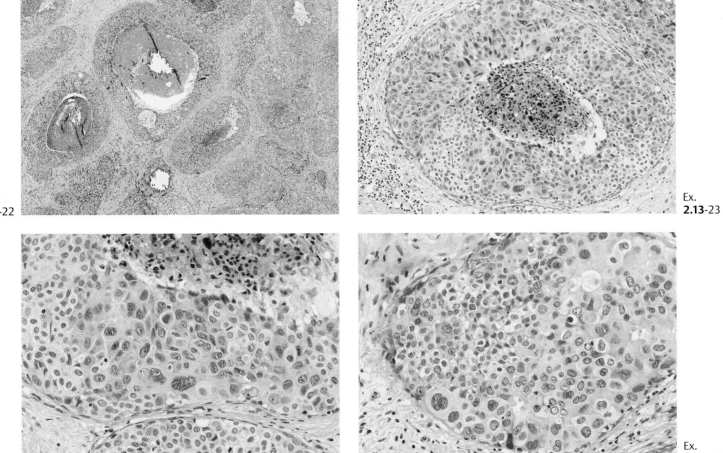

Ex. **2.13**-22

Ex. **2.13**-23

Ex. **2.13**-24

Ex. **2.13**-25

Ex. **2.13**-22 to 25   Higher-magnification histology images: high grade in situ carcinoma with solid cell proliferation and central necrosis.

Example 2.13 continued

Ex. **2.13**-26   Anti-actin staining demon-strates the maintained myoepithelial cell layer of the in situ component.

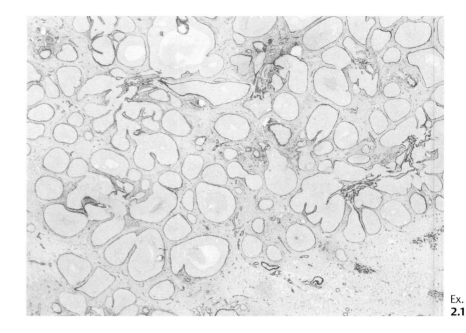

Ex.
2.1

Ex. **2.13**-27   Tenascin C immunohistochemi-cal staining.

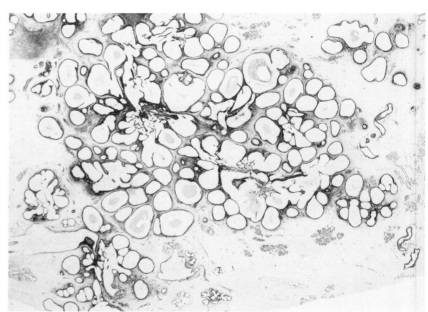

Ex.
2.1

Ex. **2.13**-28   Radiograph of one of the specimen slices with the microcalcifications.

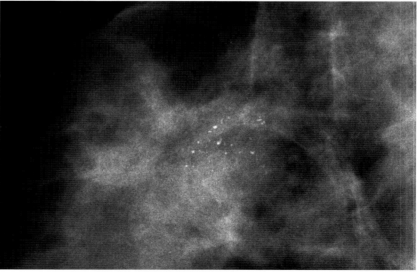

Ex.
2.1

Ex. **2.13**-29 to 31   Three histological slides showing focal Tenascin C overexpression, indicating neoductgenesis. No overexpression is seen in normal breast tissue (29, left side of the image; 31, right side of the image).

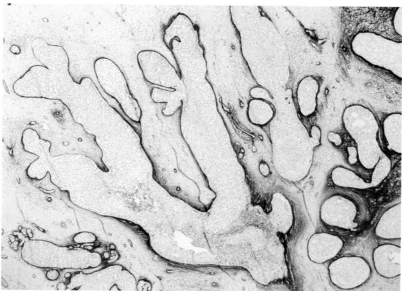

Ex.
2.13-29

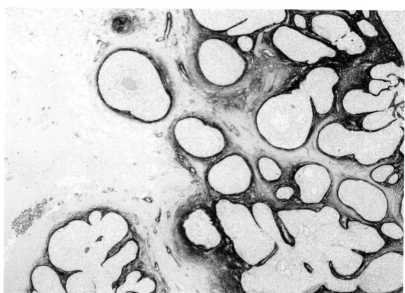

Ex.
2.13-30

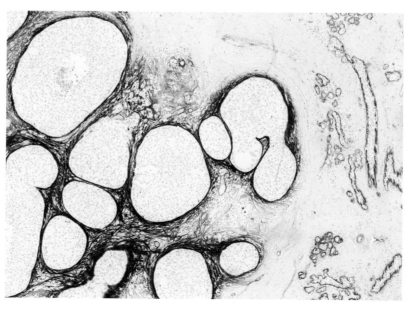

Ex.
2.13-31

Example 2.13 continued

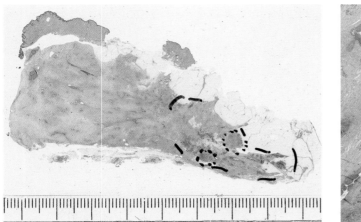

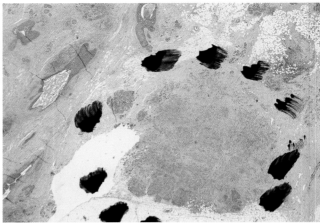

Ex.
2.13-32

Ex.
2.1

Ex. **2.13**-32 & 33   Low-power image of one of the large-section slices (32). The pathologist has marked the extent of the disease and the invasive foci (dotted lines). Medium-power histological images of one of the invasive foci (33).

3D Image

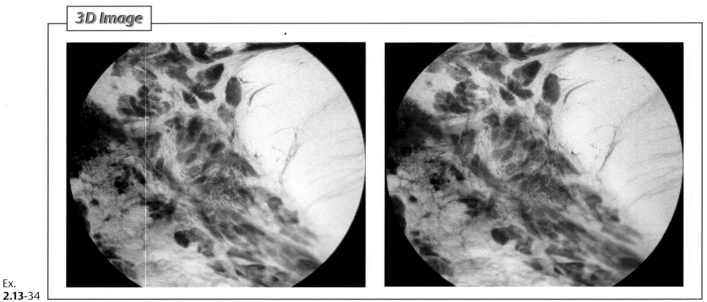

Ex.
2.13-34

Ex.
2.1

Ex. **2.13**-34 & 35   Stereoscopic subgross, thick-section (3D) histological image pair of a small invasive carcinoma surrounded by in situ components.

Treatment and outcome: Mastectomy. This is a most recent case, therfore follow-up results cannot be reported yet.

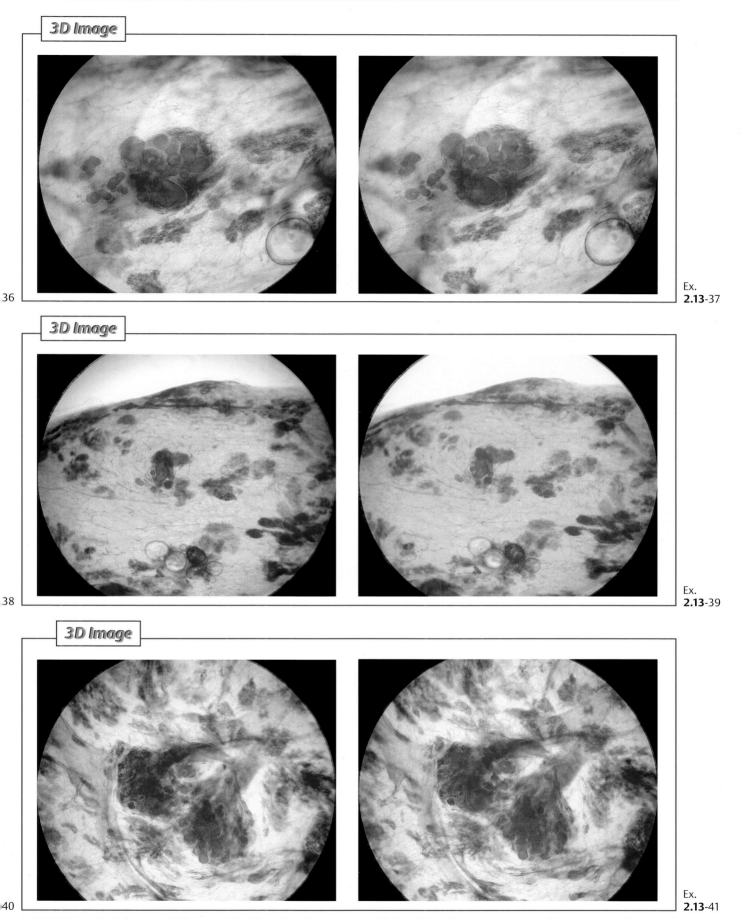

Ex. **2.13**-36 to 41   Subgross, thick-section (3D) histological image pairs of the additional in situ carcinoma foci, 10–15 mm from each other and from the main tumor focus, spread over an area measuring 50 mm × 20 mm.

■ The Long-term Outcome of Cases in Group 1B

In distinct contrast to cases in Group 1A, the mammographic image in untreated Group 1 B cases may change dramatically from a single or a few crushed stone–like calcifications to numerous crushed stone–like and casting type calcifications spread over a large part of the breast (Examples 2.11 and 2.12). Several examples of this type of progression were published in *Breast Cancer. Early Detection with Mammography, Casting Type Calcifications. Sign of a Subtype with Deceptive Features*[3] in Examples 2.2 (p. 80), 2.3 (p. 86), 2.4 (p. 90), 2.5 (p. 100), and 2.6 (p. 102). Since cases in Groups 1A and 1B cannot be mammographically distinguished from each other, despite their different underlying pathology, the practice of placing patients with crushed stone–like calcifications on follow-up, instead of performing percutaneous vacuum-assisted needle biopsy, will allow some malignant tumors to progress to an unfavorable stage. The use of functional imaging methods such as MRI of the breast, preferably prior to percutaneous biopsy, will greatly assist in the differential diagnosis and description of disease extent.

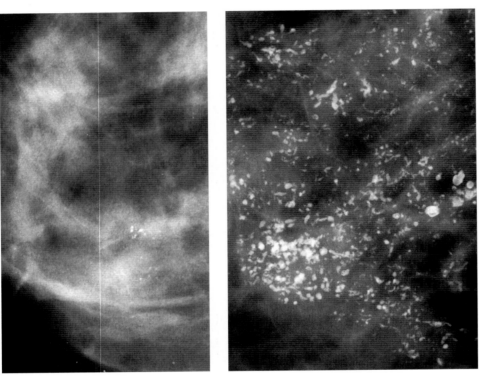

2.2-1   2.2-2

Figs. **2.2**-1 & 2   Mammograms of the same breast taken at an interval of 9 years (from Ex. **2.14**).

Example 2.14

This 88-year-old woman felt a lump in the upper-outer quadrant of her right breast. Physical examination con- firmed the finding and also showed slight skin retraction at the lateral edge of the areola.

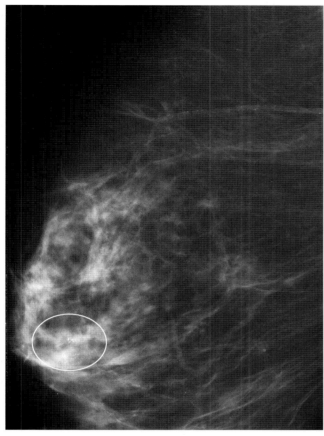

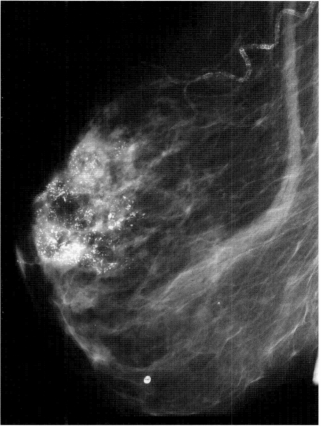

4-1

Ex.
2.14-2

Ex. **2.14**-1   Right breast, MLO projection from the previous ex- amination nine years earlier. There are two small retroareolar clusters of discernible calcifications (encircled).

Ex. **2.14**-2   Right breast, MLO projection. There is a large number of calcifications in the upper portion of the breast.

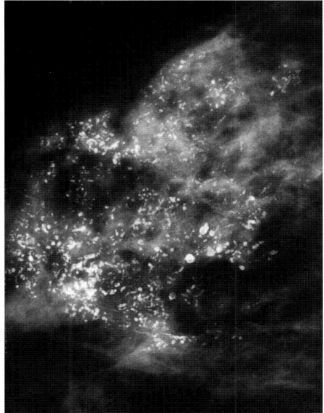

Ex. **2.14**-3   Microfocus magnification shows that calcifications are of the casting and crushed stone types, mammographically malignant. Although there is no distinct tumor mass, there is a non-specific radiopaque density confined to the area with the cal- cifications. The remainder of the breast consists mainly of adipose tissue.

Ex.
2.14-3

Example 2.14 continued

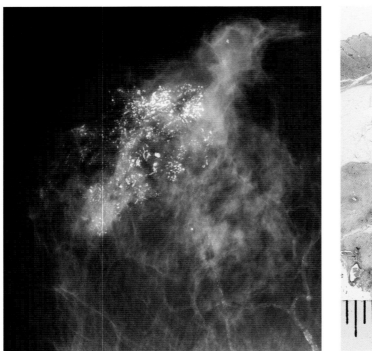

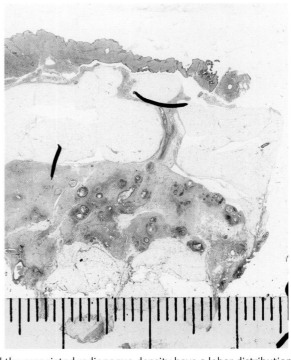

Ex.
2.14-4

Ex.
2.14-5

Ex. **2.14**-4 & 5   Right breast, CC projection (4). The calcifications and the associated radiopaque density have a lobar distribution in the lateral portion of the breast. Large-section histology (5) demonstrates the underlying pathology consisting of numerous cancerous ducts with necrosis, and calcifications and a surrounding desmoplastic reaction, corresponding to the radiopaque density on the mammogram.

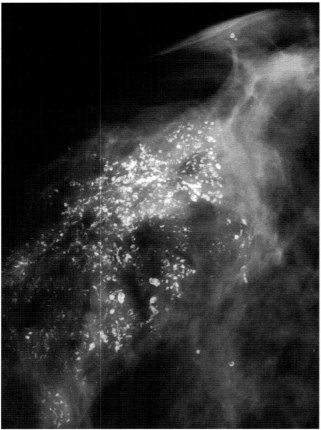

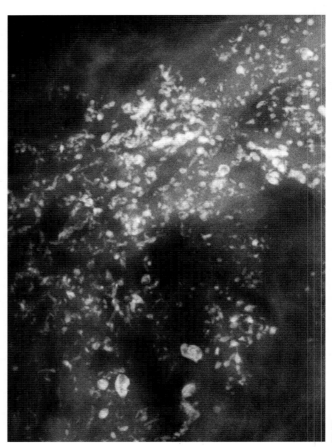

Ex.
2.14-6

Ex.
2.1

Ex. **2.14**-6 & 7   Photographic and microfocus magnification demonstrate the irregular shape and density of the crushed stone–like calcifications and how closely spaced the individual calcifications are. There are also numerous intermixed casting-type calcifications.

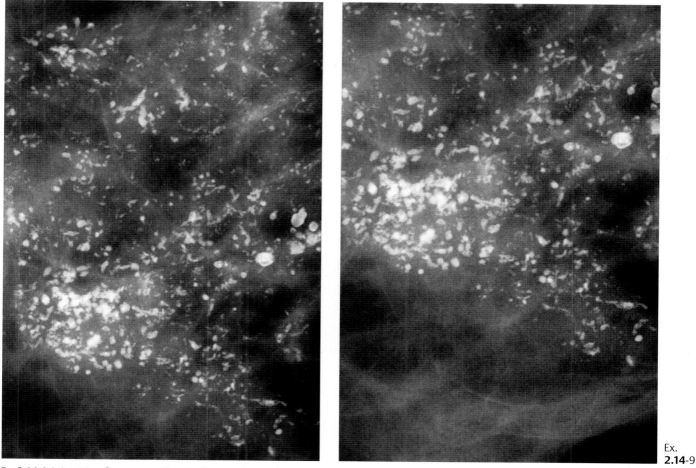

Ex. **2.14**-8 & 9   Microfocus magnification images demonstrate the mixture of the mammographically malignant crushed stone–like and casting type calcifications.

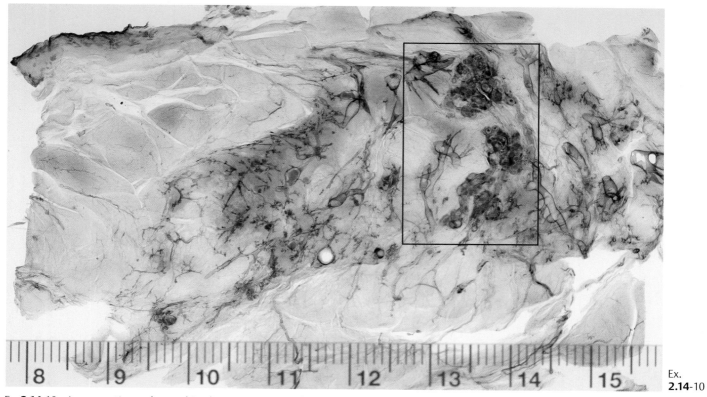

Ex. **2.14**-10   Large-section, subgross histology specimen. In this tissue slice the ducts, distended by malignant cells, necrosis, and amorphous calcifications, are within the rectangle.

Example 2.14 continued

Ex. **2.14**-11   There is a large number of faint casting type calcifications at the periphery of the calcified region. The calcifications in the central portion are much larger and have a higher density due to more extensive necrosis.

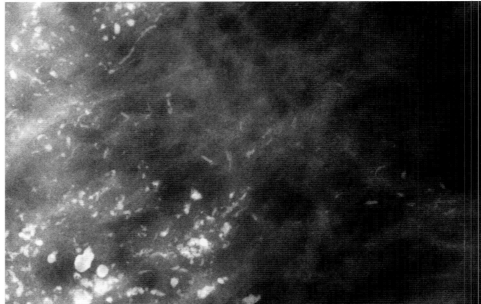

Ex. **2.1**

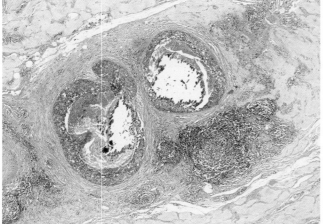

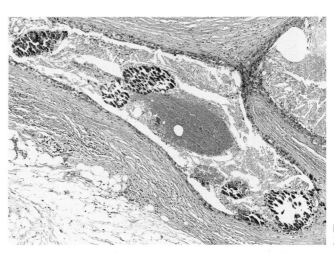

Ex. **2.14**-12

Ex. **2.1**

Ex. **2.14**-12 & 13   Histological examination of the preoperative 14-g needle core biopsy: Grade 2 and 3 in situ carcinoma with no demonstrable signs of invasion. Note the extensive desmoplastic reaction and lymphocytic infiltration surrounding the cancer-filled ducts.

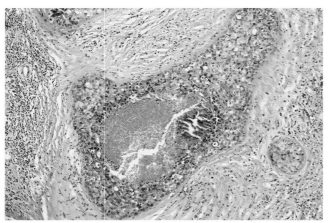

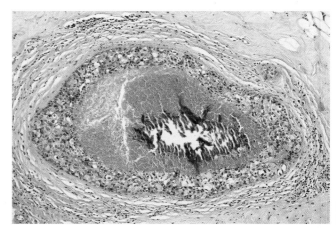

Ex. **2.14**-14

Ex. **2.1**

Ex. **2.14**-14 & 15   Histological images (H&E) of the cancerous ducts distended by Grade 3 cancer in situ with solid cell proliferation, central necrosis, and amorphous calcification.

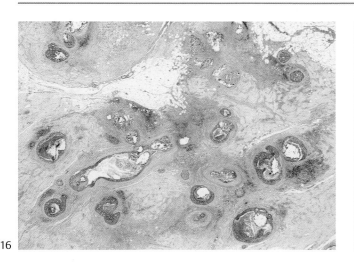

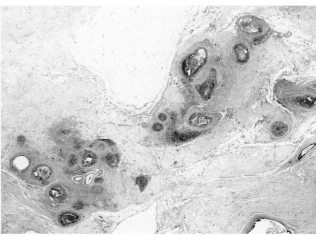

-16

Ex.
2.14-17

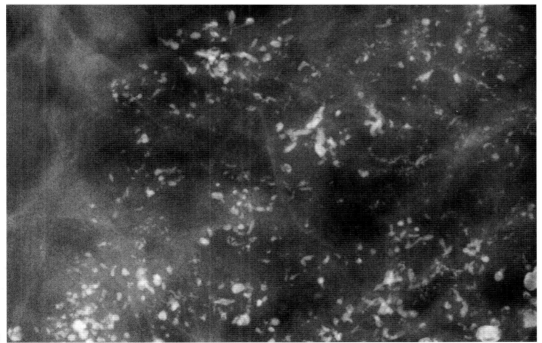

-18

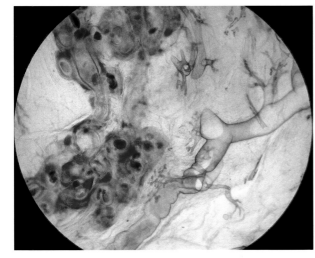

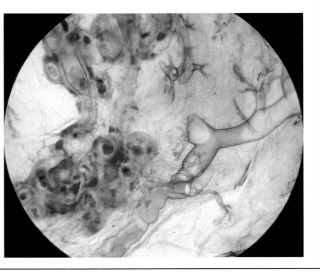

-19

Ex.
2.14-20

Ex. **2.14**-16 to 20   Comparison of histological images with a microfocus magnification mammogram. The region with Grade 3 in situ carcinoma measured 40 mm × 30 mm with no signs of invasion. No metastases were found in three removed sentinel nodes.

Example 2.14 continued

3D Image

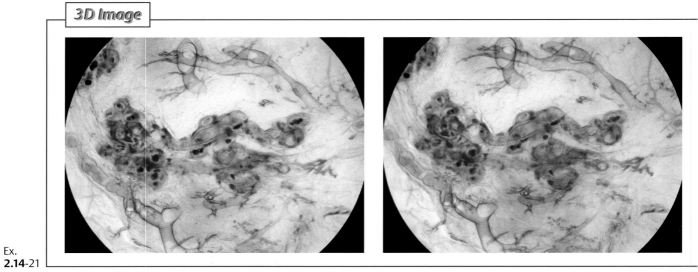

Ex. **2.14**-21

Ex. **2.1**

Ex. **2.14**-21 & 22   Subgross, thick-section (3D) image pair. On the top of the image, a fluid-filled, normal duct is seen. In the middle and lower part of the image, the ductlike structures are filled with high-grade "in situ" carcinoma, necrosis, and calcifications.

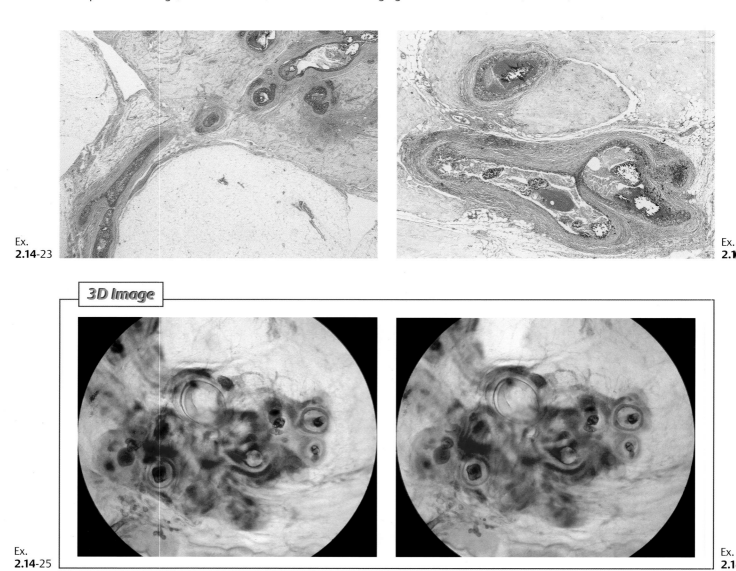

Ex. **2.14**-23

Ex. **2.1**

Ex. **2.14**-25

Ex. **2.1**

3D Image

Ex. 2.**14**-23 to 26   Comparison of conventional and subgross, thick-section (3D) histological images of the cancerous ductlike structures.

3D Image

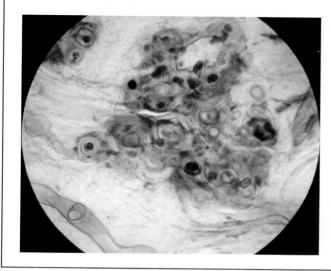 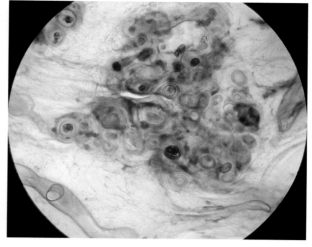

Ex.
2.14-28

Ex. **2.14**-27 to 30   Mammographic and thick-section (3D) histological image comparison in this high-grade "in situ" carcinoma case. The unnatural aggregate of the ducts containing the amorphous calcifications indicates neoductgenesis.

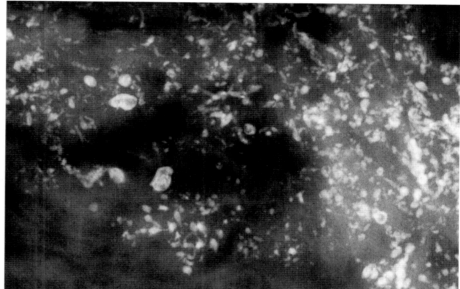

Ex.
2.14-29

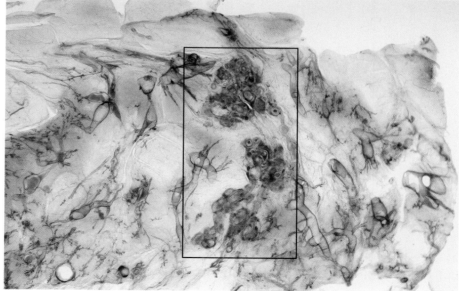

Treatment and outcome:
Mastectomy. The patient died 6 months following treatment. Cause of death: cardiac failure due to myocardial infarction.

Ex.
2.14-30

Example 2.15

This 81-year-old woman presented with left nipple discharge. Galactography showed a solitary filling defect in a dilated retroareolar duct.

Histology: Benign intraductal papilloma. The single cluster of faint crushed stone–like calcifications in the contralateral breast escaped observation.

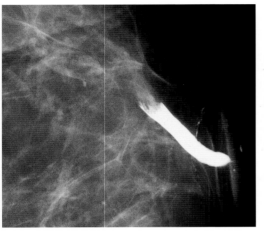

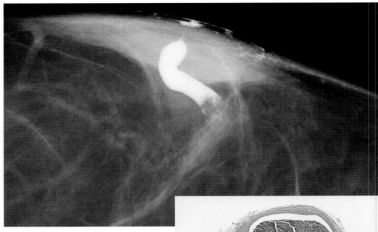

Ex.
2.1!

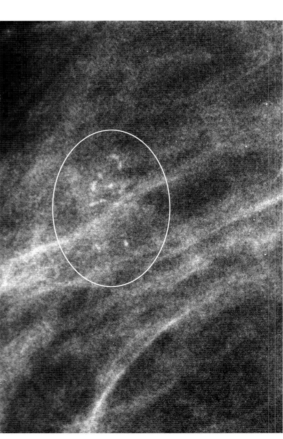

Ex.
2.1!

Ex.
2.15-1

Ex. **2.15**-1 to 3   Galactogram of the left breast. There is a filling defect in the dilated duct, which was shown to be a benign papilloma at histological examination (3).

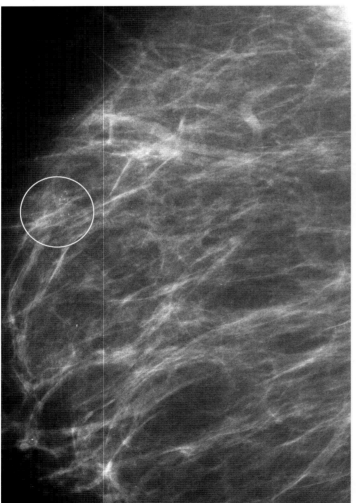

Ex.
2.15-4

Ex.
2.1!

Ex. **2.15**-4 & 5   Right breast, MLO projection and photographic magnification of the region containing the solitary cluster of calcifications.

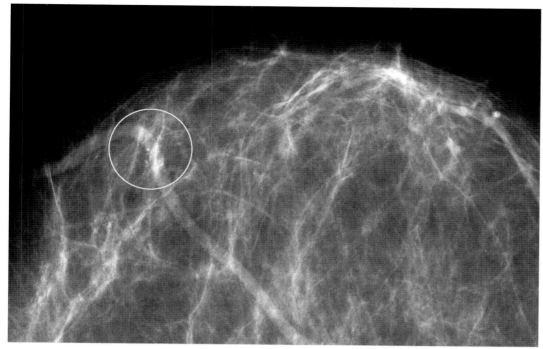

Ex. **2.15**-6

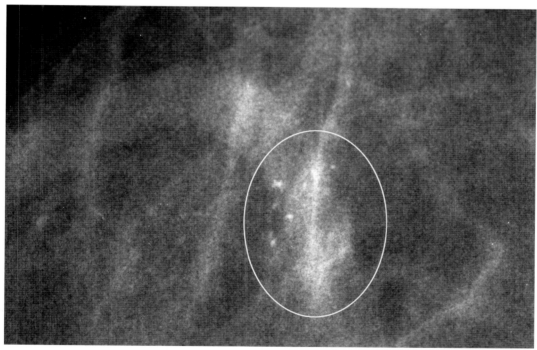

Ex. **2.15**-7

Ex. **2.15**-6 & 7 Right breast, CC projection and photographic magnification of the region containing the solitary cluster of calcifications.

Example 2.15 continued

Three and one-half years later the patient felt a tumor in the upper outer quadrant of her right breast.

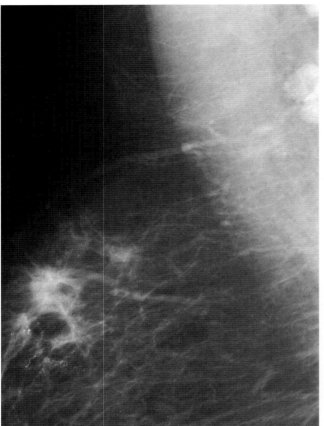 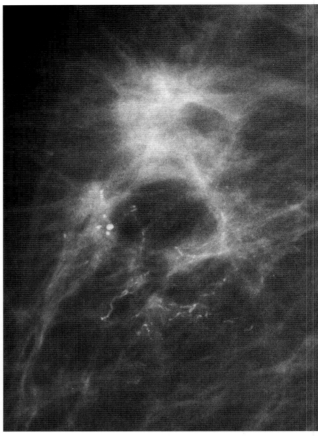

Ex. **2.15**-8

Ex. **2.1**

Ex. **2.15**-8 & 9   Right breast, detail of the MLO projection (8) and microfocus magnification (9) of the region with the palpable tumor, corresponding to a large region of architectural distortion associated with numerous casting type calcifications. Pathological axillary lymph nodes are also seen.

Ex. **2.15**-10   Right breast, CC projection. The mammographically malignant tumor and the calcifications occupy a large part of the upper-outer quadrant.

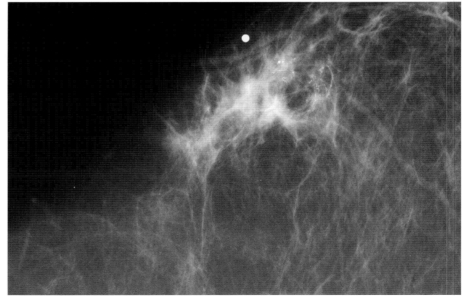

Ex. **2.1**

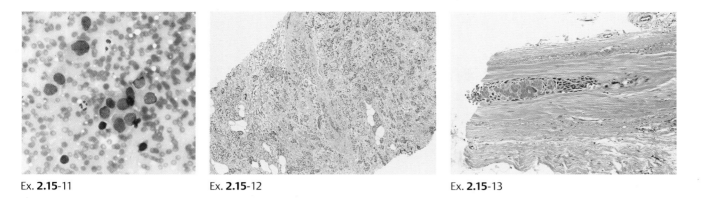

Ex. **2.15**-11   Ex. **2.15**-12   Ex. **2.15**-13

Ex. **2.15**-11 to 13   Preoperative fine-needle aspiration biopsy shows malignant cells (11). Ultrasound-guided 14-g core biopsy: Grade 2 invasive ductal carcinoma (12) associated with Grade 3 in situ carcinoma (13).

3D Image

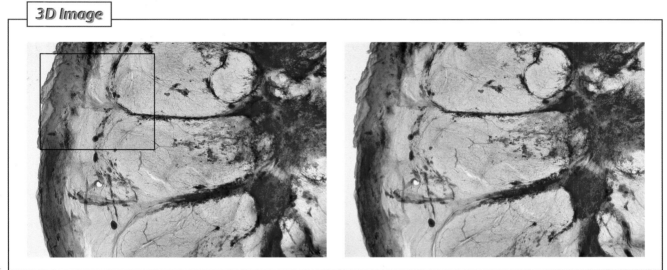

-14   Ex. **2.15**-15

Ex. **2.15**-14 & 15   Stereoscopic subgross, thick-section (3D) histology shows the multifocal invasive carcinoma infiltrating the Cooper ligaments and the superficial fascia.

3D Image

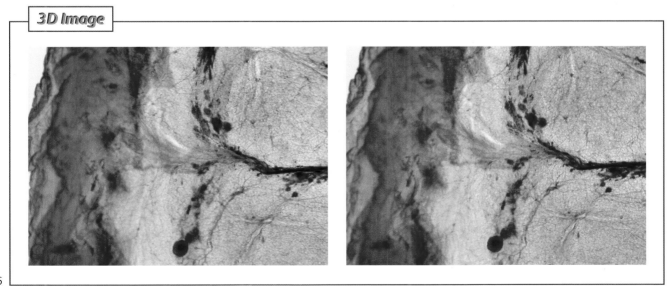

-16   Ex. **2.15**-17

Ex. **2.15**-16 & 17   Stereoscopic subgross, thick-section (3D) histological image pair of the area in the rectangle in Ex. **2.15**-14. The malignant process infiltrates the Cooper ligament and the superficial fascia.

Example 2.15 continued

3D Image

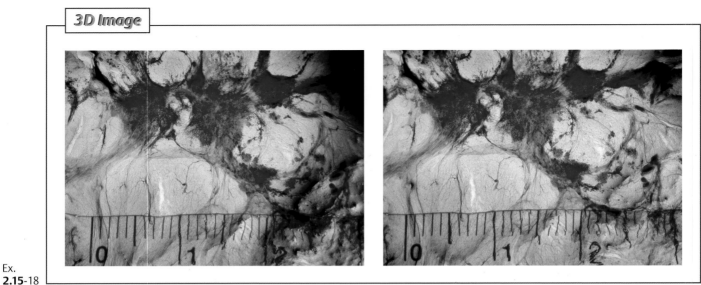

Ex.
2.15-18

Ex.
2.1

Ex. **2.15**-18 & 19   Stereoscopic subgross, thick-section (3D) histological image pair: multiple invasive foci, the largest measuring 15 mm × 10 mm, surrounded by extensive Grade 3 in situ carcinoma. Metastases were found in all 9/9 axillary lymph nodes.

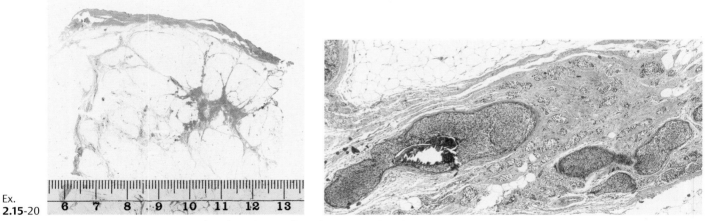

Ex.
2.15-20

Ex.
2.1

Ex. **2.15**-20 & 21   Large-section histology (20) and medium-power histological image (21) of the invasive ductal carcinoma and the associated Grade 3 in situ cancer.

Ex. **2.15**-22   Histological image of one of the metastatic lymph nodes.

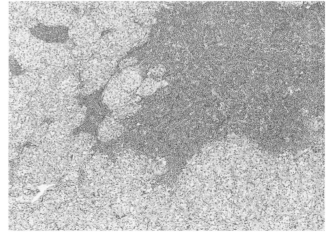

Ex.
2.1

Ex. **2.15**-23
Microfocus magnification showing extensive casting type calcifications.

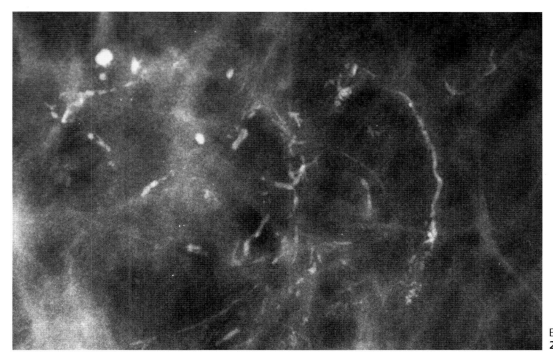

Ex. **2.15**-23

3D Image

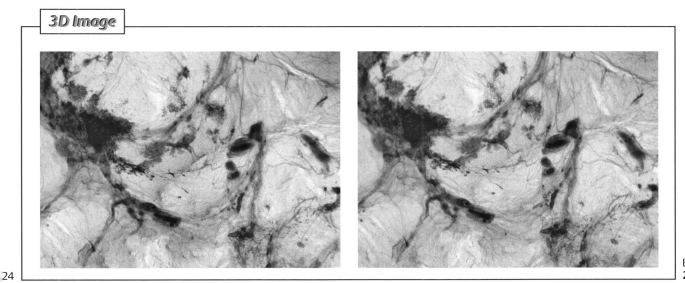

24

Ex. **2.15**-25

Ex. **2.15**-24 & 25   Stereoscopic subgross, thick-section (3D) histology of the area with casting type calcifications.

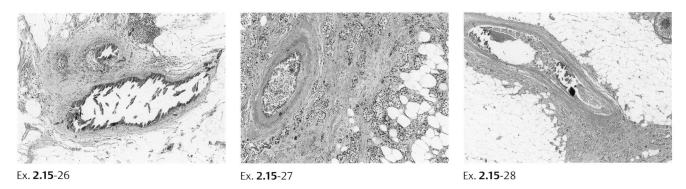

Ex. **2.15**-26   Ex. **2.15**-27   Ex. **2.15**-28

Ex. **2.15**-26 to 28   Detailed images of the histological examination illustrating the invasive ductal and Grade 3 in situ carcinoma.

Treatment and outcome: Mastectomy. Three years after treatment the patient had no evidence of disease.

Example 2.16

A 59-year-old asymptomatic woman, screening examination.

Ex. **2.16**-1
Detail of the left MLO projection. Two tiny groups of discernible calcifications have not been perceived at screening examination.

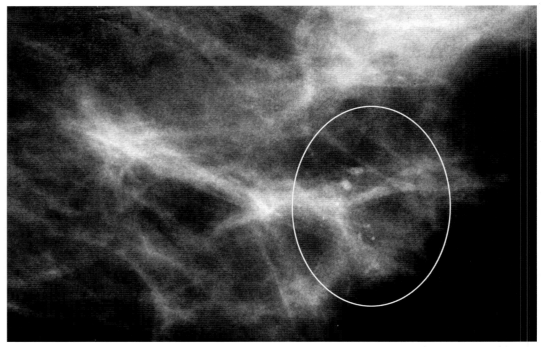

Ex. **2.16**-1

Ex. **2.16**-2   Detail of the left MLO projection 2 years later. The size of the area with calcifications (rectangle) has increased considerably since the previous examination.

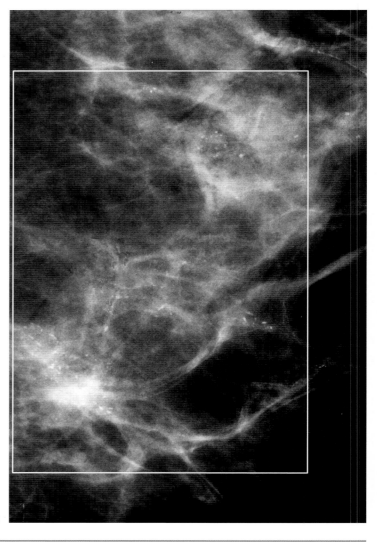

Ex. **2.16**-2

Ex. **2.16**-3
Left breast, CC projection, 2 years after the initial examination. The area with the malignant type calcifications is marked with a rectangle.

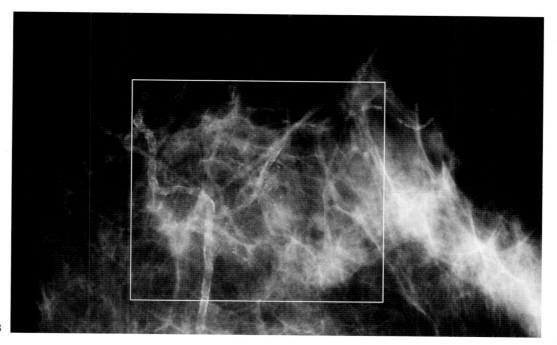

Ex. **2.16**-3

Ex. **2.16**-4
Detail of the area with the malignant type, casting-type calcifications.

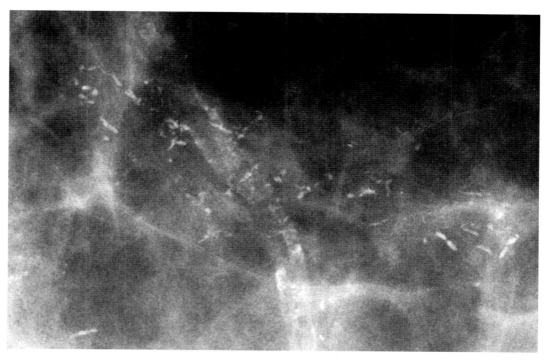

Ex. **2.16**-4

Example 2.16 continued

Treatment and outcome: Mastectomy. The patient had no signs of recurrence at the most recent follow-up 15 years after operation.

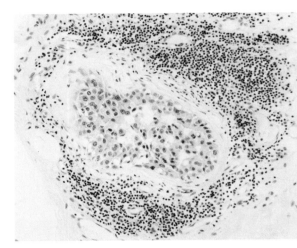

Ex. **2.16**-5   Fine-needle aspiration biopsy: malignant cells.

Ex. **2.16**-5

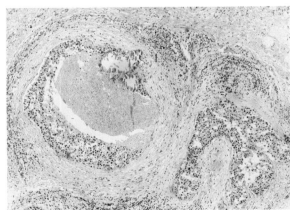

Ex. **2.16**-6

Ex. **2.16**-6 & 7   Medium-power images of ductlike structures distended by malignant cells, central necrosis and amorphous calcifications, surrounded by a thick desmoplastic reaction and lymphocytic infiltration, resembling the histological image of neoductgenesis.

Ex. **2.16**-7

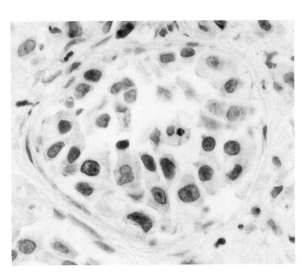

Ex. **2.16**-8   High magnification of the Grade 3 cancer in situ (van Gieson staining). Extent of the disease is > 60 mm. Histological images courtesy of Peter Karolyi, M.D., Central Hospital, Västerås, Sweden.

Ex. **2.16**-8

Chapter 3 Multiple Clusters of Crushed Stone–like Calcifications on the Mammogram Produced by Malignant Processes

Mammograms showing **multiple clusters** (or rarely a single cluster) of crushed stone–like calcifications that represent only a portion of the underlying disease can be subdivided by careful correlation of mammographic; large-section histological; and subgross, thick-section histological images into the following two subgroups.

Group 2A The in situ process is primarily **confined to TDLUs that are separated from each other by normal tissue,** although histology may reveal a few involved ducts. In these cases there is reasonable concordance between the mammographic and histological findings. The crushed stone–like calcifications may also be associated with powdery calcifications, seen in close proximity on the mammograms, representing Grade 2 and Grade 1 in situ carcinoma side by side.

Group 2B Although the mammographic image may show multiple clusters which appear similar to those in Group 2A, large-section histological examination demonstrates tightly packed cancerous TDLUs and ducts covering a larger area than that indicated by the calcifications detected at mammography. MRI of the breast plays an important role in revealing the true extent and confluent nature of the underlying disease. In some extreme cases very large numbers of clusters of crushed stone–like calcifications are visible on the mammogram, often associated with some casting type calcifications. The larger the number of clusters, the more difficult it is to discern the individual clusters. Correlation with large-section and subgross, 3D histology shows **a high density of tightly packed cancerous TDLUs and ducts with little, if any, normal tissue in between.** Histological signs of neoductgenesis and lymph vessel invasion are often present and may account for the occasional poor outcome.

Group 2A: Multiple Foci on Histology with Intervening Normal Tissue

Example 3.1

A 62-year-old asymptomatic woman, screening examination.

Ex. **3.1**-1 & 2   Details of the left MLO (1) and CC (2) screening mammograms. There are several clusters of microcalcifications in the lower-outer quadrant.

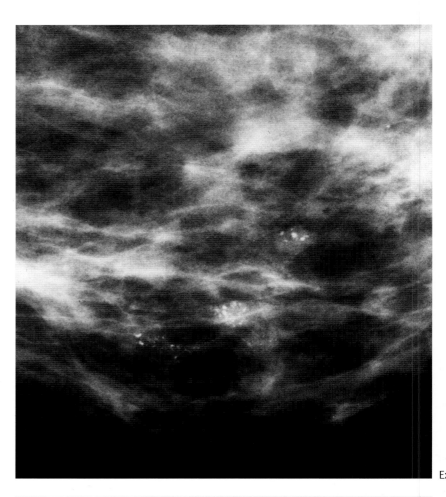

Ex

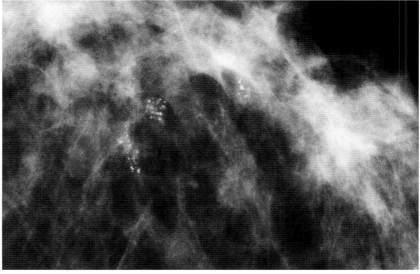

Ex

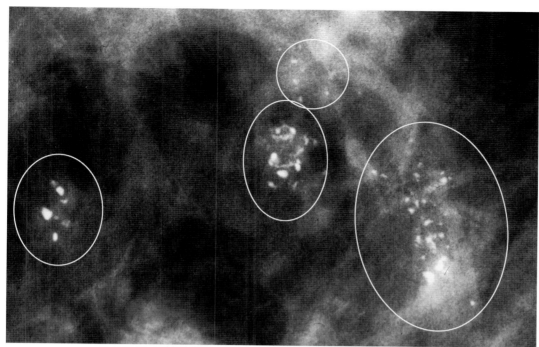

Ex. **3.1**-3

Ex. **3.1**-3 Microfocus magnification, left CC projection. There is normal breast tissue separating the clusters of calcifications from each other. The first step in calcification analysis is to determine their distribution. When they are clustered and the individual calcifications are discernible, the probability of malignancy increases with an increasing number of clusters. The second step is to evaluate the shape and density of the individual calcifications. The greater their variation in shape and density, the higher the probability that they are malignant type calcifications.

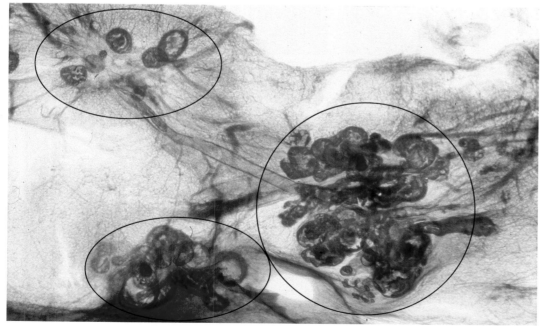

Ex. **3.1**-4

Ex. **3.1**-4 Subgross 3D histology confirms that the malignant type calcifications arise within the TDLUs which are distended by the cancer cells. The terminal ducts do not contain malignant cells. Although the current terminology is "DCIS," in reality the disease process is confined to the lobules and does not appear in the ducts in this case.

A more precise term would be Grade 2 in situ carcinoma confined to several lobules.

Example 3.1 continued

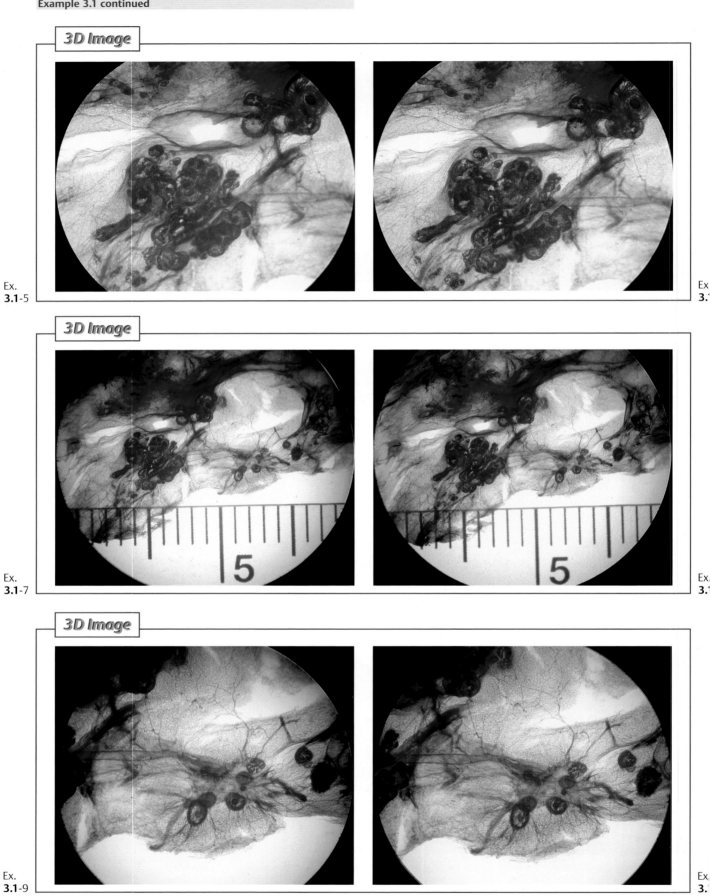

Ex. **3.1**-5 to 10   Stereoscopic image pairs of subgross, 3D histology showing several TDLUs distended by in situ carcinoma. The individual acini are larger than normal-sized TDLUs.

3D Image

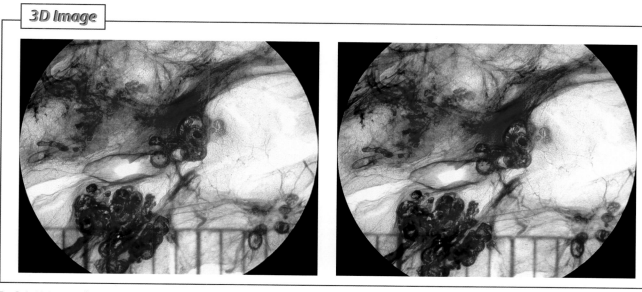

11

Ex.
3.1-12

Ex. **3.1**-11 & 12   This stereoscopic image pair demonstrates that the distended TDLU containing the malignant type calcifications measures 4 mm. Stereotactic technique is required for accurate preoperative percutaneous biopsy.

Treatment and outcome: Sector resection and postoperative irradiation. The patient died of acute leukemia 12 years after treatment. During the follow-up period there was no evidence of breast cancer recurrence.

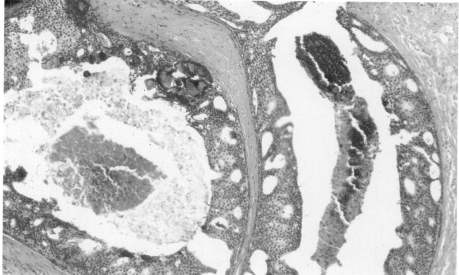

Ex.
3.1-13

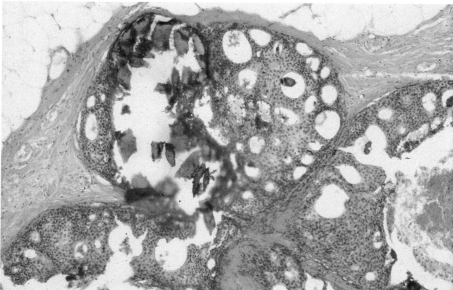

Ex. **3.1**-13 & 14   Histological diagnosis: Grade 2 in situ carcinoma with a cribriform pattern, central necrosis, and amorphous calcifications.

Ex.
3.1-14

Example 3.2

A 55-year-old asymptomatic woman, screening examination. She was called back for further assessment of the calcifications detected on the screening mammograms.

Ex. **3.2**-1   Microfocus magnification mammography of the right breast, CC projection. Multiple clusters of crushed stone–like calcifications are seen without an associated tumor mass. The calcifications vary in size and density, and some are triangular, arrowhead-shaped, and mammographically malignant.

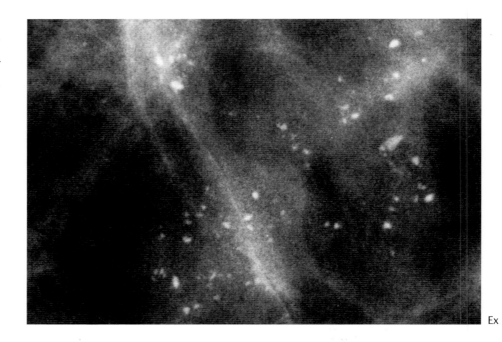

Ex

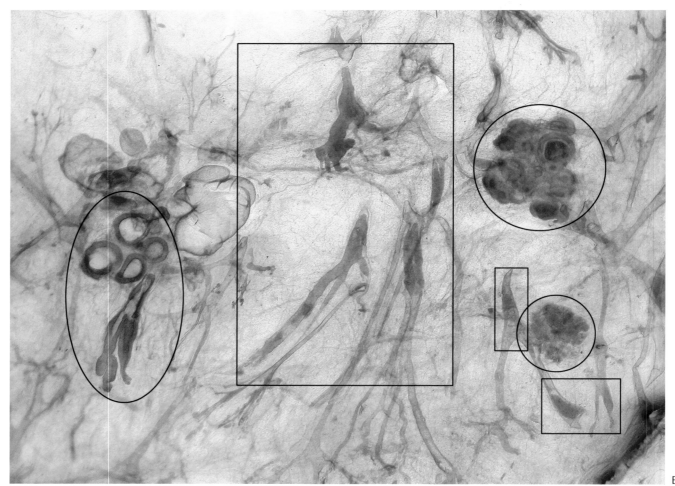

Ex.

Ex. **3.2**-2   Subgross, thick-section histology. The TDLUs distended by in situ carcinoma and containing the crushed stone–like calcifications are encircled. Foci of in situ carcinoma not containing calcifications, and thus occult to mammography, are seen within the rectangles.

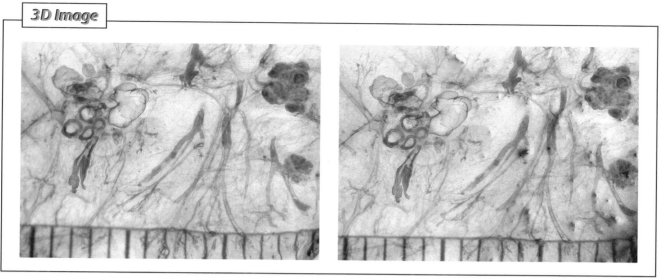

2-3   Ex. **3.2**-4

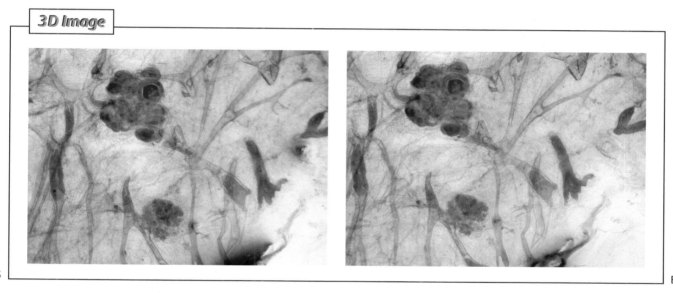

2-5   Ex. **3.2**-6

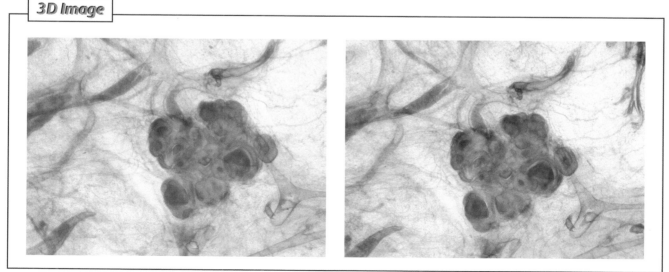

-7   Ex. **3.2**-8

Ex. **3.2**-3 to 8   Progressively enlarged stereoscopic views of this subgross, 3D specimen. These images demonstrate that the multiple clusters of calcifications are restricted to the distended TDLUs, but also show noncalcified malignant foci nearby.

Example 3.2 continued

3D Image

Ex.
3.2-9

Ex.
3.2

Ex. **3.2**-9 to 11   Stereoscopic image pair (9 & 10) and medium-power conventional histological image (11) of a single cancerous TDLU, with the terminal duct also involved.

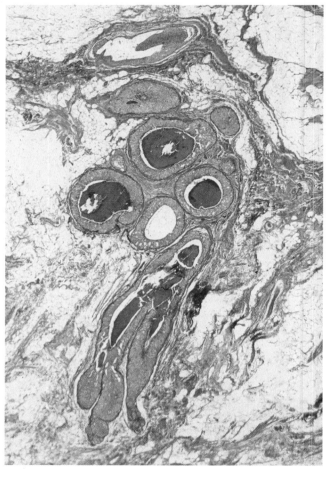

Ex.
3.2

Final histology: Grade 2 in situ carcinoma over an area measuring 50 mm in diameter. Cancer cells were demonstrated at the resection margin.

Treatment and outcome: Sector resection. Histological examination has found cancer foci on the margin. Mastectomy: no residual tumor, pNX. The patient was symptom-free at the most recent follow-up examination 12 years after operation.

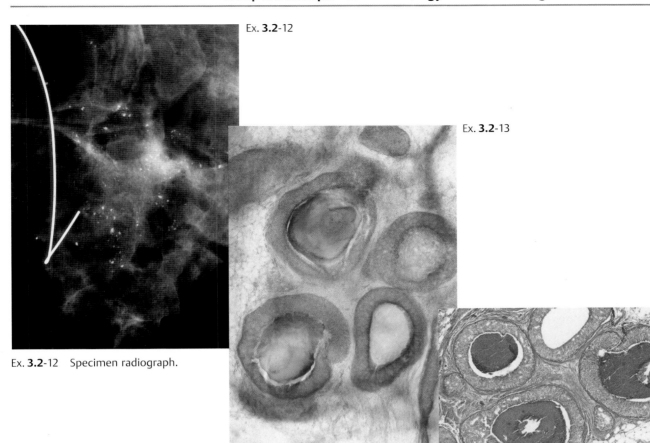

Ex. **3.2**-12

Ex. **3.2**-12   Specimen radiograph.

Ex. **3.2**-13

Ex. **3.2**-13   Subgross, 3D histologic image.

Ex. **3.2**-14

Ex. **3.2**-14   Low-power histological image of the cancer-filled acini. The extent of the Grade 2 in situ carcinoma is 50 mm.

Ex. **3.2**-15

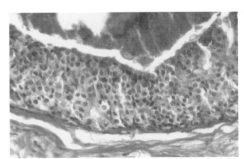

Ex. **3.2**-12 to 15   The gap between the mammogram with its lower resolution and conventional histology with its exquisite higher resolution can be bridged by subgross, thick-section histology for better mammographic–histological correlation, as illustrated in this step wedge.

Ex. **3.2**-15   Medium-power histological image: Grade 2 in situ carcinoma.

Comment

The multiple clusters on the mammogram reflect the multiple cancerous TDLUs. Unlike the contiguous tumor growth characteristic of casting type calcification cases and the subgroup 2B, the multiple cluster crushed stone–like calcification cases described at the beginning of this chapter originate in individual TDLUs that are separated from each other by a few millimeters of intervening normal tissue. Viewing the large thick-section/3D histological slices not only provides excellent correlation with the mammographic findings but also unearths additional, valuable information, such as mammographically occult cancer foci. In this particular example, the distance between two of the calcified TDLUs was 8 mm. These observations suggest that the term "close" surgical margin may be an unreliable description when the finding on the mammogram consists of multiple clusters of crushed stone–like calcifications.

Example 3.3

This 65-year-old woman was called back from mammography screening for assessment of multiple clusters of calcifications in the right breast.

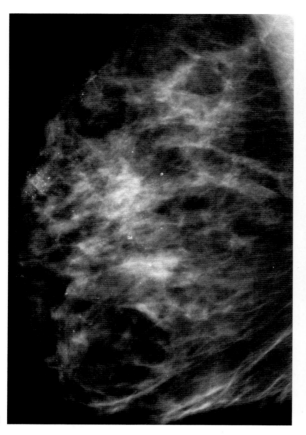

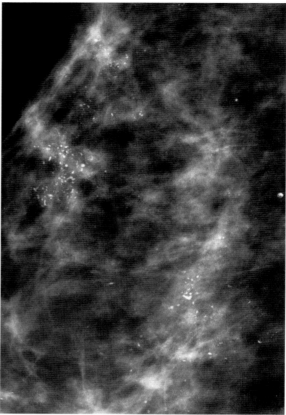

Ex. **3.3**-1

Ex. **3.3**-2

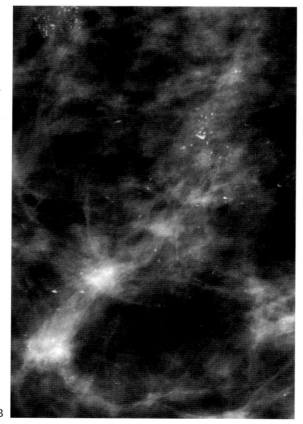

Ex. **3.3**-1 to 3 Right breast, MLO projection. Contact (1) and microfocus magnification (2, 3) images. Many clusters of crushed stone–like calcifications are scattered throughout much of the breast.

Ex. **3.3**-3

Ex. **3.3**-4 to 6   Right breast, CC projection (4). The microfocus magnification images (5 & 6) reveal the diversity of the individual calcifications within the clusters.

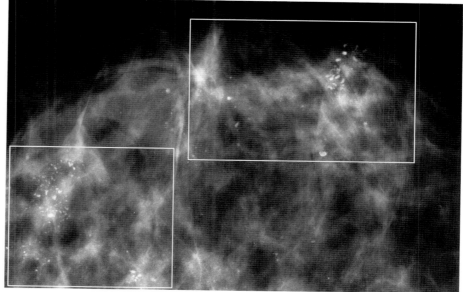

Ex. **3.3**-4

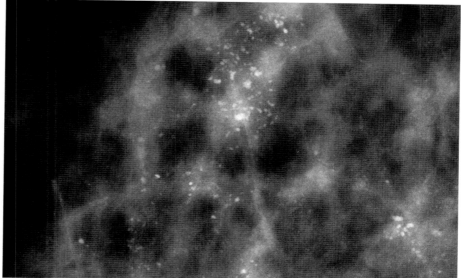

Ex. **3.3**-5

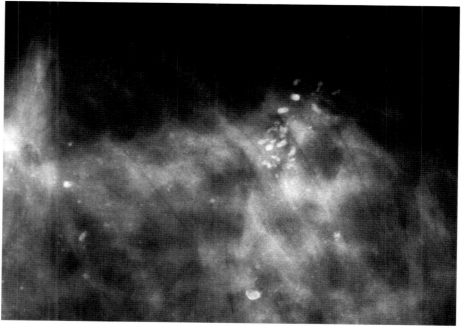

Ex. **3.3**-6

Example 3.3 continued

Ex. **3.3**-7 to 9   Right breast, CC projection, microfocus magnification images at increasing enlargement.

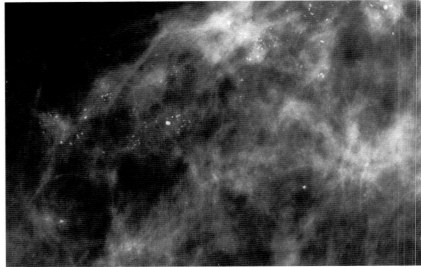

Ex.

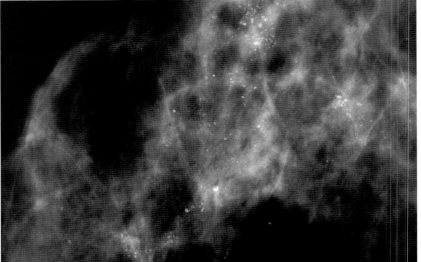

Ex.

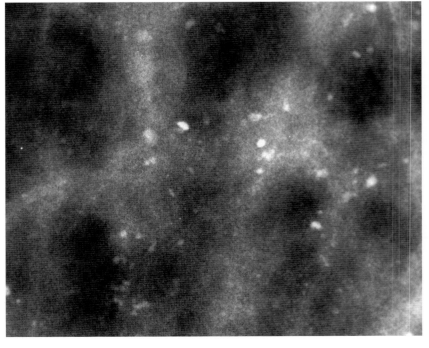

Ex.

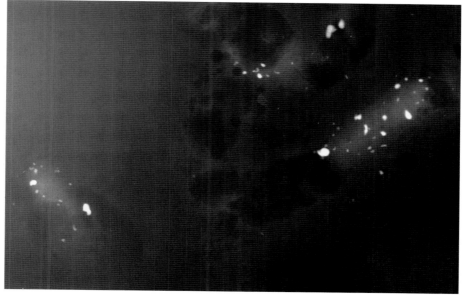

Ex.
3.3-10

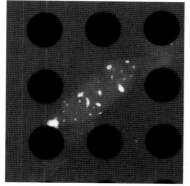

Ex. **3.3**-11

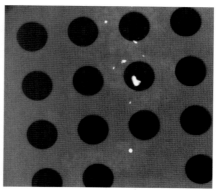

Ex. **3.3**-12

Ex. **3.3**-13

Ex. **3.3**-10 to 13   Radiographs of the preoperative vacuum-assisted biopsy specimen.

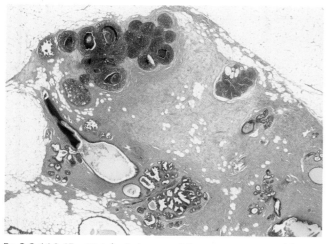

-14

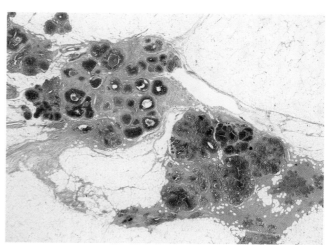

Ex.
3.3-15

Ex. **3.3**-14 & 15   Histologic image of the vacuum-assisted biopsy specimen (H & E): in situ carcinoma.

Example 3.3 continued

Ex. **3.3**-16
Radiograph of one
of the operative
specimen slices.

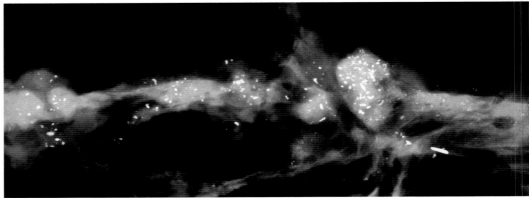

Ex.
3.3

3D Image

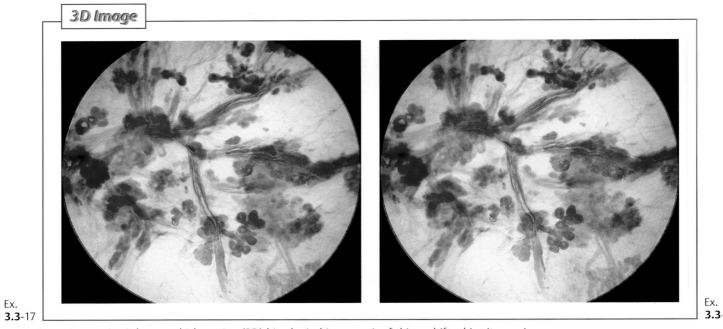

Ex.
3.3-17

Ex.
3.3

Ex. **3.3**-17 & 18   Subgross, thick-section (3D) histological image pair of this multifocal in situ carcinoma.

Ex. **3.3**-19
Magnification of the
left half of the
specimen radio-
graph in Ex. **3.3**-16.

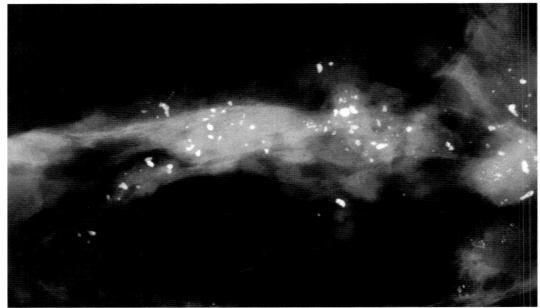

Ex.
3.3

Ex. **3.3**-20   Magnification of the remaining half of the specimen radiograph in Ex. **3.3**-16.

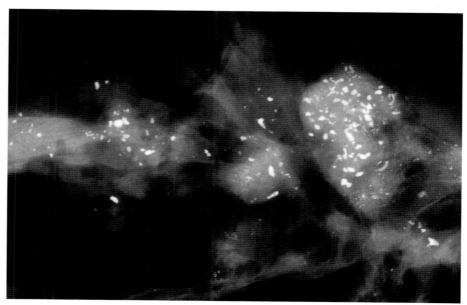

Ex. **3.3**-20

Ex. **3.3**-21   Large-section histology
image shows the extensive multifocal in situ carcinoma involving individual, separate TDLUs.

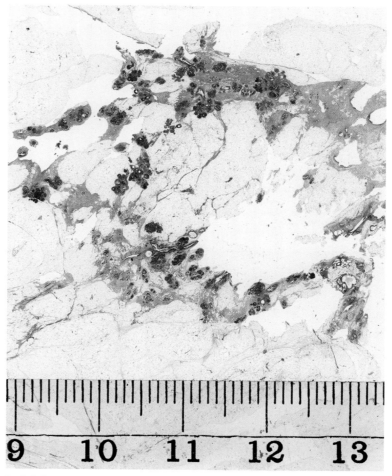

Ex. **3.3**-21

Example 3.3 continued

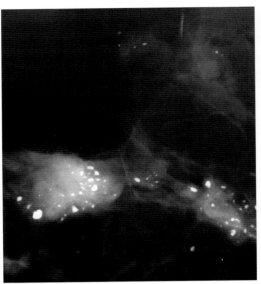

Ex. **3.3**-22

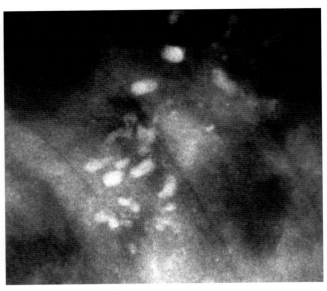

Ex. **3.3**-23

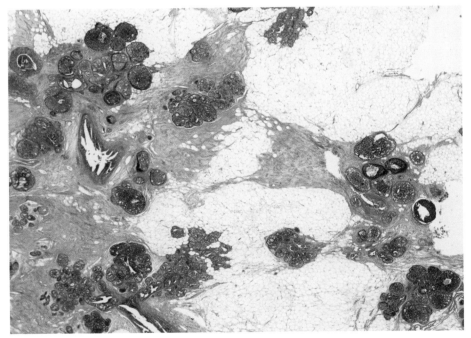

Ex. **3.3**-24

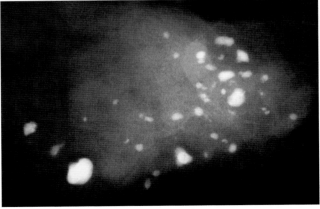

Ex.
3.3-25

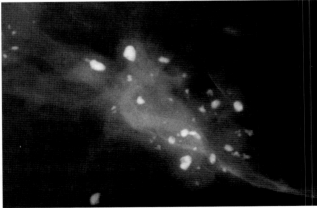

Ex.
3.3

Ex. **3.3**-22 to 26   Histological–mammographic correlation of the multiple clusters of cancerous TDLUs containing the crushed stone–like calcifications

Ex. **3.3**-27 to 29   The histological image shows a single TDLU distended by in situ carcinoma, central necrosis and amorphous calcifications. This corresponds to one of the many clusters of crushed stone–like calcifications on the mammogram.

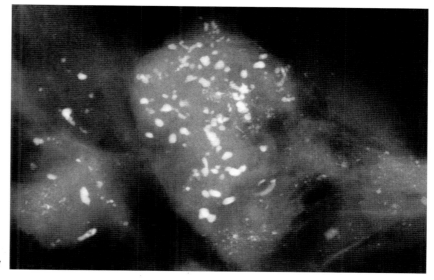

Ex. **3.3**-27

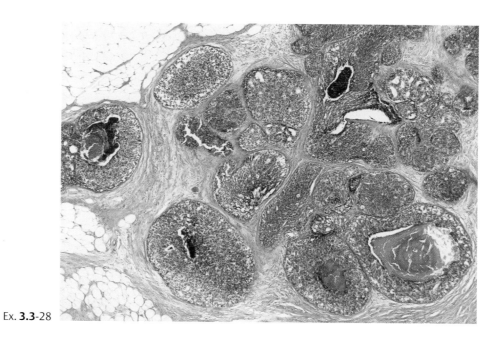

Ex. **3.3**-28

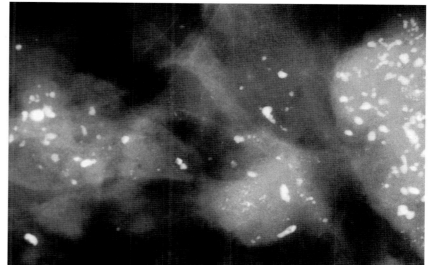

Ex. **3.3**-29

Example 3.3 continued

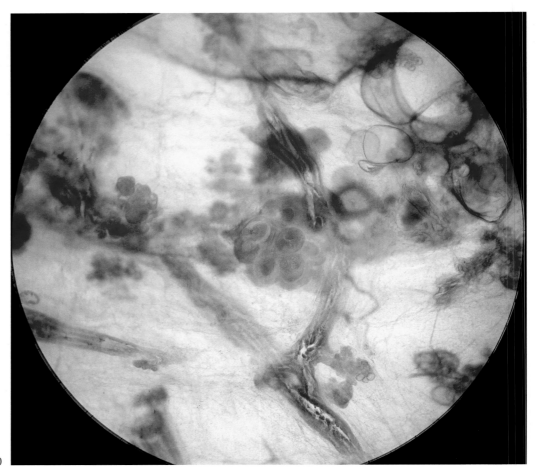

Ex. **3.3**-30

Ex. **3.3**-30 & 31　The in situ carcinoma distending several TDLUs and a duct is demonstrated in comparative subgross, thick-section (3D) (30) and low-power conventional (31) histological sections.

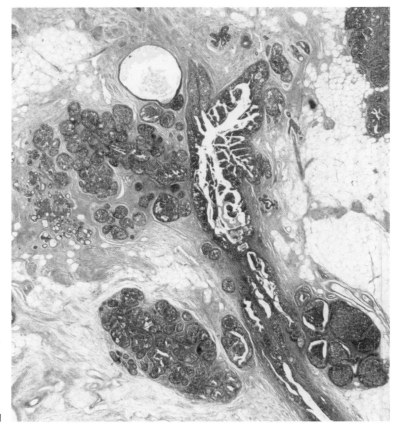

Ex. **3.3**-31

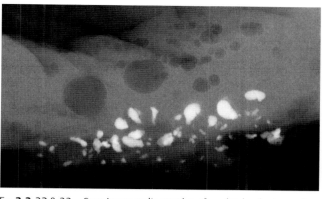

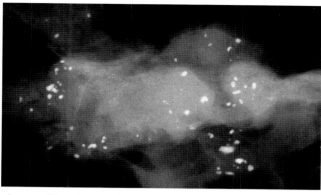

Ex. **3.3**-32

Ex. **3.3**-33

Ex. **3.3**-32 & 33   Specimen radiographs of multiple clusters of crushed stone–like, pleomorphic calcifications.

3D Image

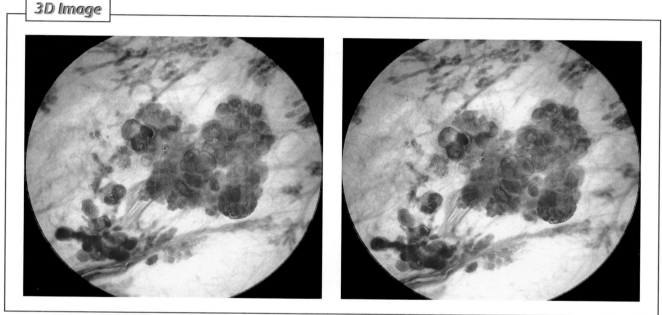

-34

Ex. **3.3**-35

Ex. **3.3**-34 & 35   Subgross, thick-section (3D) histological image of one of the TDLUs distended by Grade 2 in situ carcinoma, containing the crushed stone–like calcifications.

Ex. **3.3**-36   The Grade 2 in situ carcinoma is associated with the amorphous calcifications. These are seen on the mammogram as crushed stone–like, pleomorphic calcifications.

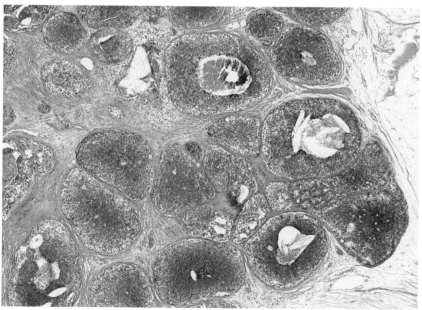

Ex. **3.3**-36

Example 3.3 continued

3D Image

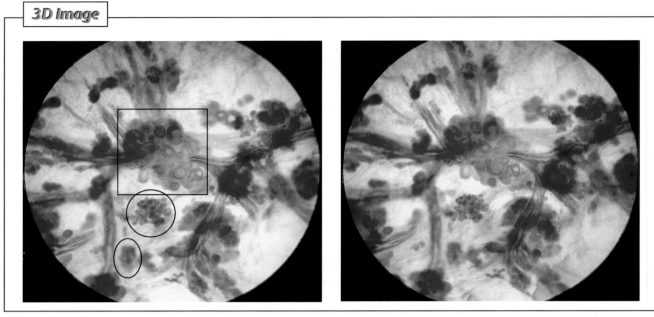

Ex.
3.3-37

Ex.
3.3

Ex. **3.3**-37 & 38   Subgross, thick-section (3D) image pair of several cancerous TDLUs and ducts.

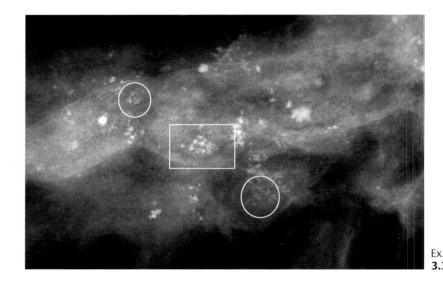

Ex. **3.3**-39   Radiograph of a specimen slice showing the crushed stone–like calcifications (rectangle) and the powdery calcifications (circles). Compare with the corresponding subgross (37 & 38) and conventional (40) histological images.

Ex.
3.3

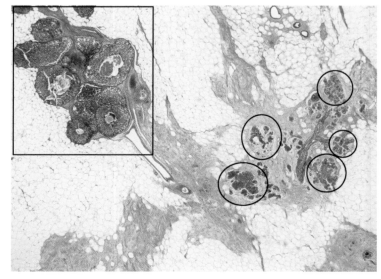

Ex. **3.3**-40   Mammographic–histological correlation (39 & 40) of adjacent TDLUs containing Grade 2 and Grade 1 in situ carcinoma. The Grade 2 in situ process (rectangle) distends the TDLU to a greater extent and contains the crushed stone–like calcifications, while the Grade 1 in situ carcinoma distends the TDLU considerably less and contains the powdery calcifications, if there is any calcification at all associated with it.

Ex.
3.3

3D Image

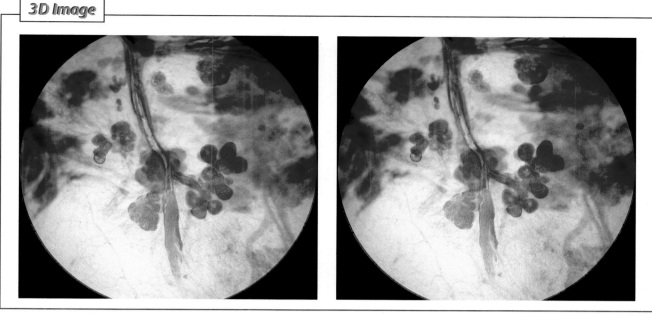

Ex. **3.3**-41 & 42   Subgross histological image pair of several TDLUs and a subsegmental duct distended by in situ carcinoma.

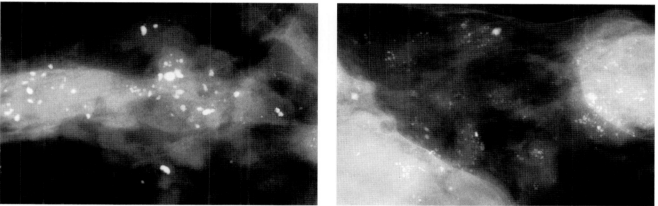

Ex. **3.3**-43 & 44   Specimen radiographs containing crushed stone–like (43) and multiple clusters of powdery (44) calcifications.

3D Image

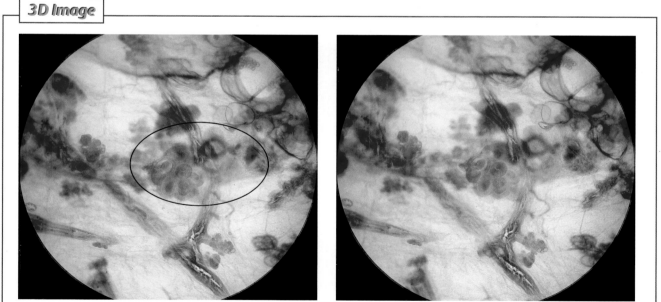

Ex. **3.3**-45 & 46   Stereotactic image pair showing acini greatly distended by Grade 2 in situ carcinoma and intraluminal amorphous calcifications (oval) and less distended acini containing Grade 1 in situ cancer, interconnected by cancerous ducts.

Example 3.3 continued

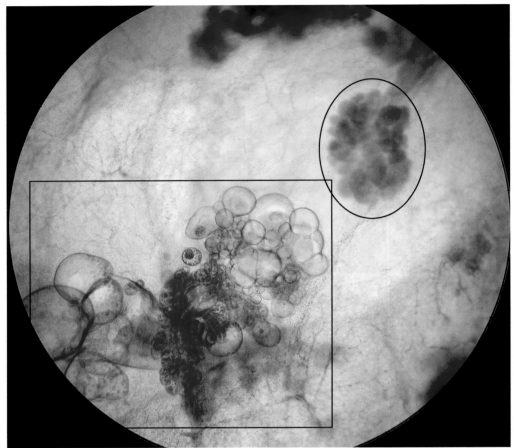

Ex. **3.3**-47

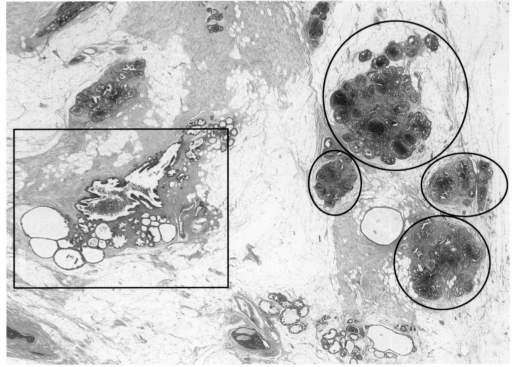

Ex. **3.3**-48

Ex. **3.3**-47 to 48   Subgross, thick-section (3D) and large-section histological images of several adjacent TDLUs. The cystically dilated TDLU (rectangle) contains psammoma body–like calcifications that are shown on the mammogram as powdery and teacup–like microcalcifications. Also the Grade 1 in situ carcinoma (circles) contain powdery calcifications, mammographically indistinguishable from those seen in cystically dilated TDLUs or in sclerosing adenosis.

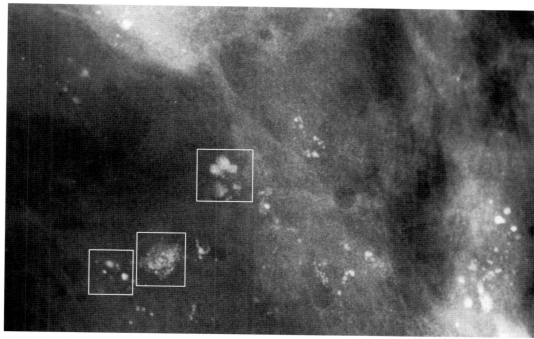

Ex. **3.3**-49

Ex. **3.3**-49   Specimen radiograph demonstrating powdery and teacup–like calcifications in benign fibrocystic change.

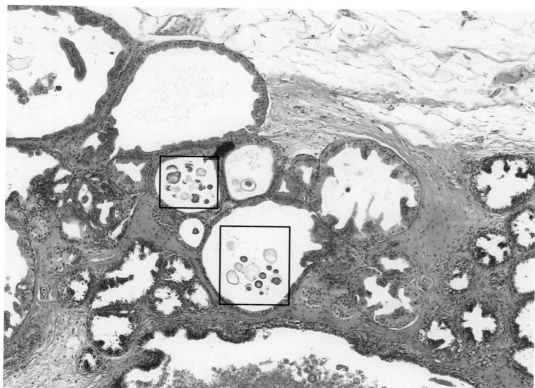

Ex. **3.3**-50

Ex. **3.3**-50   Low-power histological image of cystically dilated acini lined with apocrine metaplasia. The summation of the psammoma body–like calcifications can be seen on the mammogram as either powdery or teacup–like calcifications.

Example 3.4

A 54-year-old asymptomatic woman, screening examination. Her sister had breast cancer at age 59 years.

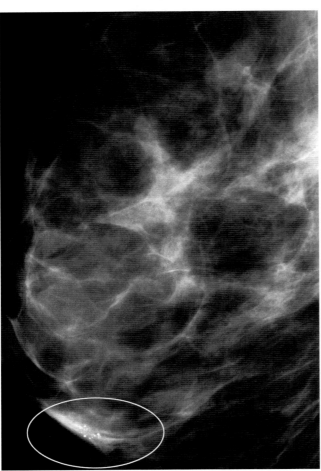

Ex. **3.4**-1

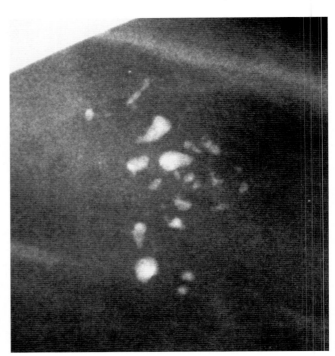

Ex.

Ex. **3.4**-3 Microfocus magnification: the calcifications are closely spaced, irregularly shaped and vary in size and density. These microcalcifications are of a mammographically malignant type.

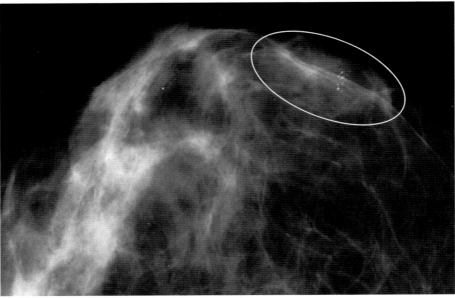

Ex. **3.4**-2

Ex. **3.4**-1 & 2 Screening mammograms, right breast, MLO (1) and CC (2) projections. There is a single cluster of crushed stone–like calcifications in the lower-inner quadrant.

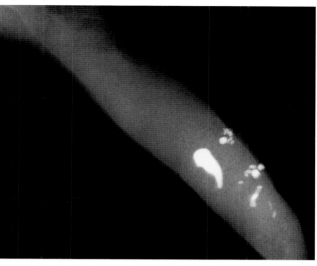
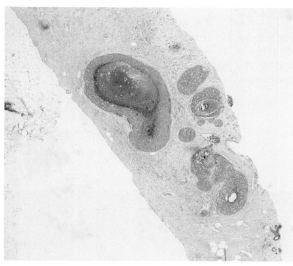

-4   Ex. **3.4**-5

Ex. **3.4**-4 & 5   Specimen radiograph (4) and low-power histological image of the vacuum-assisted biopsy specimen (5).
Histology: in situ carcinoma.

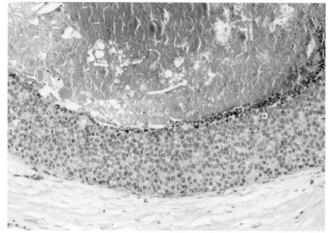
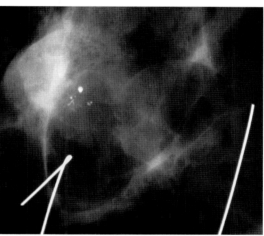

-6   Ex. **3.4**-7

Ex. **3.4**-6   Higher-power histological image of this Grade 2 in situ
carcinoma.

Ex. **3.4**-7   Operative specimen radiograph. The remaining calcifications have been removed with good margins.

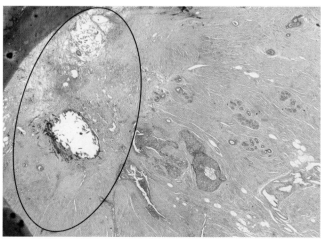
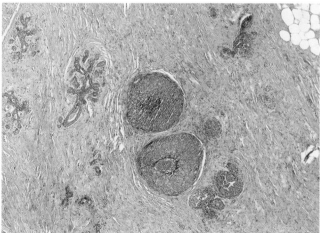

-8   Ex. **3.4**-9

Ex. **3.4**-8 & 9   Histological findings: 15 mm × 8 mm Grade 2 in situ carcinoma associated with central necrosis and amorphous calcifications. There were no signs of invasion. A post-biopsy scar and an amorphous calcification (displaced) are seen within the oval. Histologically tumor-free margin: 8 mm. The patient declined postoperative radiotherapy.

Example 3.4 continued

Four years later, at routine follow-up mammography, two new clusters of crushed stone–like calcifications were detected at the site of operation. The patient was still asymptomatic.

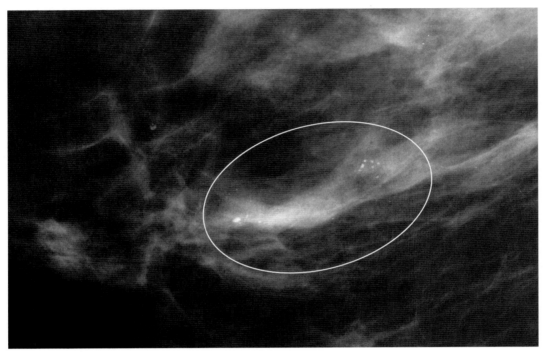

Ex. **3.4**-10

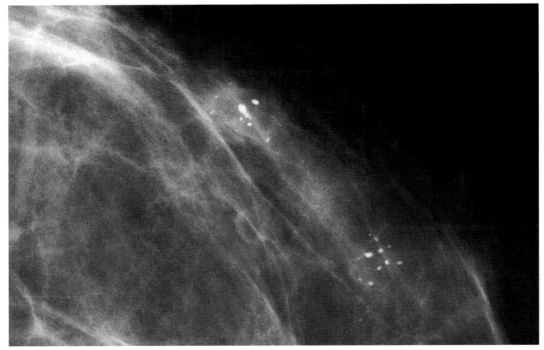

Ex. **3.4**-11

Ex. **3.4**-10 & 11   Right breast, microfocus magnification images in the MLO (9) and CC (10) projections. The newly developed clusters of crushed stone–like calcifications resemble the calcifications previously removed from this site. There is no associated tumor mass.

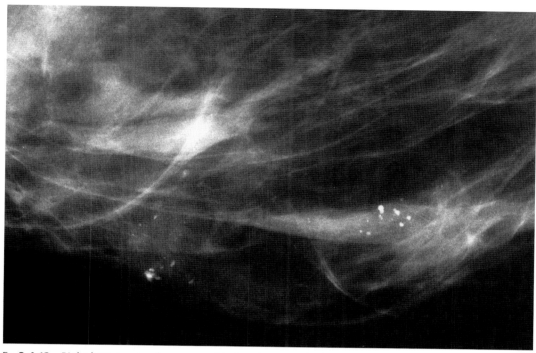

Ex. **3.4**-12

Ex. **3.4**-12   Right breast, microfocus magnification image in the lateromedial horizontal projection.

Ex. **3.4**-13   Vacuum-assisted biopsy specimen radiograph.

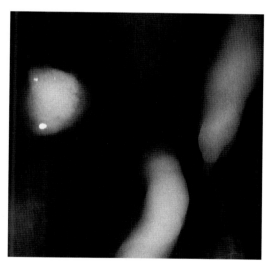

Ex. **3.4**-13

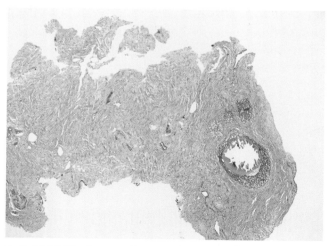

14

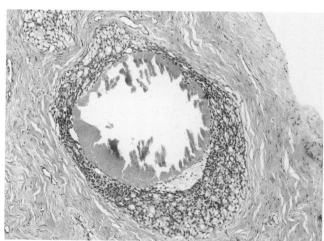

Ex. **3.4**-15

Ex. **3.4**-14 & 15   Low- and intermediate-power histological images of the biopsy specimen: in situ carcinoma with necrosis and amorphous calcification.

Example 3.4 continued

Ex. **3.4**-16 Operative specimen radiograph following preoperative localization using the bracketing technique.

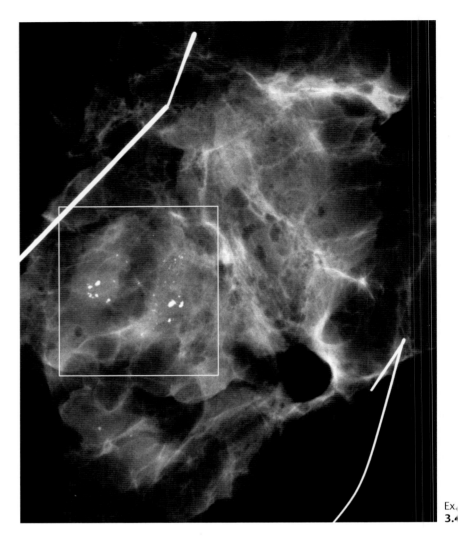

Ex. 3.4

Ex. **3.4**-17 Large-section histology. The TDLUs containing the in situ carcinoma are within the rectangle.

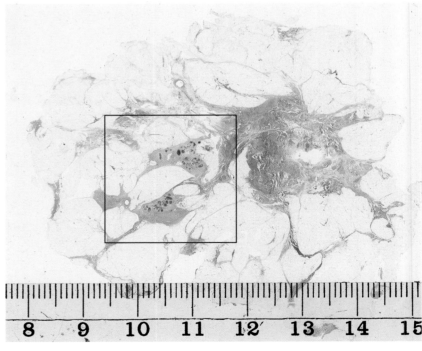

Ex 3.4

Ex. **3.4**-18 Operative specimen radiograph using microfocus magnification technique. Due to the increased image resolution, additional calcifications can now be visualized, suggesting the presence of more extensive disease.

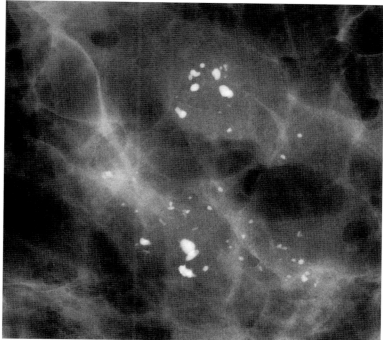

Ex. **3.4**-18

Ex. **3.4**-19 Sliced specimen radiograph.

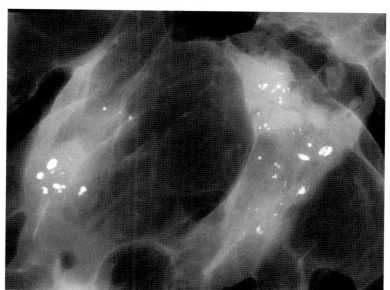

Ex. **3.4**-19

Ex. **3.4**-20 Paraffin block radiograph showing the multiple clusters of calcifications.

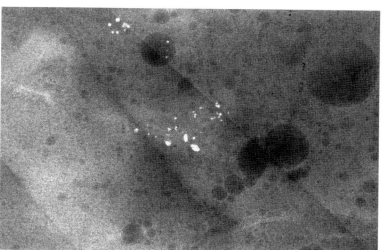

Ex. **3.4**-20

Example 3.4 continued

Ex. **3.4**-21   Low-power histological image. Numerous acini are filled with malignant cells, but only few of them contain calcifications.

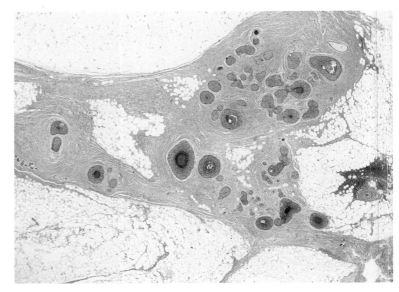

Ex.
3.4

Ex. **3.4**-22   An additional focus of calcified and noncalcified in situ carcinoma.

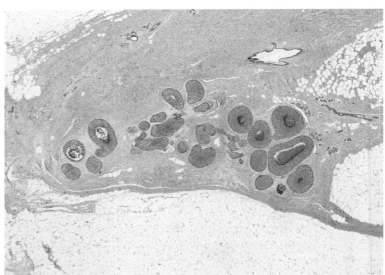

Ex.
3.4

Ex. **3.4**-23   Medium-power histological image.

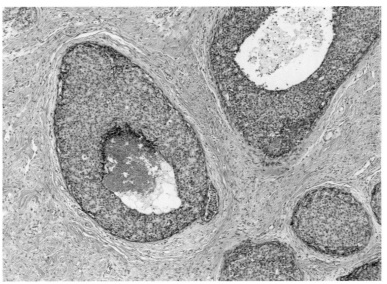

Ex.
3.4

Ex. **3.4**-24 to 26   Mammographic–histological correlation of this in situ carcinoma.

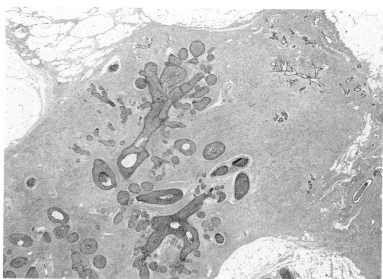

Ex. **3.4**-24

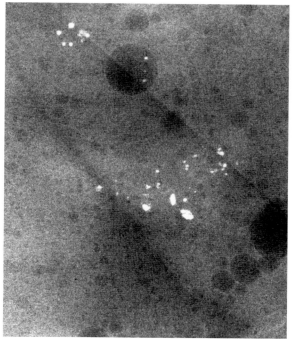

Ex. **3.4**-25

Treatment and outcome: Sector resection and postoperative irradiation following the diagnosis of recurrence. The patient had no evidence of disease at the most recent follow-up examination 2 years after her second operation.

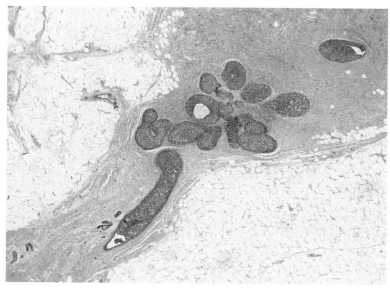

Ex. **3.4**-26

Example 3.5

A 57-year-old asymptomatic woman, screening examination.

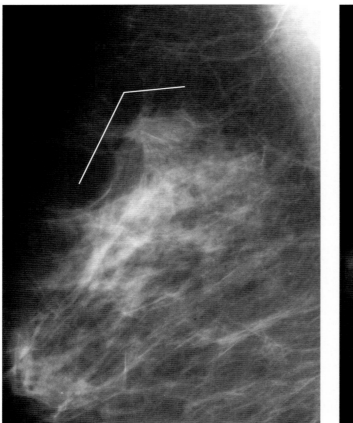

Ex. **3.5**-1

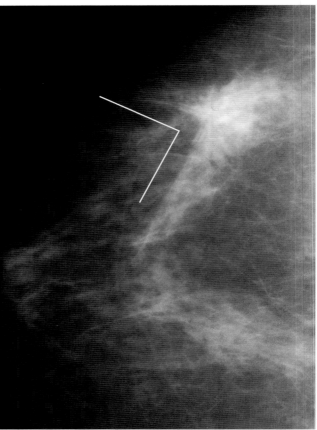

Ex.

Ex. **3.5**-1 & 2   Right breast, MLO (1) and CC projections (2). The "elbow sign" on the MLO projection and the "tent sign" on the CC projection indicate the presence of a pathological abnormality in the upper-outer quadrant of the breast.

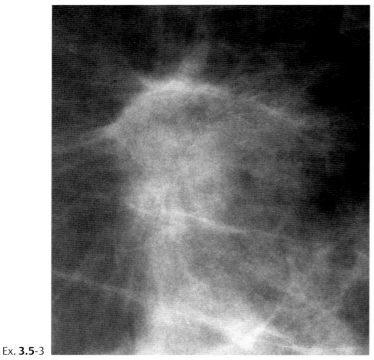

Ex. **3.5**-3

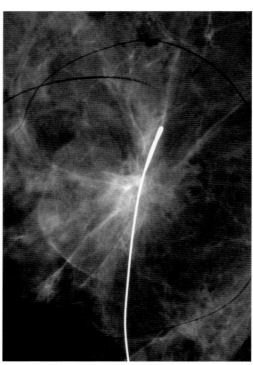

Ex. **3.5**-4

Ex. **3.5**-3   Microfocus magnification combined with spot compression reveals a spiculated (stellate) lesion without associated calcifications. Mammographically malignant tumor.

Ex. **3.5**-4   Specimen radiograph of the surgically removed tumor.

Follow-up examination 6 years after surgery.

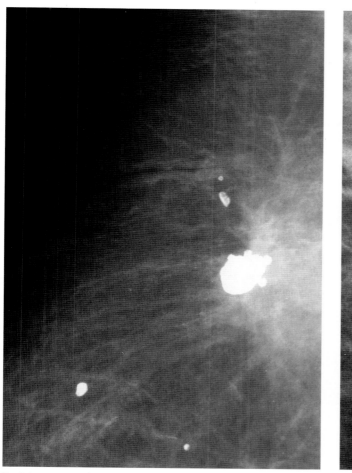

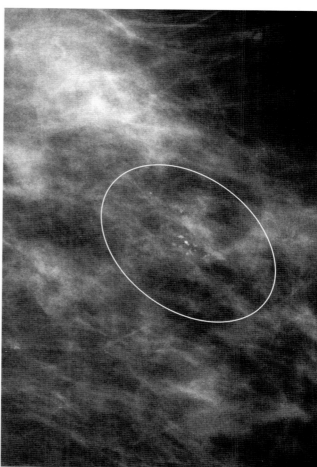

5-5

Ex. **3.5**-6

Ex. **3.5**-5 & 6   Right and left breasts, detailed views in the MLO projection. Postsurgical scar with calcified oil cysts are seen in the right breast (5). A few clusters of de-novo crushed stone–like calcifications have developed in the lateral portion of the left breast (6).

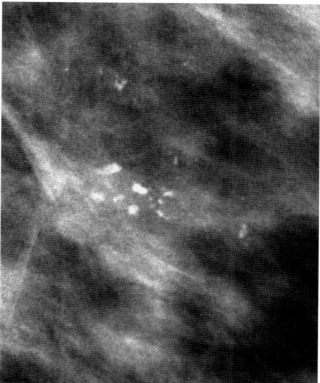

Ex. **3.5**-7   Microfocus magnification of the de-novo calcification clusters: the individual particles are in close proximity to each other, vary in density, size and shape, and are mammographically of the malignant type.

Ex. **3.5**-7

Example 3.5 continued

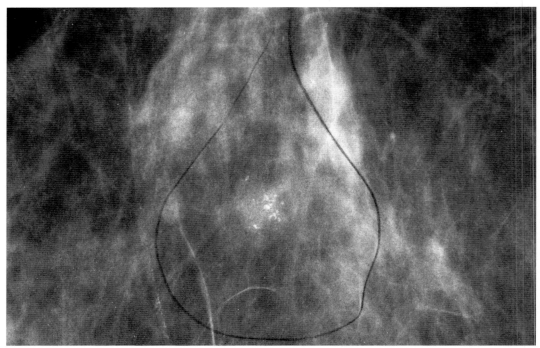

Ex. **3.5**-8

Ex. **3.5**-8   Left breast, CC projection, showing the cluster of calcifications.

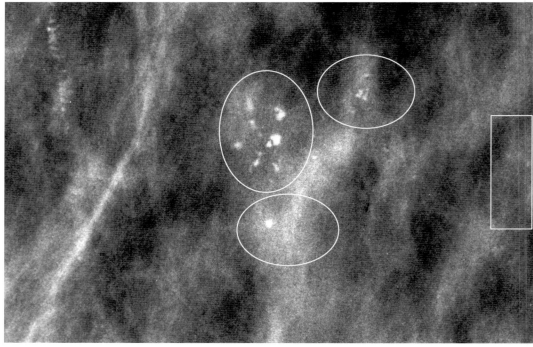

Ex. **3.5**-9

Ex. **3.5**-9   Microfocus magnification demonstrates that there are multiple clusters of calcifications.

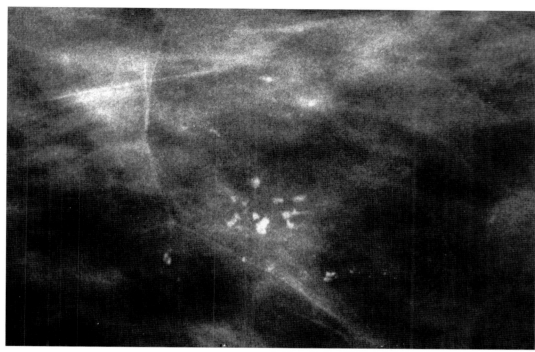

Ex. **3.5**-10

Ex. **3.5**-10 Microfocus magnification in the lateromedial horizontal projection.

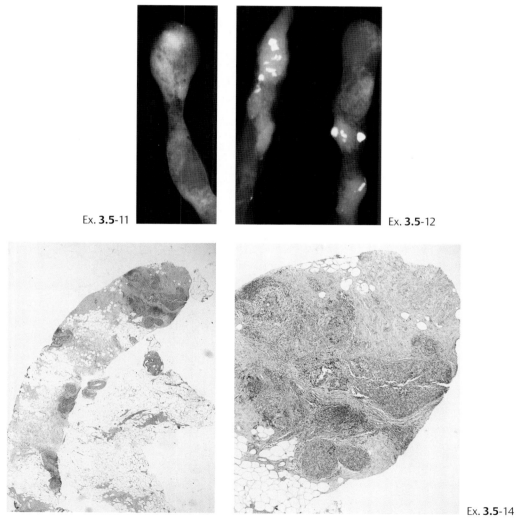

Ex. **3.5**-11   Ex. **3.5**-12

Ex. **3.5**-13   Ex. **3.5**-14

Ex. **3.5**-11 to 14   Vacuum-assisted specimen radiographs without (11) and with (12) calcifications. Histological examination reveals in situ carcinoma in the noncalcified sample as well (13, 14).

Example 3.5 continued

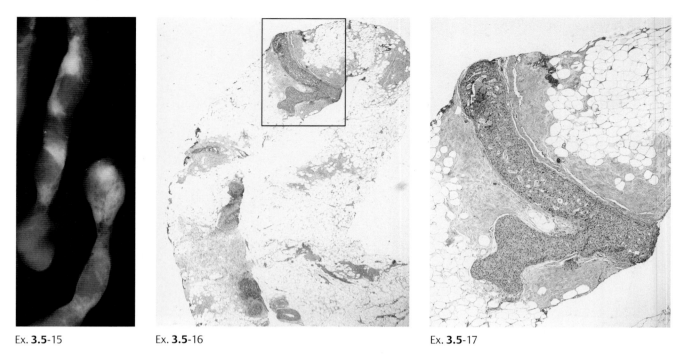

Ex. **3.5**-15   Ex. **3.5**-16   Ex. **3.5**-17

Ex. **3.5**-15 to 17   Vacuum-assisted specimen radiograph without calcifications correlated with histology. The preoperative biopsy establishes the diagnosis of in situ carcinoma.

Ex. **3.5**-18 & 19   Radiographs of the operative specimen slices.

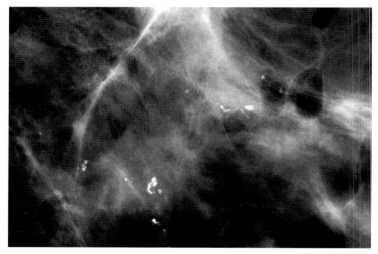

Ex. **3.5**-18

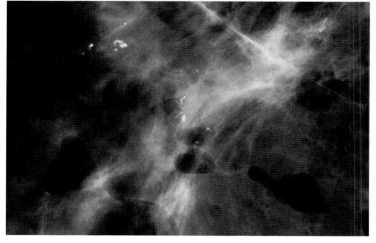

Ex. **3.5**-19

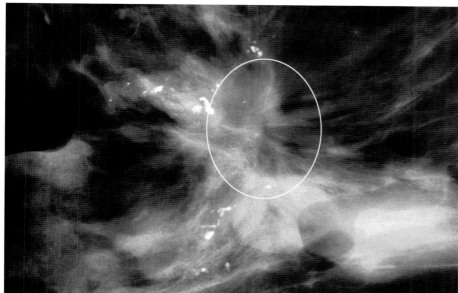

Ex. **3.5**-20

Ex. **3.5**-20   In this specimen slice there appears to be a spiculated lesion (encircled) adjacent to the malignant type calcifications.

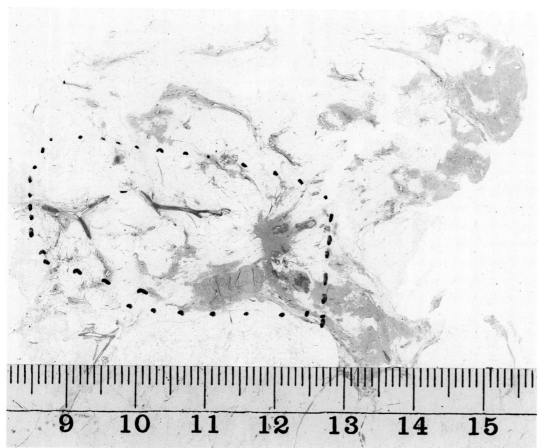

Ex. **3.5**-21

Ex. **3.5**-21   The large-section histological image can be correlated with the specimen radiograph. The area containing in situ carcinoma foci and the spiculated lesion has been outlined by the pathologist.

Example 3.5 continued

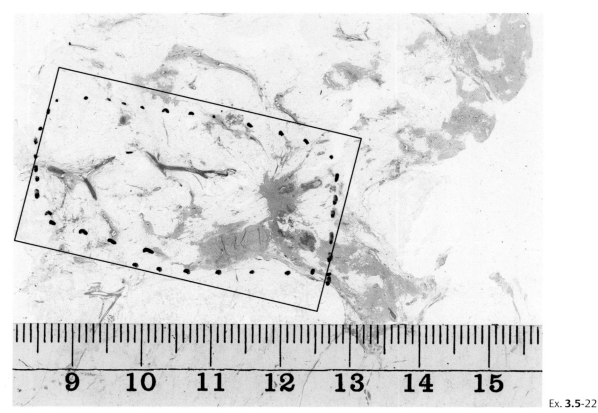

Ex. **3.5**-22

Ex. **3.5**-22   The large-section histology image can be compared with the detailed photomicrographs on these two pages (Ex. **3.5**-23 to 29).

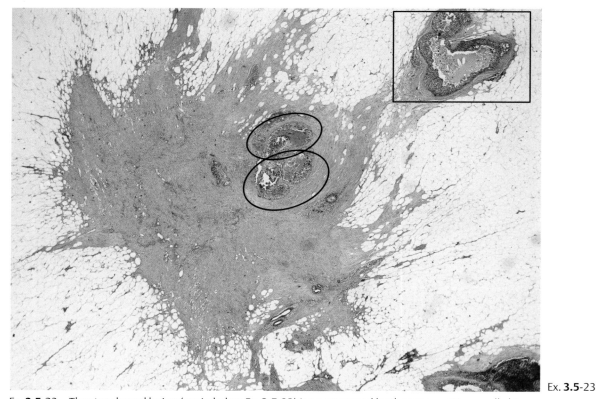

Ex. **3.5**-23

Ex. **3.5**-23   The star-shaped lesion (encircled on Ex. **3.5**-22) is a scar caused by the preoperative needle biopsy performed 3 weeks earlier. There are in situ carcinoma foci (ovals) entrapped within the scar. Another in situ focus is outlined by a rectangle.

The photomicrographs on this page are higher-power views of the in situ foci within the rectangle on Ex. **3.5**-22.

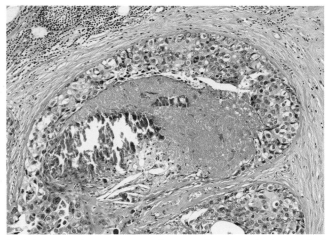

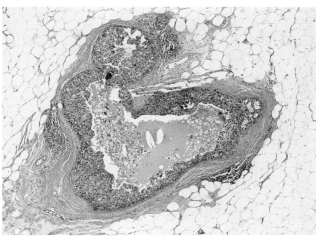

Ex. **3.5**-24   High-power magnification of one of the in situ foci (upper oval on Ex. **3.5**-23) with solid cell proliferation, central necrosis, and amorphous calcification.

Ex. **3.5**-25   Higher magnification of another focus of in situ carcinoma, seen on Ex. **3.5**-23 within the rectangle.

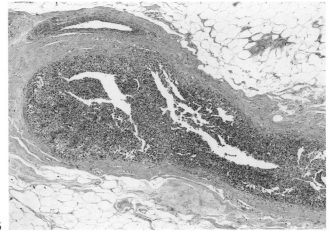

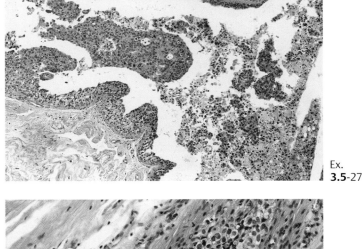

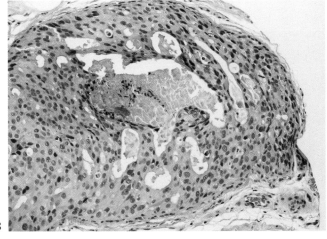

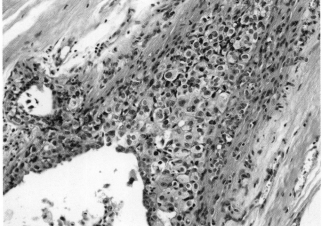

Ex. **3.5**-26 to 29   Four enlarged images of the noncalcified in situ carcinoma foci within the rectangle on Ex. **3.5**-22. The area with in situ carcinoma measured 40 mm × 15 mm, considerably larger than the area with crushed stone–like calcifications on the mammogram.

Treatment and outcome: Right breast: sector resection and postoperative irradiation. **Left breast** (6 years later): mastectomy. The patient had no signs of recurrence 2 years following mastectomy of the left breast.

Example 3.6

A 47-year-old asymptomatic woman, screening examination. She was called back for further assessment of the small cluster of calcifications detected on the screening mammograms.

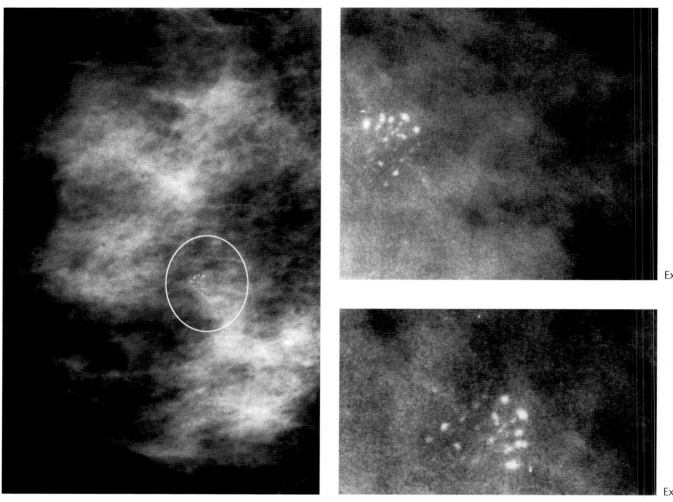

Ex. **3.6**-1

Ex.

Ex. **3.6**-1 to 3   Right breast, MLO projection and microfocus magnification views of the cluster of calcifications. These crushed stone–like calcifications are closely spaced and vary in size, shape, and density. Some of them resemble broken needle tips. The cluster is composed of mammographically malignant type calcifications.

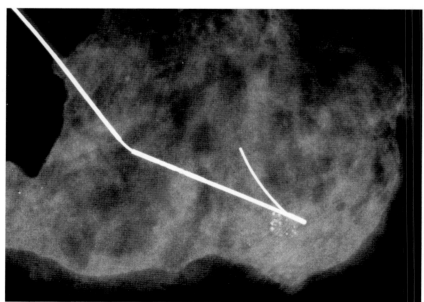

Ex. **3.6**-4   Specimen radiograph showing the cluster calcifications.

Ex.

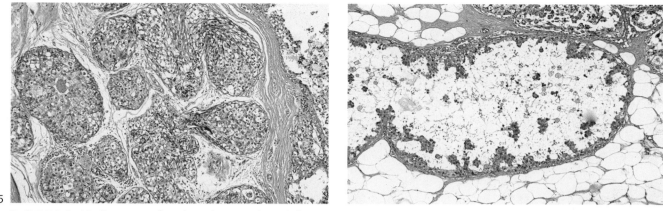

5   Ex.
                                                                                                                                    3.6-6

Ex. **3.6**-5 & 6   Medium-power histological images (H & E) demonstrating in situ carcinoma with solid and micropapillary cell proliferation, but with no associated calcifications, so that these foci were occult on the mammograms.

3D Image

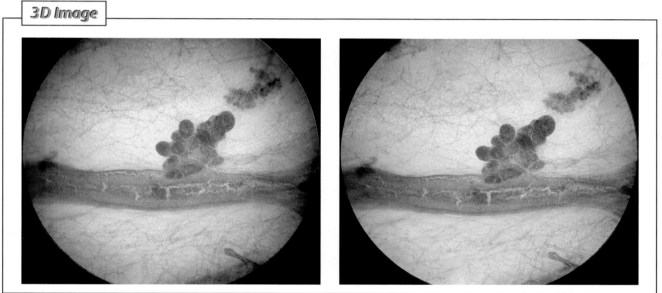

7   Ex.
                                                                                                                                    3.6-8

Ex. **3.6**-7 & 8   Stereoscopic subgross 3D images of a section of a cancerous duct and an associated TDLU with in situ carcinoma. The conventional histological image of this TDLU is seen in Ex. **3.6**-5.

3D Image

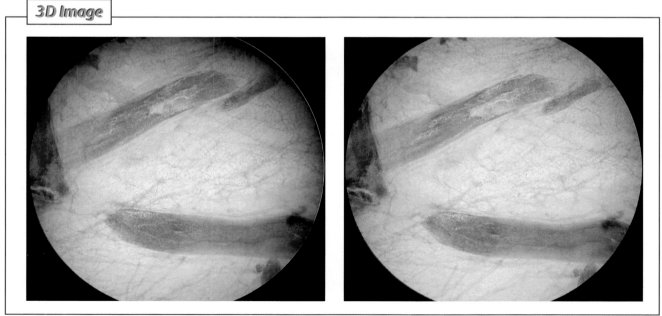

9   Ex.
                                                                                                                                    3.6-10

Ex. **3.6**-9 & 10   Cancer-filled ducts without calcifications are seen in these stereoscopic 3D images.

Example 3.6 continued

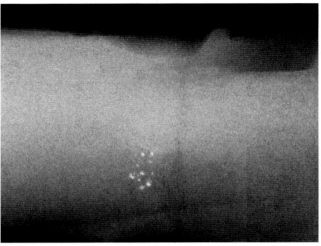
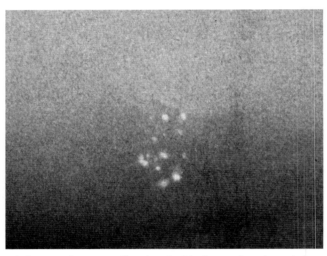

Ex.
3.6-11

Ex.
3.

Ex. **3.6**-11 & 12   Paraffin block specimen radiographs reveal that the calcification cluster is still within the block. New histological slices were taken at the level of the calcifications.

3D Image

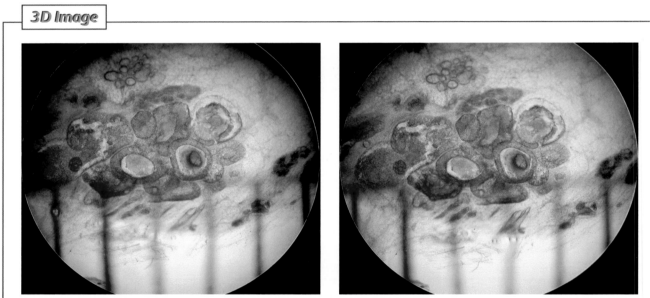

Ex.
3.6-13

Ex.
3.

Ex. **3.6**-13 & 14   Stereoscopic images of a slice through the single dilated TDLU containing the in situ carcinoma. Many layers of viable tumor cells line the walls of the acini. The center of each acinus is filled with necrosis, and one of the acini in this slice contains an amorphous calcification.

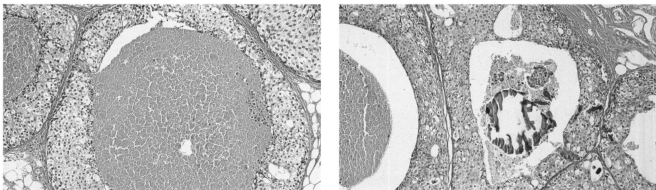

Ex.
3.6-15

Ex.
3.

Ex. **3.6**-15 & 16   Medium-power histological images (H & E) of some of the acini distended by in situ carcinoma cells, central necrosis, and amorphous calcifications. Since the Grade 2 in situ carcinoma is localized to the TDLU, the term "ductal" carcinoma in situ is erroneous; the proper description is Grade 2 in situ carcinoma within the TDLU.

3D Image

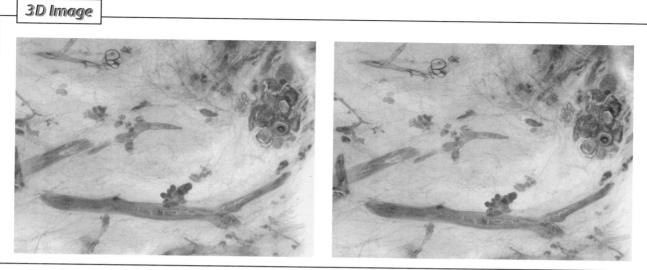

Ex. **3.6**-17 & 18   Stereoscopic image pair: the mammographically detected calcifications are found in the TDLU (on the right) distended by in situ carcinoma. In the surrounding tissue, over an area of 35 mm diameter, there are ducts filled with noncalcified, mammographically occult Grade 2 in situ carcinoma.

3D Image

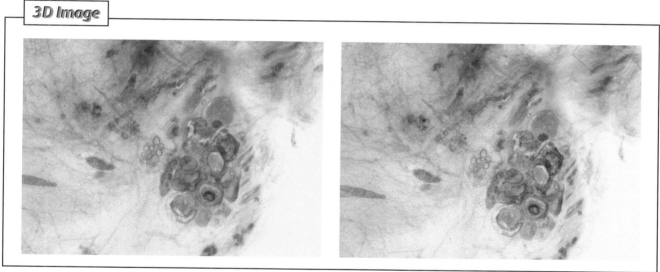

Ex. **3.6**-19 & 20   Stereoscopic image pair of the TDLU extremely distended by in situ carcinoma with associated central necrosis and amorphous calcifications. For comparison, there are normal sized and cystically dilated TDLUs in the surrounding tissue.

Treatment and outcome: Sector resection with no post-operative radiotherapy. The patient was without evidence of breast cancer at the most recent follow-up examination 10 years after surgery.

Comment
This case reflects the uncertainty always associated with crushed stone–like calcifications on the mammogram. Contrary to the cases in the previous section (Group 1A cases), occult, noncalcified in situ carcinoma was found over a large area surrounding the single calcified cluster.

Example 3.7

A 59-year-old asymptomatic woman attended mammographic screening and was called back for assessment of a cluster of microcalcifications in the left breast.

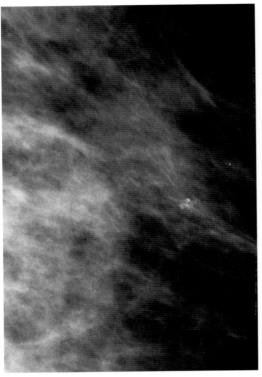

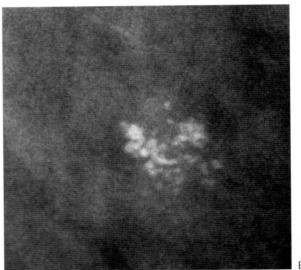

Ex. **3.7**-2

Ex. **3.7**-1

Ex. **3.7**-1 to 3   Detailed views of the left MLO and CC projections and microfocus magnification showing a single cluster of discernible calcifications with no associated tumor mass. They are closely spaced and appear irregular in shape and density, suspicious for malignancy.

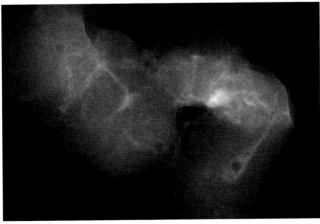

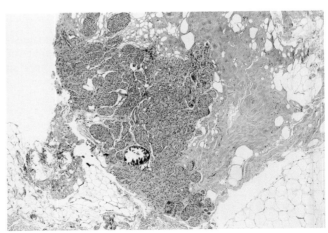

Ex. **3.7**-3

Ex. **3.7**-4

Ex

Ex. **3.7**-4 & 5   Radiograph and histological image of the preoperative vacuum-assisted biopsy specimen. The calcification appears to be surrounded by malignant cells.

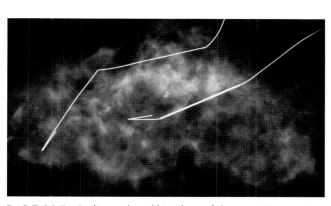

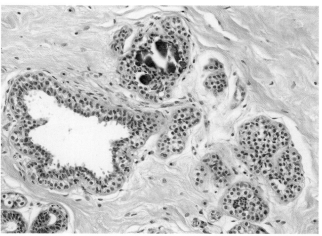

-6

Ex. **3.7**-6 & 7   Radiograph and histology of the operative specimen. The cluster of calcification has been removed with good margin.

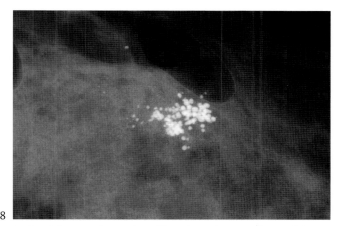

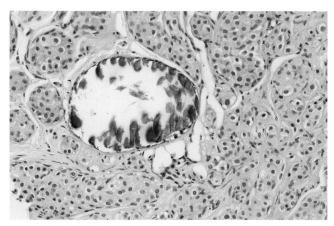

-8

Ex. **3.7**-8 & 9   Radiograph and histological image of one of the specimen slices. The calcifications appear to be spherical and regular and no longer resemble the crushed stone type.

3D Image

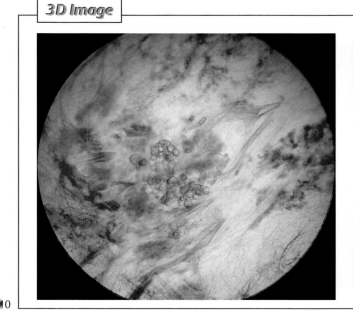

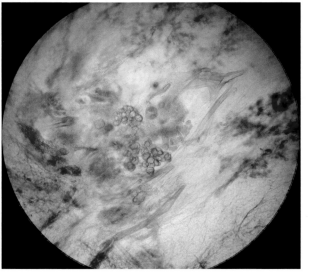

0

Ex. **3.7**-10 & 11   Subgross, thick-section (3D) histological image pair demonstrating that the round/oval calcifications (corresponding to the calcifications seen on the mammogram) are localized within the stroma and not contained within the TDLU that is involved with LCIS.

Example 3.7 continued

3D Image

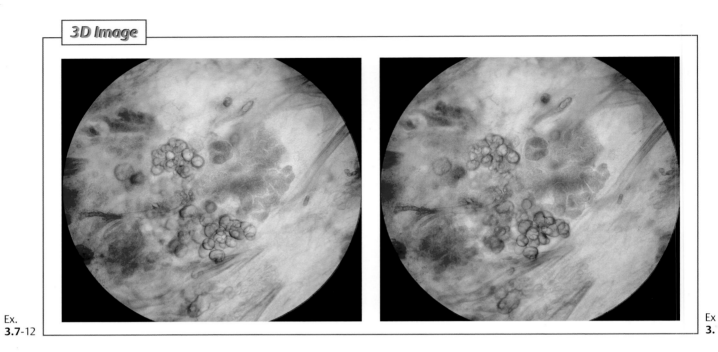

Ex.
3.7-12

Ex
3.

3D Image

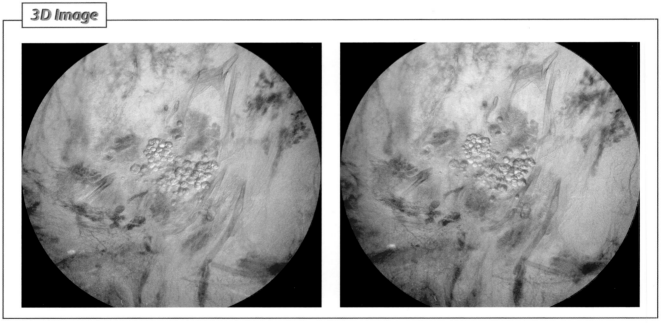

Ex.
3.7-14

Ex
3.

Ex. **3.7**-12 to 15   Subgross, thick-section (3D) histological image pairs of the same TDLU and calcifications as on Ex. **3.7**-10 & 11, but with different magnification and light.

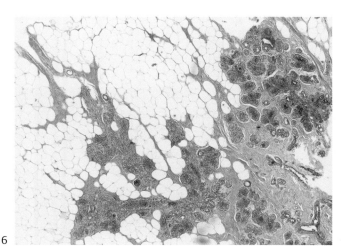

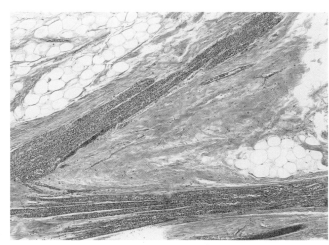

-16

Ex.
3.7-17

Ex. **3.7**-16 & 17   Low-power histological images demonstrate the noncalcified portion of this 60 mm × 50 mm Grade 1 & 2 in situ carcinoma, including LCIS.

Treatment and outcome: Mastectomy. The patient had no signs of recurrence at the first-year follow-up examination after surgery.

Comment
This case demonstrates the discordance between the subtle mammographic findings and the extensive histological finding in Group 2A cases. In addition, the round/oval calcifications are an incidental finding in the vicinity of the TDLU distended by lobular carcinoma in situ (LCIS).

Example 3.8

This 49-year-old asymptomatic woman was called back after mammography screening for assessment of the cluster of calcifications found in the left breast.

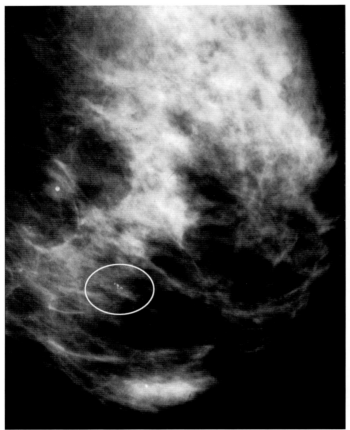

Ex. **3.8**-1

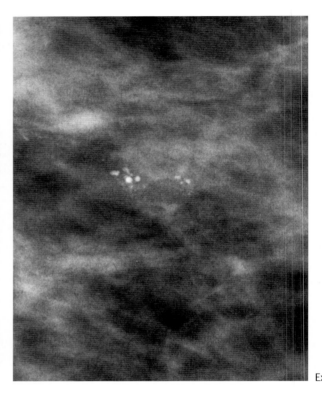

Ex.

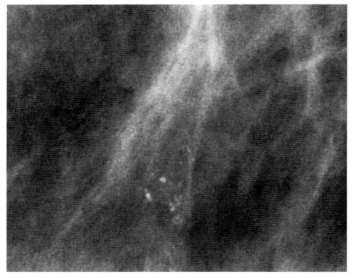

Ex. **3.8**-2

Ex. **3.8**-1 to 3 Left breast, MLO projection (1): there is a tiny cluster of calcifications in the lower portion of the breast. Microfocus magnification images (2 & 3) reveal two small adjacent clusters containing crushed stone–like calcifications.

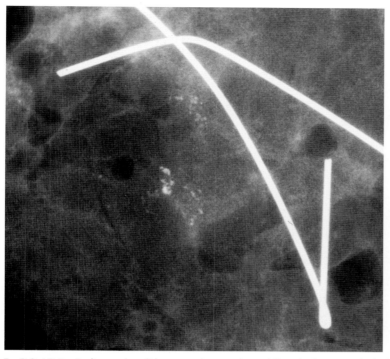
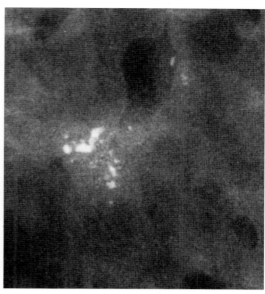

8-4 Ex. **3.8**-5

Ex. **3.8**-4 & 5   Radiographs of the operative specimen (4) and of a 5 mm thick slice from the operative specimen (5). Some of the calcifications appear to be of the powdery type, in close proximity to the crushed stone–like calcifications.

3D Image

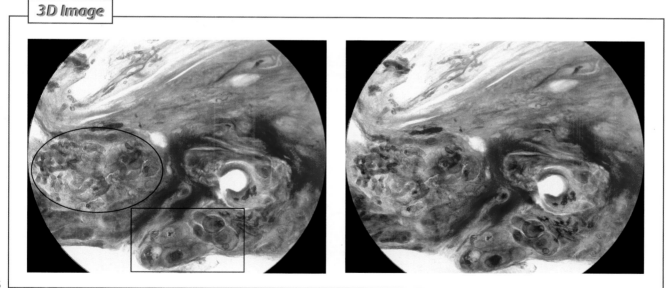

8-6 Ex. **3.8**-7

Ex. **3.8**-6 & 7   Subgross, thick-section histological image pair where the two different types of calcifications are present: the amorphous at the left (crushed stone–like on the mammogram) and the psammoma body–like at the lower border of the image pair (powdery on the mammogram).

Example 3.8 continued

3D Image

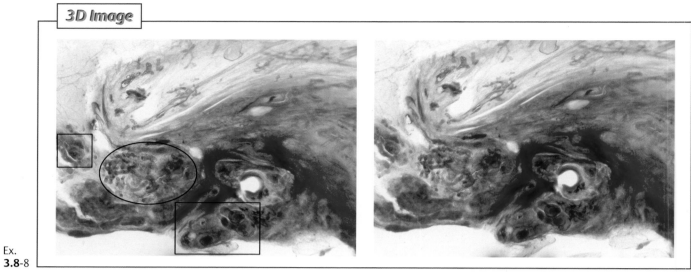

Ex. **3.8**-8

Ex. 3.

Ex. **3.8**-8 & 9 Subgross, thick-section histological image pair of the region with the calcifications. The central tissue defect results from the core needle biopsy. Hemorrhage surrounds the biopsy site.

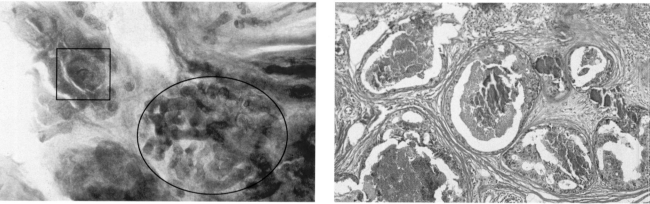

Ex. **3.8**-10

Ex. 3.8

Ex. **3.8**-10 & 11 The Grade 2 in situ carcinoma with amorphous calcifications is seen both on the subgross, thick-section image (10, in the rectangle) and on conventional histology (11). The Grade 1 in situ carcinoma associated with psammoma body–like calcifications appears within the oval.

3D Image

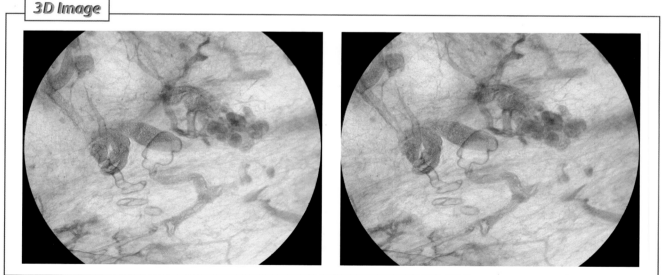

Ex. **3.8**-12

Ex. **3.8**

Ex. **3.8**-12 & 13 Subgross, thick-section (3D) image pair demonstrates tortuous ducts filled with in situ carcinoma, cribriform type. These malignant changes are not visible mammographically.

3D Image

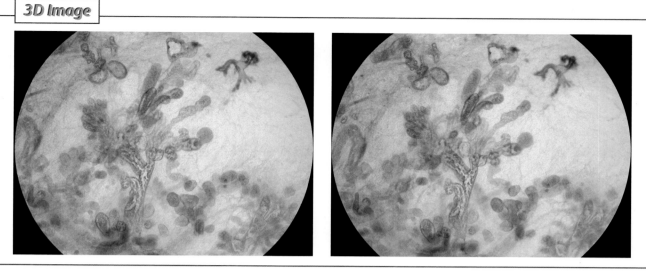

Ex. **3.8**-14 & 15   In this subgross, thick-section (3D) image pair the in situ carcinoma with micropapillary and solid architecture is demonstrated.

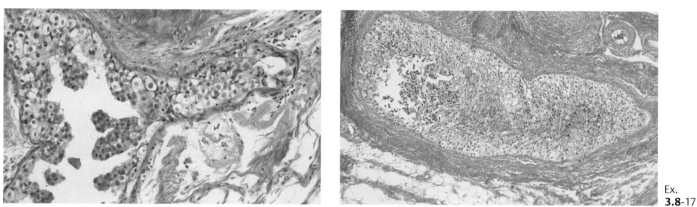

Ex. **3.8**-16 & 17   Conventional histological images of the in situ carcinoma with micropapillary (16) and solid (17) architecture without associated calcifications.

3D Image

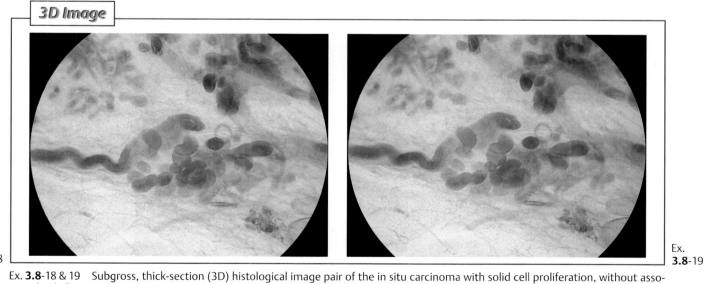

Ex. **3.8**-18 & 19   Subgross, thick-section (3D) histological image pair of the in situ carcinoma with solid cell proliferation, without associated calcifications.

Treatment and outcome: The patient underwent segmental resection and received postoperative radiation therapy. There was no evidence of breast cancer at 10 years of follow-up.

Comment
The extent of in situ carcinoma was 60 mm × 50 mm in this case, but only a small (< 10 mm) cluster of calcifications was visible on the mammogram.

Example 3.9

This 41-year-old asymptomatic woman was called back after her first mammography screening for assessment of the cluster of calcifications found in her left breast.

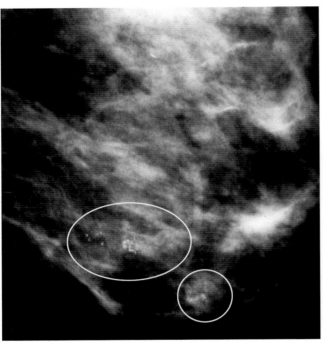

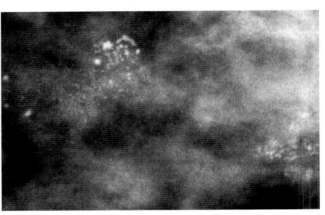

Ex. **3.9**-1   Ex.

Ex. **3.9**-1 & 2   Left breast, detail of the MLO projection (1) and microfocus magnification view (2). There are several clusters of calcifications in the lower half of the breast (encircled); some of them are pleomorphic, crushed stone–like, others are powdery calcifications. No associated tumor mass is demonstrable.

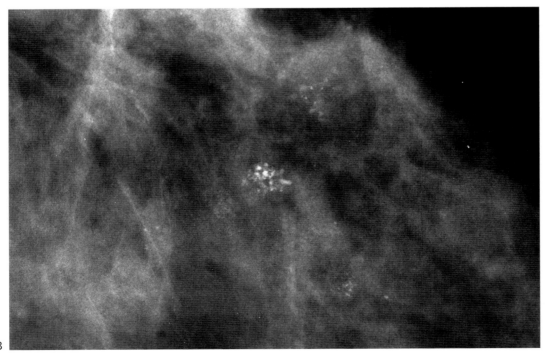

Ex. **3.9**-3

Ex. **3.9**-3   Left breast, detail of the CC projection. Microfocus magnification view, CC projection.

Ex. **3.9**-4 Magnification radiograph of one of the specimen slices. Two kinds of calcification clusters can be differentiated: the crushed stone–like (in rectangles) and the powdery type (in ovals).

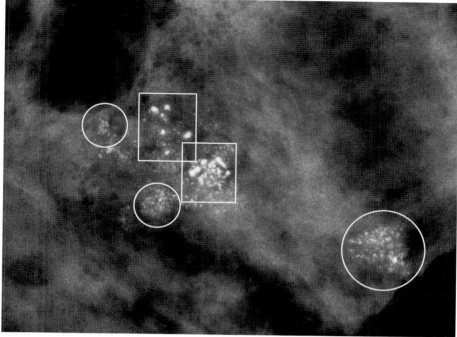

Ex. **3.9**-4

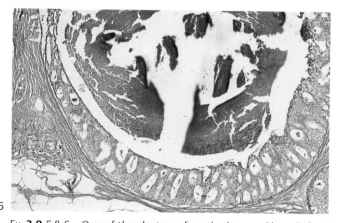

.9-5

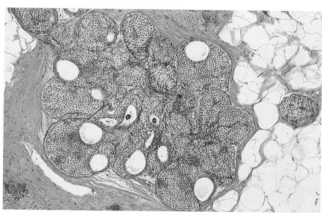

Ex. **3.9**-6

Ex. **3.9**-5 & 6 One of the clusters of crushed stone–like calcifications is localized within an acinus distended by a Grade 2 in situ carcinoma with cribriform architecture (5). On (6) there is a single TDLU containing Grade 1 in situ carcinoma and psammoma body–like calcifications, corresponding to the powdery calcifications on the mammogram.

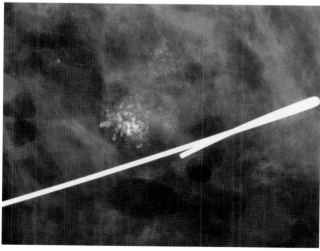

9-7

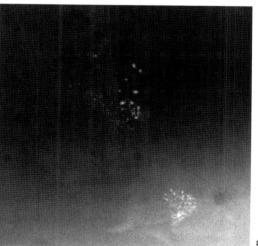

Ex. **3.9**-8

Ex. **3.9**-7 & 8 Operative specimen and paraffin block radiographs.

Example 3.9 continued

Ex. **3.9**-9   Operative specimen radiograph.

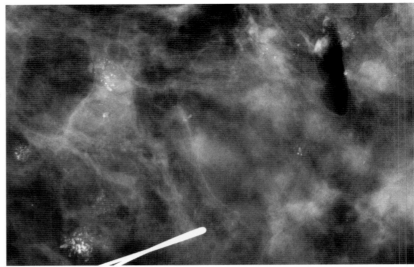

Ex. **3.9**

3D Image

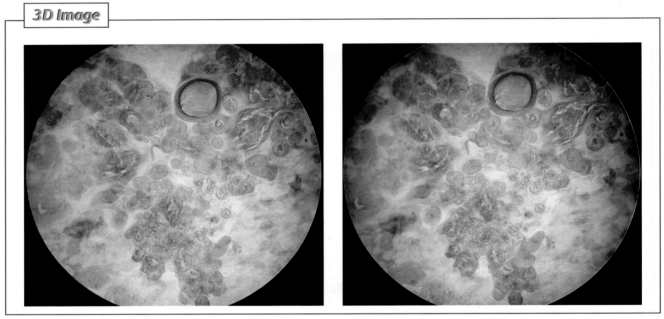

Ex. **3.9**-10

Ex. **3.9**

Ex. **3.9**-10 & 11   Subgross, thick-section (3D) histological image pair shows neighboring TDLUs where the cribriform in situ carcinoma is associated with numerous psammoma body–like (powdery) calcifications.

Ex. **3.9**-12   Specimen slice radiograph. The clusters of crushed stone–like and powdery calcification clusters are intermixed.

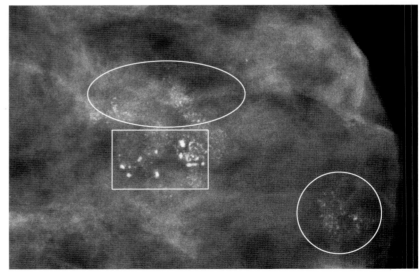

Ex. **3.9**

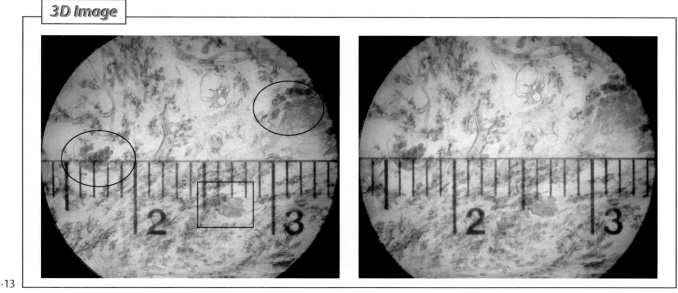

Ex. **3.9**-14

Ex. **3.9**-13 to 18   The subgross histological image pair (13, 14) demonstrates the separate, noncalcified TDLUs containing in situ carcinoma with intervening normal tissue. The malignant foci are separated from each other by distances of 1 cm. The in situ focus within the rectangle is magnified in (15, 16) and the in situ focus within the left-hand oval is magnified in (17, 18).

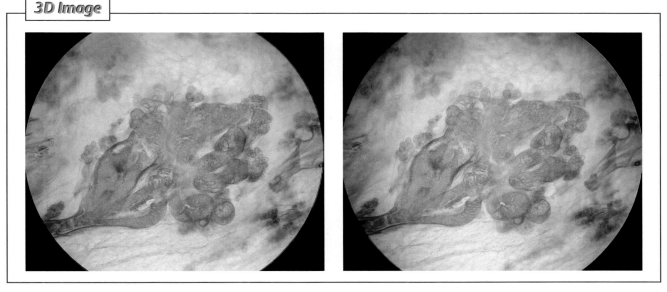

Ex. **3.9**-16

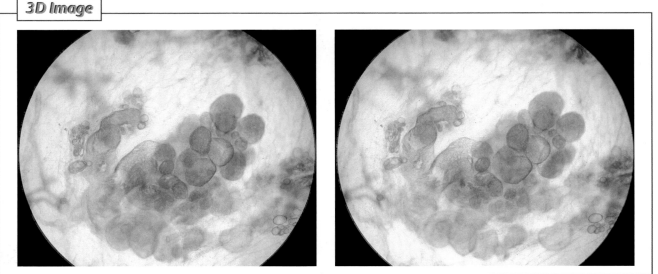

Ex. **3.9**-18

Example 3.9 continued

Ex. **3.9**-19 to 22   Histology images with medium (19) and high (20) magnification as well as sub-gross, thick-section (3D) histology (21 & 22) images of a TDLU with Grade 1 cribriform in situ carcinoma associated with psammoma body–like (powdery) calcifications (rectangle). There are neighboring normal TDLUs for comparison (oval) (19).

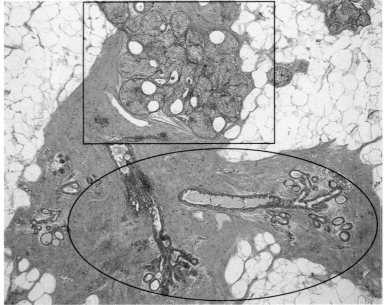

Ex. **3.9**

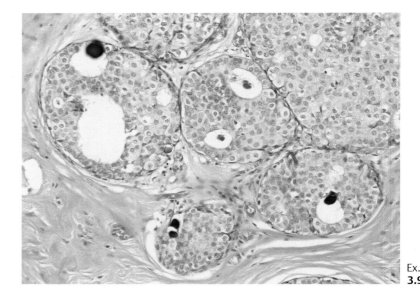

Ex. **3.9**

Treatment and outcome: Sector resection with no postoperative irradiation. The patient was symptom-free, without evidence of recurrence 11 years following surgical treatment.

3D Image

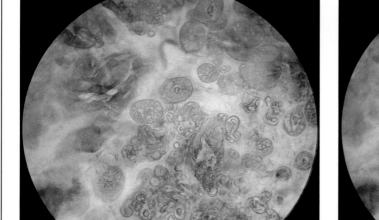
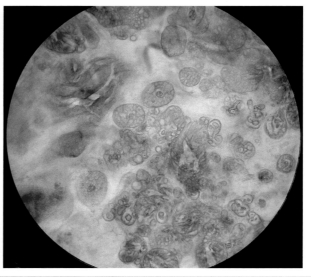

Ex. **3.9**-21

Ex. **3.9**

Example 3.10

A 54-year-old asymptomatic woman, screening examination.

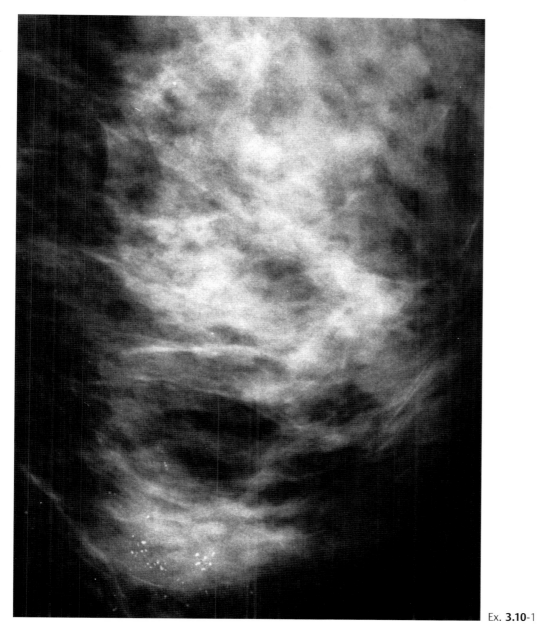

Ex. **3.10**-1

Ex. **3.10**-1   Left breast, detail of the MLO projection (1) and magnified image over the area with calcifications (1a). There are multiple clusters of crushed stone–like calcifications in the lower portion of the breast with no associated tumor mass.

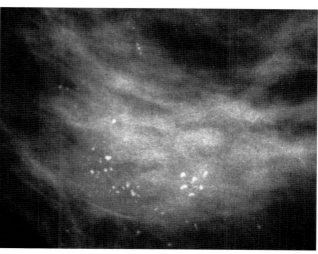

Ex.
3.10-1a

Example 3.10 continued

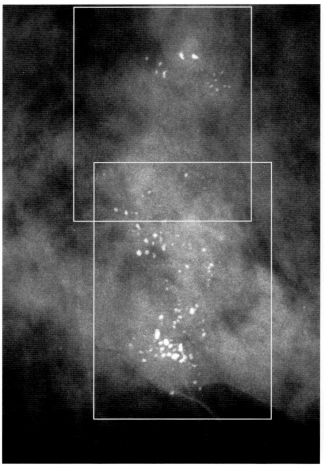

Ex.
3.10-2

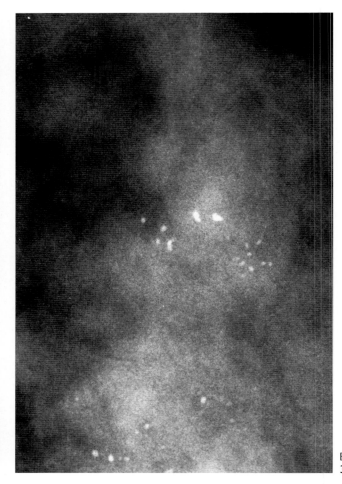

Ex.
3.1

Ex. **3.10**-2 to 4   Detail of the CC projection (2) and two micro-focus magnification images (3, 4) showing the multiple clusters of crushed stone–like calcifications outlined within rectangles on Ex. **3.10**-2.

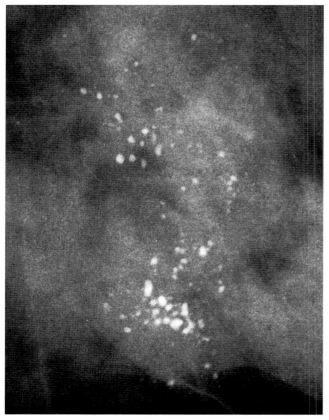

Ex.
3.1

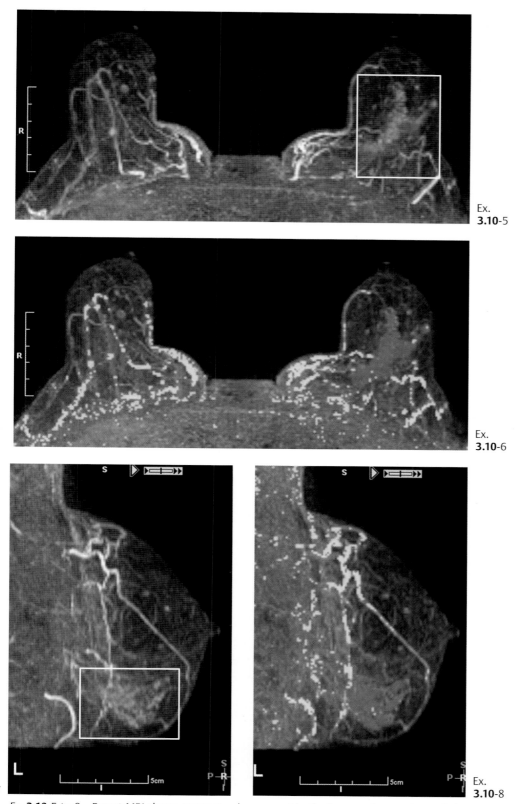

Ex. **3.10**-5

Ex. **3.10**-6

Ex. **3.10**-8

Ex. **3.10**-5 to 8   Breast MRI shows contrast enhancement in the lower-outer quadrant of the left breast, suggesting malignancy over an area measuring 60 mm × 35 mm.

Example 3.10 continued

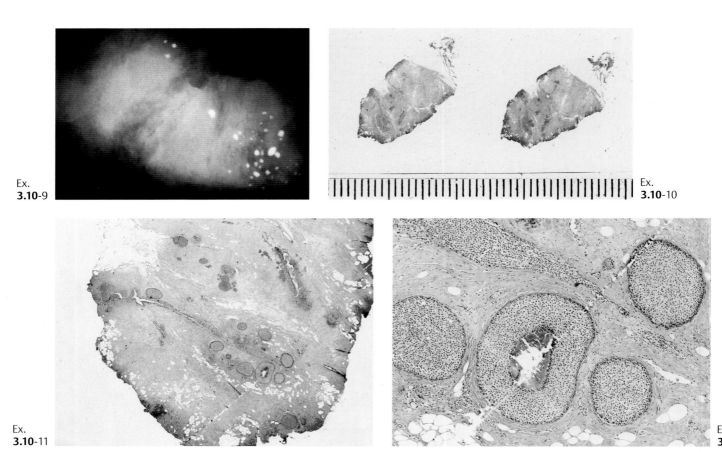

Ex.
3.10-9

Ex.
3.10-10

Ex.
3.10-11

Ex.
3.1

Ex. **3.10**-9 to12   Preoperative vacuum-assisted biopsy. Radiograph (9) and low-power histological images of the specimen at increasing magnification. **Histological diagnosis:** lobular carcinoma in situ with associated central necrosis and amorphous calcification.

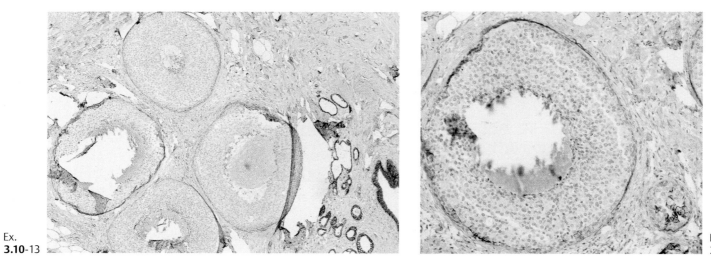

Ex.
3.10-13

Ex.
3.1

Ex. **3.10**-13 & 14   Immunohistochemical staining demonstrates total loss of E-cadherin expression in the tumor in contrast to normal glands and hyperplasia. This confirms the diagnosis of LCIS.

Ex. **3.10**-15 Radiograph of the operative specimen. In addition to the calcifications, there is a region with architectural distortion (rectangle).

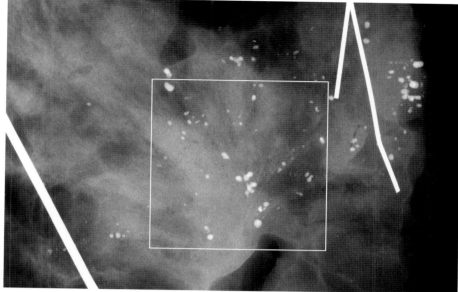

Ex. **3.10**-15

Ex. **3.10**-16 Large-section histological image. The pathologist has marked the area with the necrotic LCIS. The architectural distortion seen on the specimen radiograph corresponds to a large preoperative vacuum biopsy scar.

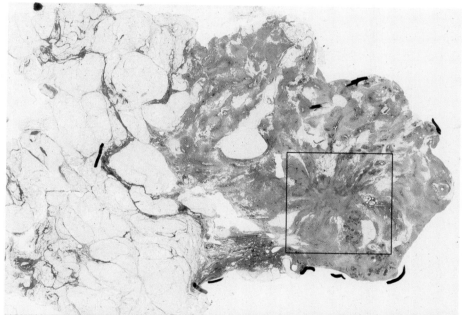

Ex. **3.10**-16

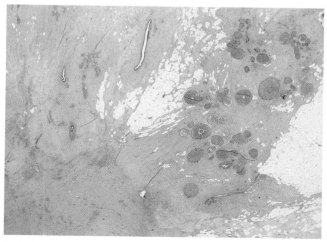

17

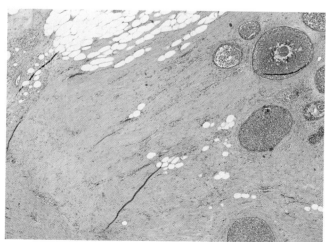

Ex. **3.10**-18

Ex. **3.10**-17 & 18 Medium-power images of the post-biopsy scar and adjacent LCIS.

Example 3.10 continued

Ex. **3.10**-19   Specimen radiograph with multiple cluster crushed stone–like calcifications.

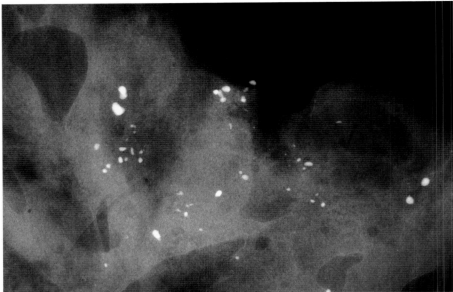

Ex. **3.1**

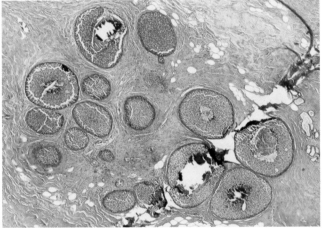

Ex. **3.10**-20

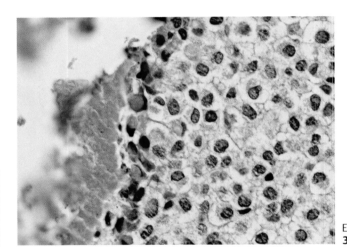

Ex. **3.1**

Ex. **3.10**-20 & 21   Medium- and high-magnification histological images of this special form of LCIS.

Comment

Lobular carcinoma in situ is infrequently associated with central necrosis and amorphous calcifications. This rare variant has recently been recognized. Sapino et al. reported 10 cases and described the mammographic–histological features.[1] This is the only variant of LCIS that is detectable on the mammogram due to the presence of crushed stone–like calcifications. Its characteristic histological features are a noncohesive, monotonous cell-population and the loss of E-cadherin expression. The diagnosis of this variant of LCIS is being made with increasing frequency.[2, 3] The long-term outcome of these cases is still unknown, but the presence of amorphous calcification suggests a different natural history from that of the majority of LCIS cases without calcifications. MRI of the breast is expected to be positive in this subtype of LCIS. The question is whether we will be able to distinguish which among the different subtypes of LCIS has the potential to become invasive cancer during follow-up.

Ex. **3.10**-22 & 25   Mammographic–histological correlation of LCIS with necrosis.

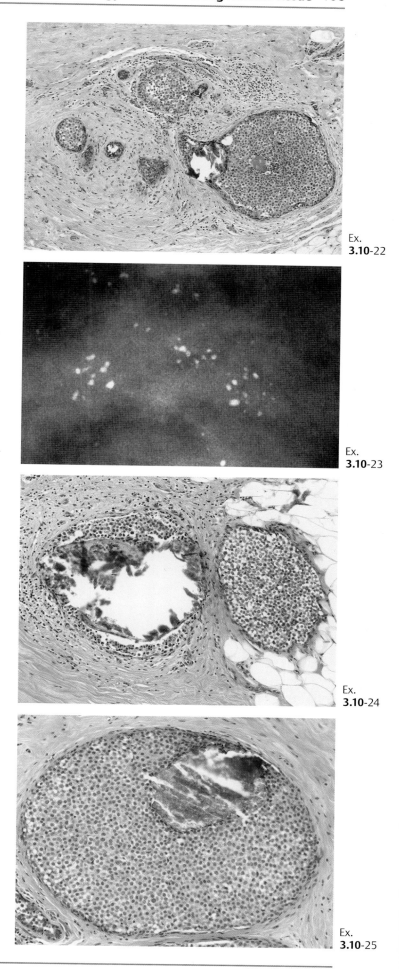

Ex.
3.10-22

Ex.
3.10-23

Ex.
3.10-24

Ex.
3.10-25

Example 3.10 continued

This variant of LCIS, although mainly localized within the TDLUs, may also show Pagetoid spread in larger ducts (Ex. 3.10–26 to 29).

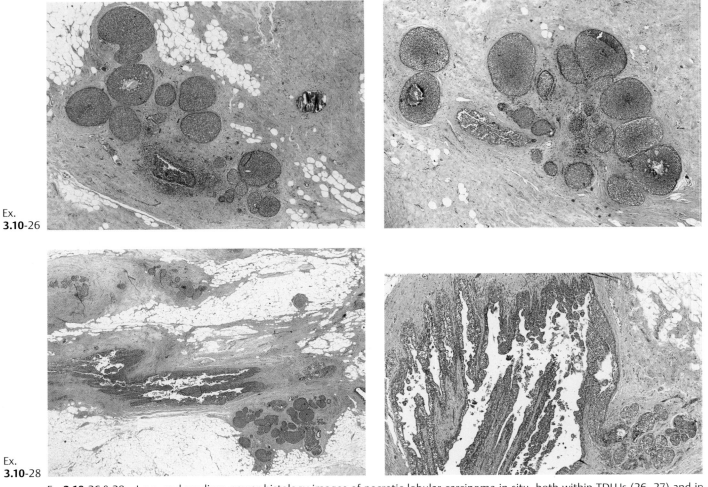

Ex. **3.10**-26

Ex. 3.1

Ex. **3.10**-28

Ex. 3.1

Ex. **3.10**-26 & 29   Low- and medium-power histology images of necrotic lobular carcinoma in situ, both within TDLUs (26, 27) and in larger ducts (28, 29).

Treatment and outcome: This is a recent case. The patient had sector resection and postoperative irradiation.

Group 2B: Contiguous and Extensive Disease on Histology

Although the mammographic image may show multiple clusters which appear similar to those in Group 2A, large-section histological examination demonstrates tightly packed cancerous TDLUs and ducts contiguously covering a larger area than that indicated by the calcifications detected at mammography. MRI of the breast plays an important role in revealing the true extent and confluent nature of the underlying disease. In some extreme cases very large numbers of clusters of crushed stone–like calcifications are visible on the mammogram, often associated with some casting type calcifications. The larger the number of clusters, the more difficult it is to discern the individual clusters. Correlation with large-section and subgross, 3D histology shows a high density of tightly packed cancerous TDLUs and ducts with little, if any, normal tissue in between. Histological signs of neoductgenesis and lymph vessel invasion are often present and may account for the occasional poor outcome.

Example 3.11

[Case courtesy of David Beatty, M.D., FACS, Swedish Hospital, Seattle, WA, USA.]

A 39-year-old woman of Ashkenazi Jewish ancestry and with a family history of breast cancer has been undergoing routine mammography at 1–2-year intervals. A previous biopsy of the left breast was benign.

Ex. **3.11**-1 & 2   Right breast, MLO and CC projections, February 2005. No mammographic abnormality is seen.

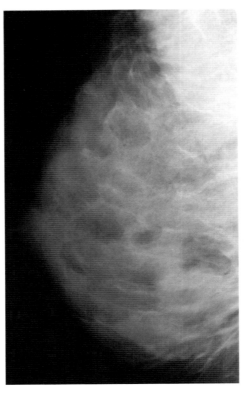

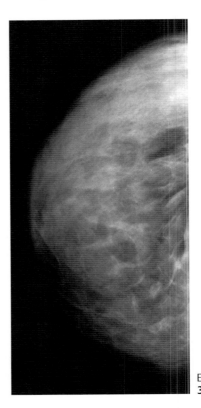

Ex. **3.11**-3 & 4   Right breast, MLO projection and comparative CC projections. There are a large number of de-novo clusters of calcifications (rectangles).
▽

Ex.
3.11-1

Ex.
3.1

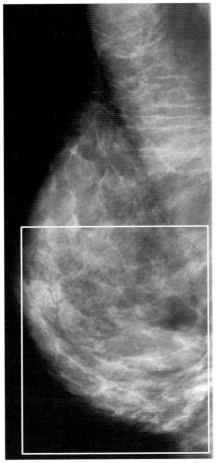

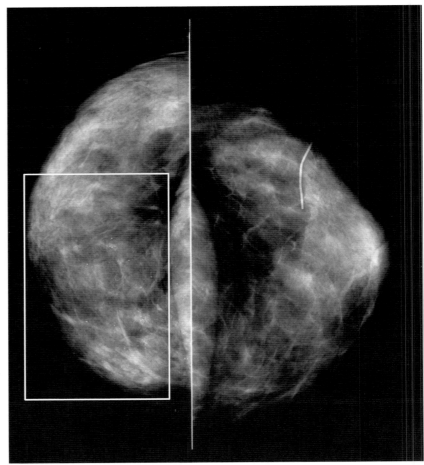

Ex.
3.11-3

Ex
3.

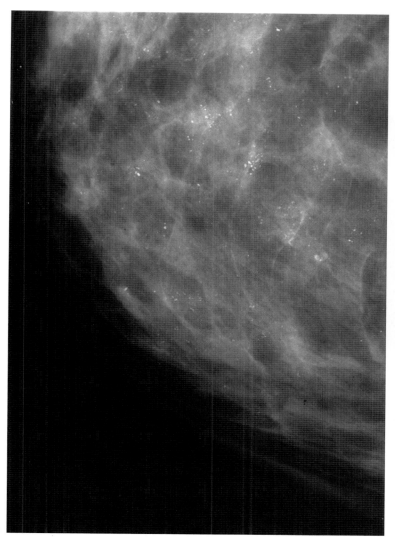

1-5

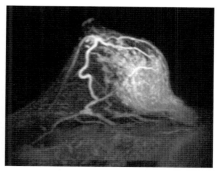

Ex. **3.11**-6

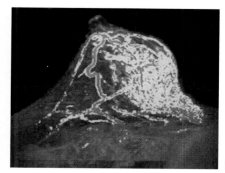

Ex. **3.11**-7

Ex. **3.11**-5   Right breast, microfocus magnification of the medial portion, CC projection. There are numerous clusters of crushed stone–like calcifications without an associated tumor mass.

Ex. **3.11**-6 & 7   MRI demonstrates intense contrast enhancement over approximately half of the breast, indicating an extensive malignant process.

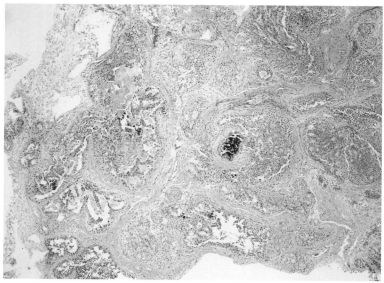

Ex. **3.11**-8

Ex. **3.11**-8   Low-power histological image of the 14-g core biopsy specimen: Grade 2 in situ carcinoma in ductlike structures that are tightly packed without intervening normal tissue. The disease extends over 18 cm with no evidence of invasion. The mastectomy specimen showed involved margins and one sentinel node had micrometastases. PET/CT was negative for distant metastases.

Example 3.12

A 49-year-old asymptomatic woman, screening examination. She was called back for assessment of the microcalcification detected on the mammogram of her right breast.

Ex. **3.12**-1 & 2 Right breast, detail of the MLO (1) and CC (2) projections. Multiple clusters of crushed stone–like calcifications can be seen in the lower-outer quadrant of the breast. There is no associated tumor mass.

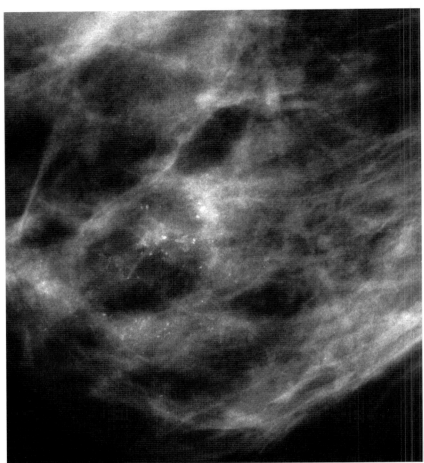

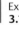

Ex.
3.1

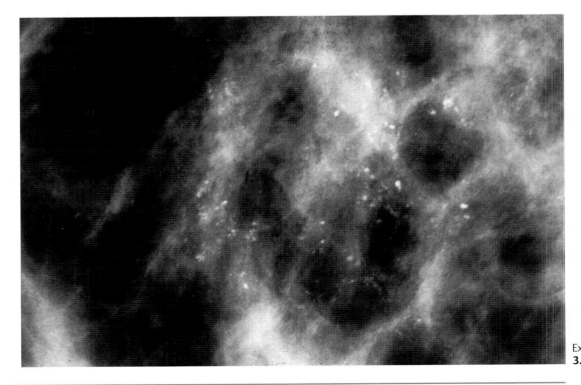

Ex
3.

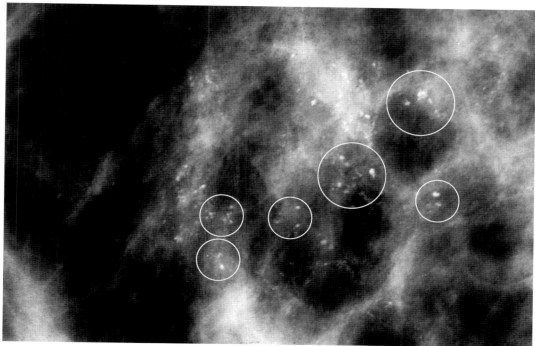

Ex. **3.12**-3

Ex. **3.12**-3   Photographic magnification of Ex. **3.12**-2 with many of the individual calcification clusters encircled to emphasize the importance of detecting and appreciating the multiple-cluster nature of the underlying disease process. **The higher the number of clusters with discernible, crushed stone–like calcifications on the mammogram, the greater the probability of malignancy.**

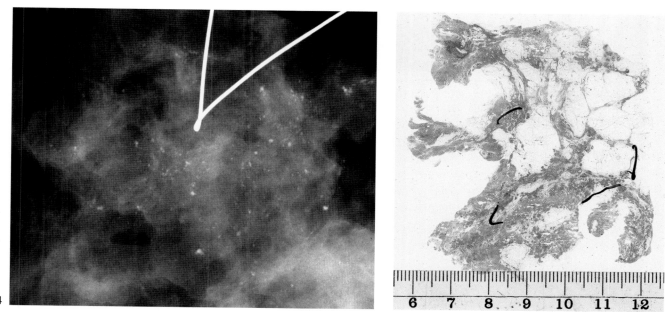

Ex.
3.12-5

2-4

Ex. **3.12**-4 & 5   Specimen radiograph and large-section histological image outlining the extent of the disease.

Example 3.12 continued

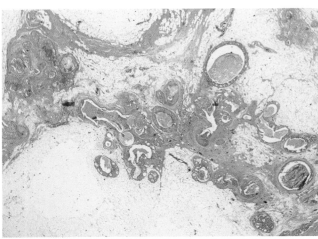

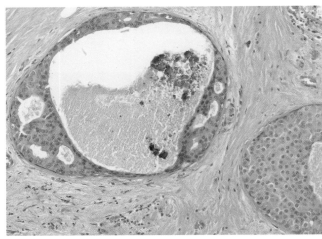

Ex.
3.12-6

Ex.
3.1

Ex. **3.12**-6 & 7   Low- (6) and higher-power (7) histological images of the area with cancer-filled, closely spaced, ductlike structures. Solid and cribriform architecture. The distended lumen has necrotic debris and calcifications (7), corresponding to the calcifications seen on the mammogram.

3D Image

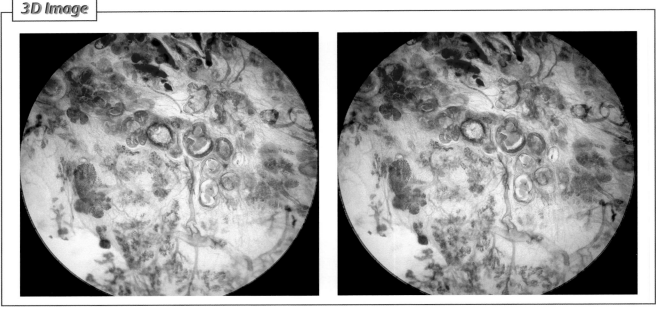

Ex.
3.12-8

Ex.
3.1

Ex. **3.12**-8 & 9   Subgross histological image pair. The TDLUs and subsegmental ducts greatly distended by in situ carcinoma (upper portion of the image) contrast with the normal size TDLUs (lower part of the picture).

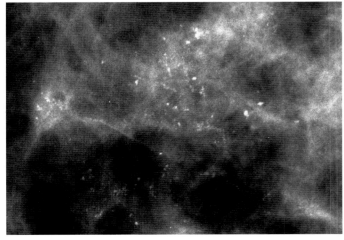

Ex. **3.12**-10   Detail of the right CC projection, microfocus magnification image.

Ex.
3.1

3D Image

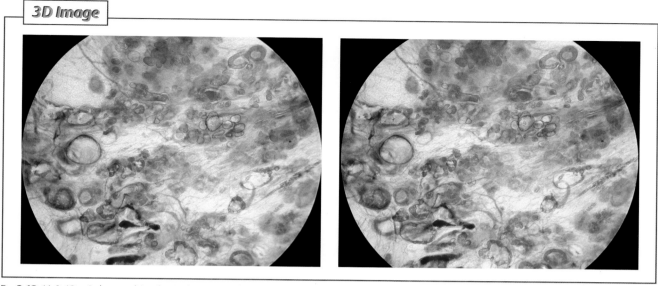

Ex. **3.12**-11 & 12   Subgross histological images. The in situ process covers the field of view and contains prominent tumor vessels.

3D Image

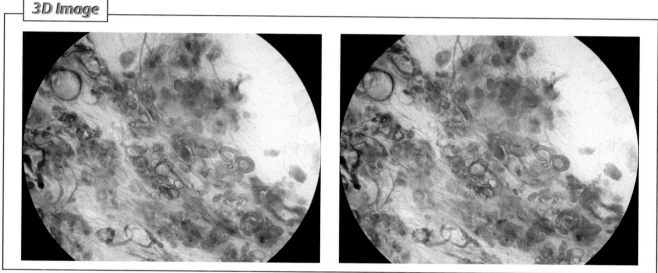

Ex. **3.12**-13 & 14   Subgross histological image pair. The 1–1.5 mm-thick tissue slices allow us to appreciate the contiguity of the affected ducts and lobules as well as the true extent of the disease in three dimensions.

3D Image

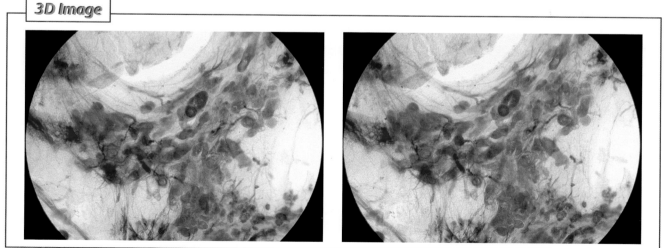

Ex. **3.12**-15 & 16   The in situ carcinoma is associated with an extensive blood supply resulting from neoangiogenesis

Treatment and outcome: Mastectomy. There was no evidence of recurrence 16 years following surgery.

Example 3.13

A 45-year-old asymptomatic woman, screening examination. She was called back for assessment of multiple clusters of calcifications in the right breast. This patient has a strong family history of breast cancer: her mother had premenopausal breast cancer and both her grandmothers also had breast cancer.

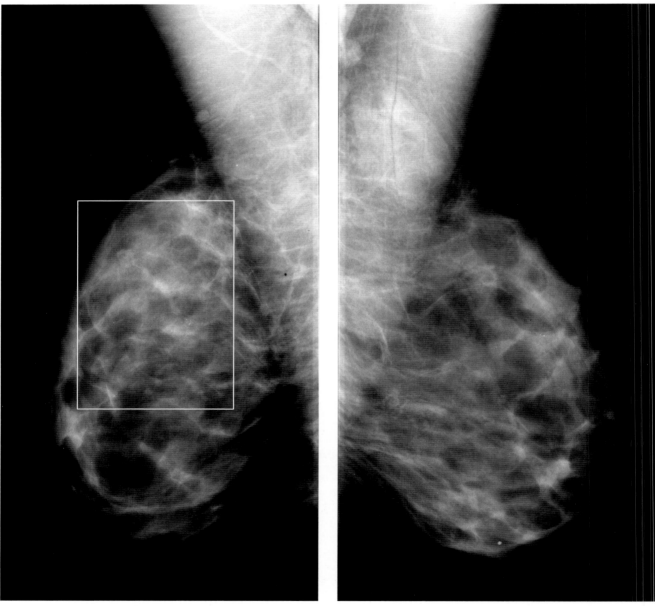

Ex.
3.13-1

Ex.
3.1

Ex. **3.13**-1 & 2   Right and left breasts, MLO projection. Faint clusters of calcifications are seen in the upper portion of the right breast. There is no demonstrable tumor mass.

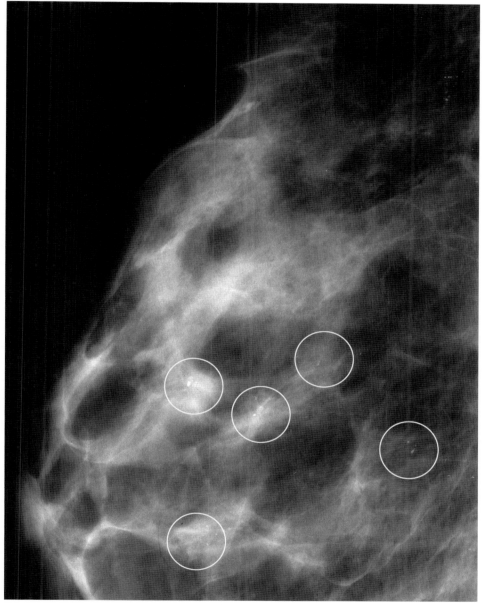

Ex. **3.13**-3

Ex. **3.13**-3 Right breast, microfocus magnification in the lateromedial horizontal projections. The clusters of calcifications are encircled.

Example 3.13 continued

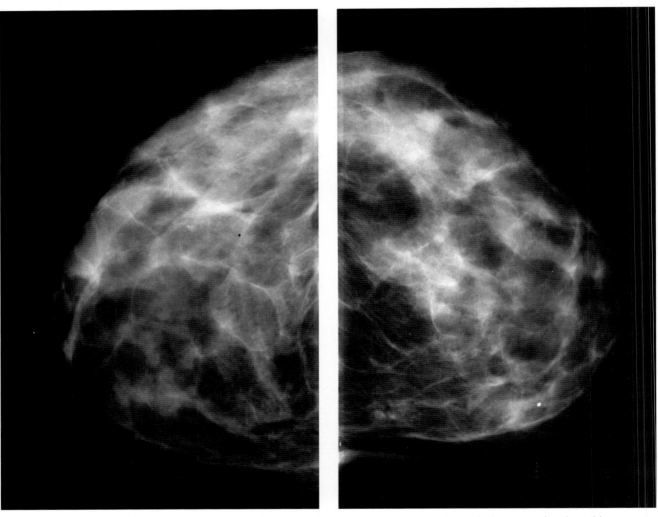

Ex.
3.13-4

Ex.
3.1

Ex. **3.13**-4 & 5   Right and left breasts, CC projection. The faint clusters of calcifications in the right breast are barely visible.

Ex. **3.13**-6   Right breast, microfocus magnification in the CC projection. The large number of clusters of calcifications are spread throughout much of the breast. Preoperative needle biopsy showed malignant cells.

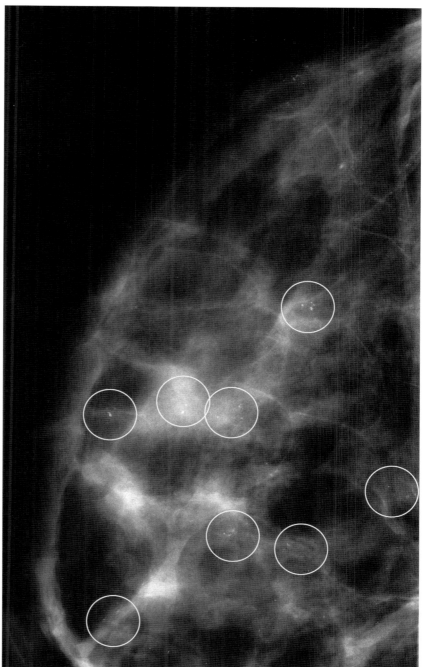

Ex.
3.13-6

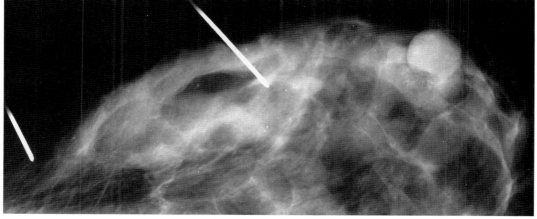

Ex.
3.13-7

Ex. **3.13**-7   Preoperative localization following the positive fine-needle aspiration biopsy.

Example 3.13 continued

Ex. **3.13**-8   Radiograph of one of the operative specimen slices.

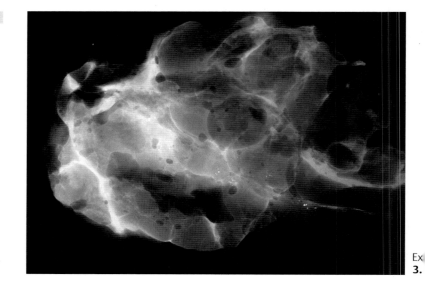

Ex. 3.

Ex. **3.13**-9   Large-section histological image, H & E staining. The pathologist has outlined the area with in situ carcinoma, showing involved margins. The area with in situ carcinoma measured more than 50 mm × 50 mm.

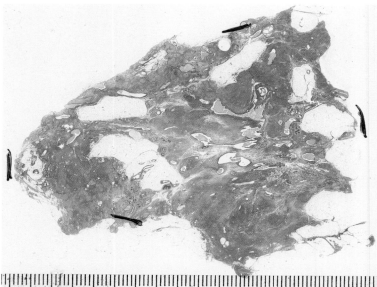

Ex. 3.1

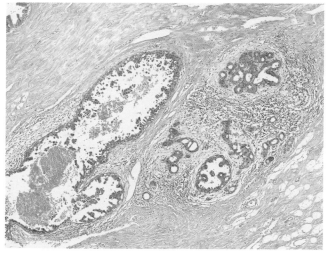

Ex. **3.13**-10

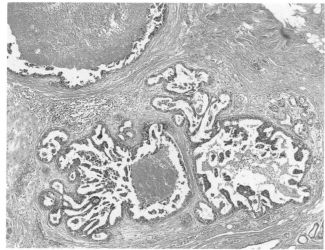

Ex. 3.

Ex. **3.13**-10 & 11   Low-power histological images. The dominant feature is high-grade micropapillary in situ carcinoma with intraluminal necrosis.

Ex. **3.13**-12 Radiograph of the operative specimen.

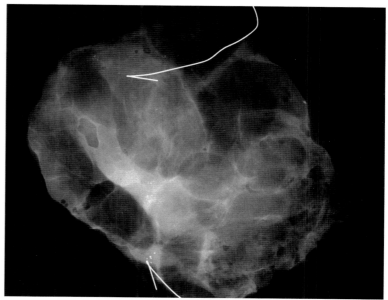

Ex.
3.13-12

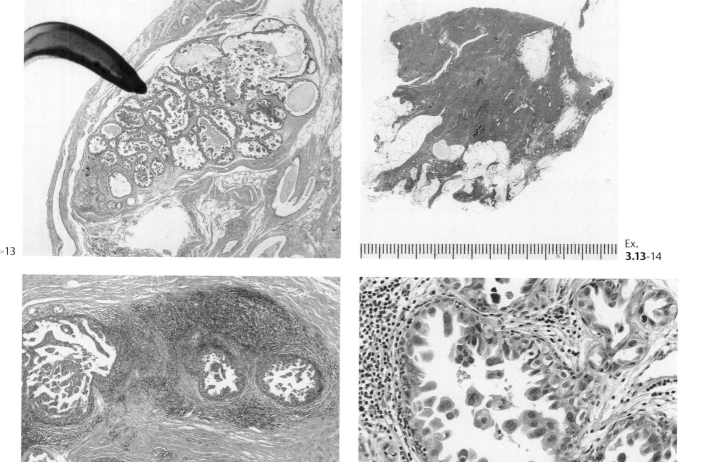

-13

15

Ex.
3.13-14

Ex.
3.13-16

Ex. **3.13**-13 to 16 Low-power histological image of the involved margin at segmentectomy (13). Large-section histological image of the mastectomy specimen (14). Histological examination revealed an additional 85 mm × 55 mm area with high-grade micropapillary carcinoma in situ (15, 16). Although no invasive foci were detected, there was extensive lymphocytic infiltration and desmoplastic reaction surrounding some of the ductlike structures, resembling neoductgenesis.

Treatment and follow-up: Mastectomy with reconstruction. The patient was without signs of recurrence at the most recent follow-up examination 8 years after surgery.

Example 3.14

A 51-year-old woman, who had been taking hormone replacement treatment (HRT) for 6 months, noted a lump in the central portion of her right breast.

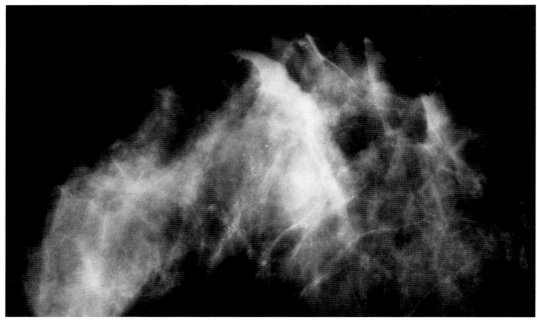

Ex. **3.14**-1

Ex. **3.14**-1 Right breast, CC projection. There are several clusters of calcifications in the central portion of the breast.

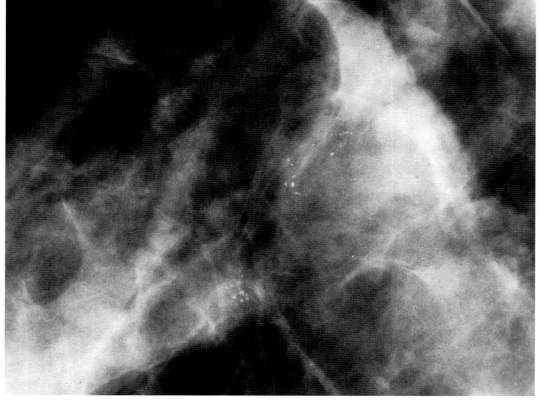

Ex. **3.14**-2

Ex. **3.14**-2 Microfocus magnification: the clustered calcifications are of the crushed stone–like, mammographically malignant type. No associated tumor mass is seen.

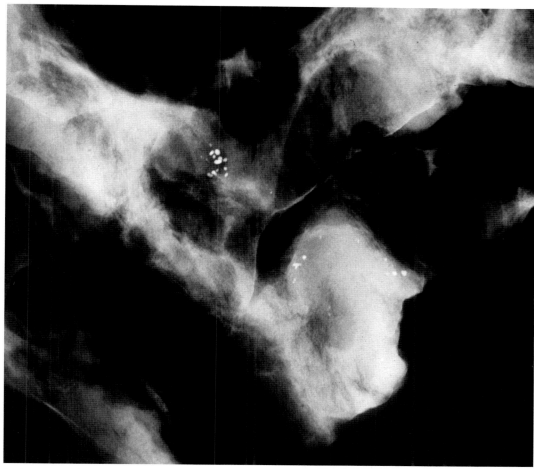

Ex. **3.14**-3

Ex. **3.14**-3   Radiograph of one of the specimen slices containing parts of the clusters.

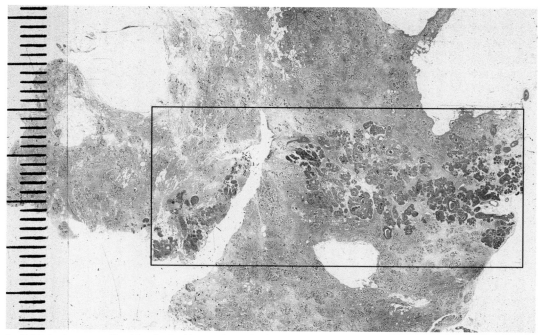

Ex. **3.14**-4

Ex. **3.14**-4   Large-section histological image (H & E). The in situ malignant process is contiguous and extensive (rectangle). The in situ foci are tightly packed together with little or no normal tissue among them. The margin is involved.

Example 3.14 continued

Ex. **3.14**-5 & 6   Low-power views showing normal sized TDLUs (encircled) adjacent to TDLUs and terminal ducts grossly distended by the malignant in situ process, which occupies the remainder of the field.

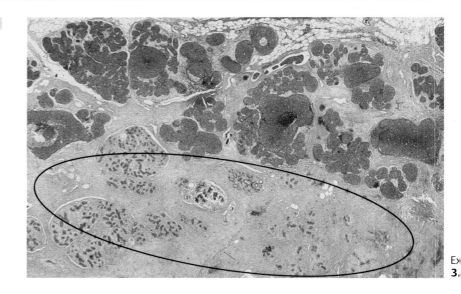

Ex
3.

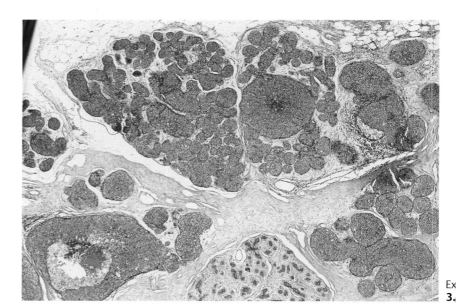

Ex
3.

Ex. **3.14**-7   Immunohistochemical staining with anti-actin outlines the continuous myoepithelial cell layer. The same was seen in the entire specimen, confirming the diagnosis of in situ carcinoma.

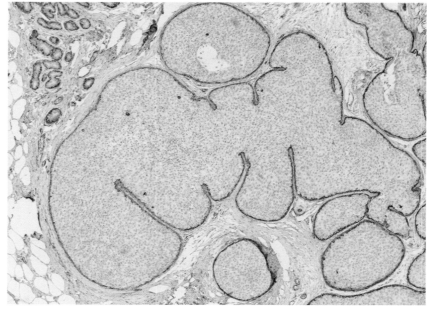

Ex
3.

Ex. **3.14**-8 Most of the acini in this single, enlarged lobule are massively distended by the in situ malignant process, but a few uninvolved normal acini also co-exist within the same lobule (encircled).

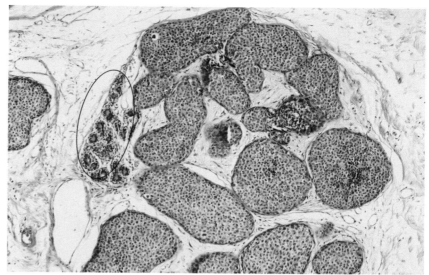

Ex.
3.14-8

Ex. **3.14**-9 Medium-power magnification image shows spots of amorphous calcification within individual acini. This case serves to demonstrate the commonly observed discrepancy between the sparse finding on the mammogram and the extensive disease process seen at histological examination.

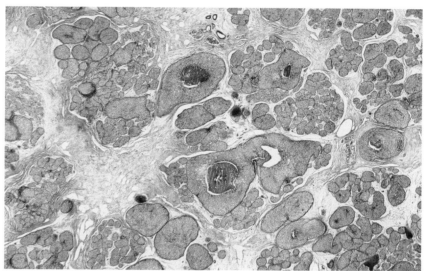

Ex.
3.14-9

Ex. **3.14**-10 Higher-power magnification shows a terminal duct in cross-section with solid cell proliferation, central necrosis, and amorphous calcification. The adjacent cancerous acini are distended with viable cells, but contain no demonstrable necrosis or calcifications.

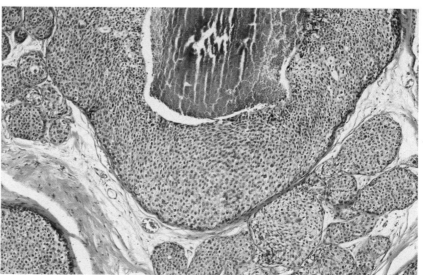

Histological diagnosis: Two areas of Grade 2 in situ carcinoma measuring 40 mm × 17 mm and 10 mm × 3 mm with no signs of invasion.

Ex.
3.14-10

Example 3.14 continued

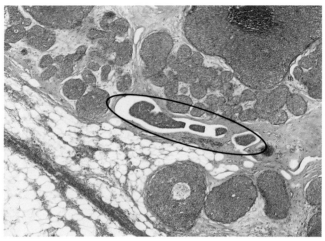

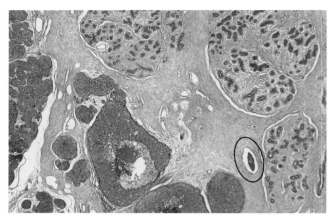

Ex. **3.14**-11

Ex. **3.14**-11 & 12   Histological examination of the operative specimen from the second sector resection reveals lymph vessel invasion at multiple sites.

Ex. **3.14**-13   Six years after operation and breast reconstruction the patient felt a large supraclavicular node. Fine-needle aspiration of the pathological supraclavicular node shows malignant cells.

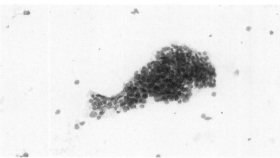

Ex. **3.14**-13

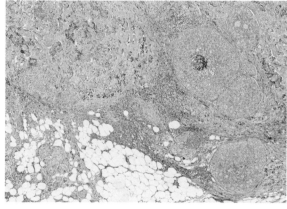

Ex. **3.14**-14

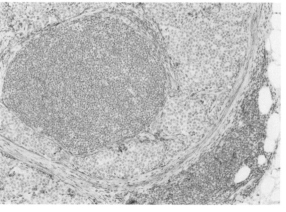

Ex. **3.14**-15

Ex. **3.14**-14   Histological image of the surgically removed lymph node shows ductlike structures mimicking in situ carcinoma and periglandular tumor growth.

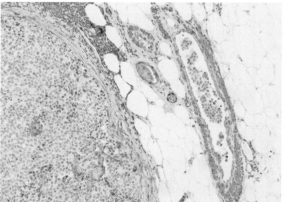

Ex. **3.14**-15 & 16   Anti-actin staining of the lymph node and its surrounding. One large vessel in the vicinity of the lymph node contains cancer cells.

Ex. **3.14**-16

Treatment and outcome: Two sector resections followed by mastectomy and immediate reconstruction. Six years later, axillary and supraclavicular node metastases were diagnosed containing tissue "very similar to the original breast cancer." After 3 more years, skeletal metastases were found at MRI examination.

Comment
No foci of invasive carcinoma were found at thorough histological examination and at the external review of the large-section histological slides. Neoductgenesis is a plausible explanation for the unexpected appearance of cancer foci in the axillary and supraclavicular nodes, foci which also mimicked in situ carcinoma.

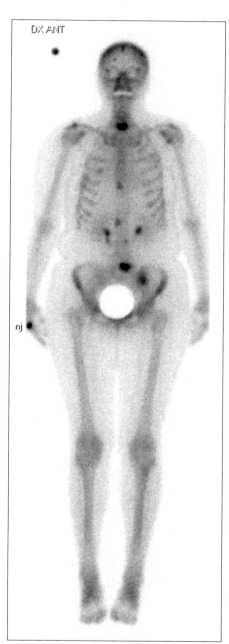

Ex. **3.14**-17

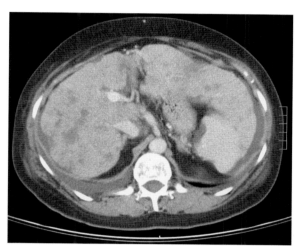

Ex. **3.14**-18

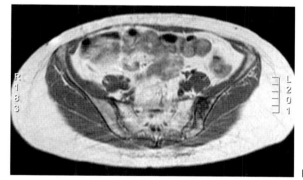

Ex. **3.14**-19

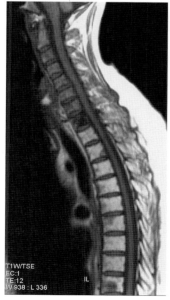

Ex. **3.14**-20

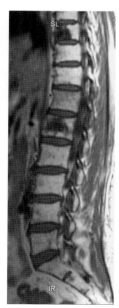

Ex. **3.14**-21

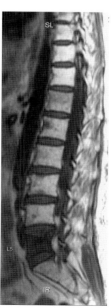

Ex. **3.14**-22

Ex. **3.14**-17 to 22　Technetium bone scan, CT and MR images demonstrate multiple lytic and blastic bone metastases.

Example 3.15

A 35-year-old woman complained of "swollen breasts." The mammograms of the right breast showed no abnormality, but there were a large number of calcifications on the mammograms of the left breast.

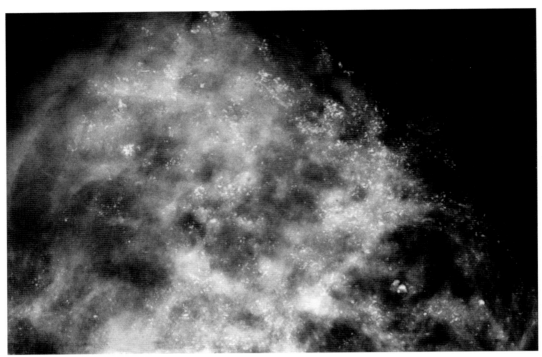

Ex. **3.15**-1

Ex. **3.15**-1   Left breast, CC projection. A large number of clustered calcifications are seen over most of the breast.

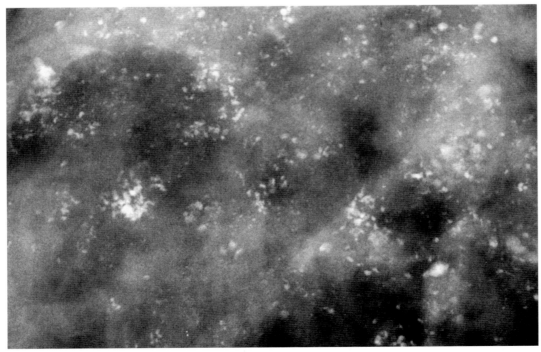

Ex. **3.15**-2

Ex. **3.15**-2   Microfocus magnification, CC projection. There are many clusters of crushed stone–like, mammographically malignant type calcifications superimposed over each other. No tumor mass is demonstrable.

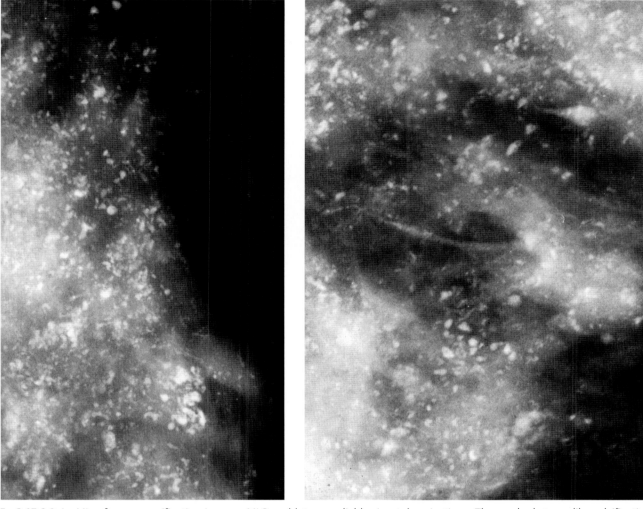

-3

Ex. **3.15**-3 & 4   Microfocus magnification images, MLO and lateromedial horizontal projections. The crushed stone–like calcifications dominate the image, but there are also casting type calcifications present.

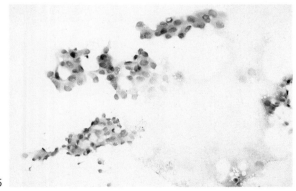

-5

Ex. **3.15**-5   Fine-needle aspiration biopsy: malignant cells.

Example 3.15 continued

Ex. **3.15**-6   Portion of the large-section histological slide. There is an unnaturally large number of cancerous ducts which are tightly squeezed together with no intervening normal tissue. The malignant cell proliferation is a mixture of the solid, cribriform and micropapillary types.

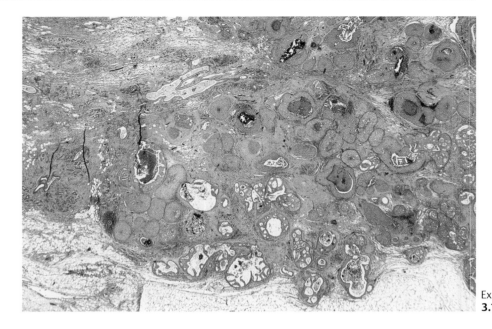

Ex. **3.15**-7   Medium-power magnification shows solid cell proliferation, central necrosis, and amorphous calcification.

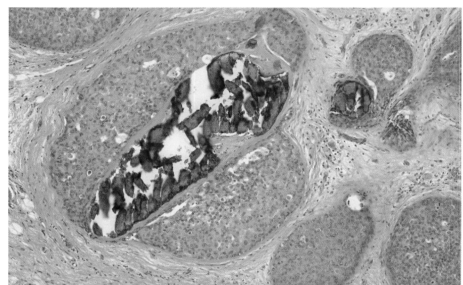

Ex. **3.15**-8   High-power magnification image with cribriform cell proliferation.

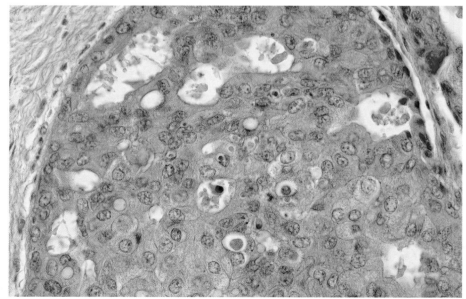

Ex.
3.1

3D Image

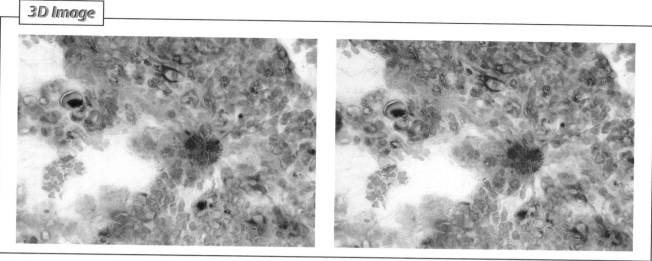

Ex. **3.15**-9 & 10   The spiculated invasive carcinoma at the center of the image is surrounded by an unnaturally large number of ducts and TDLUs distended by cancer cells.

3D Image

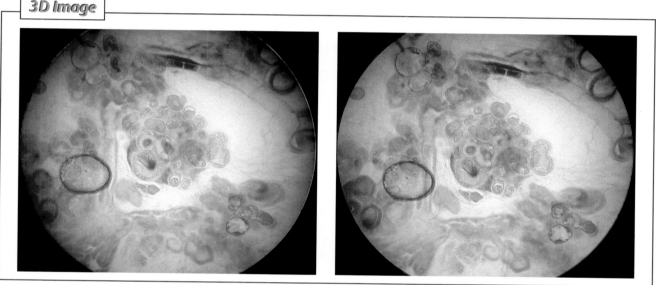

Ex. **3.15**-11 & 12   A greatly distended TDLU containing a cluster of amorphous calcifications appears in the foreground and is surrounded by several other cancerous TDLUs. A large blood vessel crosses the top of the image.

3D Image

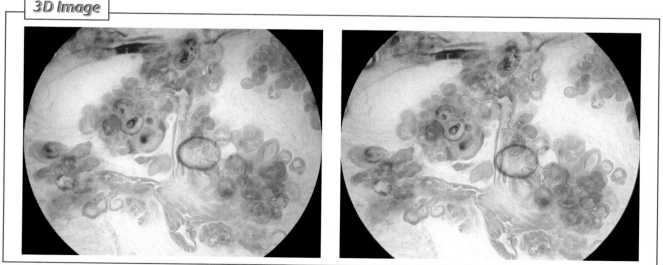

Ex. **3.15**-13 & 14   The same image pair as in Ex. **3.14**-11 & 12, but the 1 mm-thick tissue slice has been photographed from the opposite side, in order to bring the cancer-filled ducts into the foreground.

Example 3.15 continued

3D Image

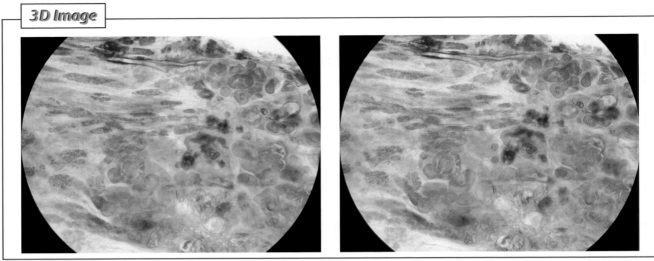

Ex.
3.15-15

Ex.
3.1

Ex. **3.15**-15 & 16   Normal TDLUs (in the left upper part of the image) contrast with the cancer-filled ducts and TDLUs in the remainder of the image. The calcifications are scattered at various depths.

3D Image

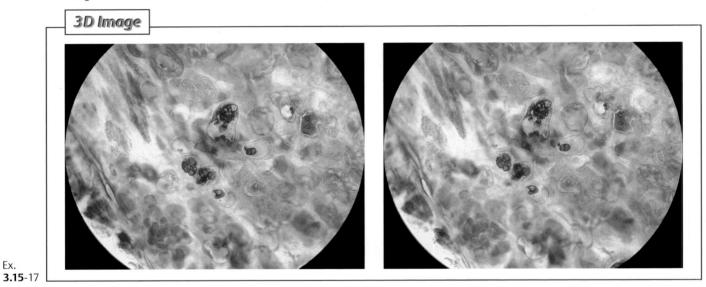

Ex.
3.15-17

Ex.
3.1

Ex. **3.15**-17 & 18   Subgross, 3D histological image pair of cavities containing clusters of crushed stone–like calcifications.

3D Image

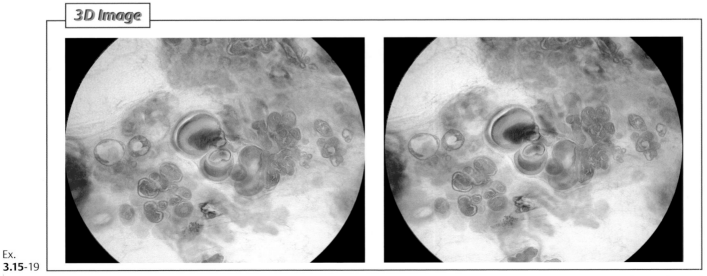

Ex.
3.15-19

Ex.
3.1

Ex. **3.15**-19 & 20   Subgross histological image pair of numerous acini greatly distended by the proliferating cancer cells, intraluminal necrosis, and amorphous calcifications.

3D Image

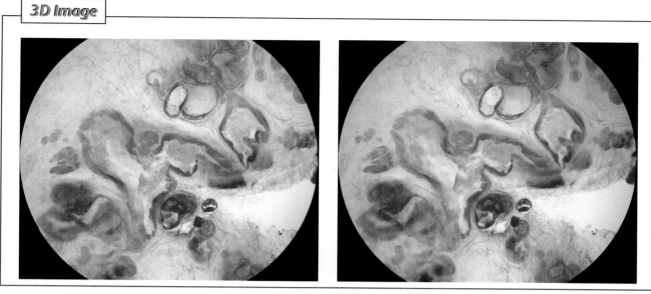

5-21

Ex.
3.15-22

Ex. **3.15**-21 & 22   Tortuous ducts with a thick lining of cancer cells and intraluminal necrosis.

3D Image

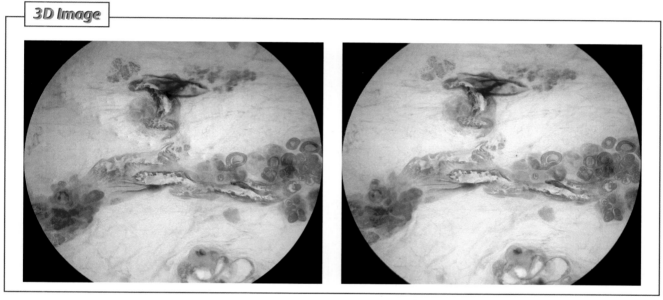

5-23

Ex.
3.15-24

Ex. **3.15**-23 & 24   In this 3D image pair the ducts contain micropapillary cancer cell proliferation and central necrosis.

Histological diagnosis: A 20 mm × 16 mm Grade 2 invasive ductal carcinoma was found in the retroareolar region. Another focus of Grade 2 invasive carcinoma, measuring 28 mm × 18 mm, was located in the medial portion of the breast, close to the chest wall. Five out of the 13 surgically removed axillary lymph nodes contained metastases.

Treatment and outcome: Mastectomy. The patient **died of metastatic breast cancer** 3¹/₂ years after treatment.

Example 3.16

A 58-year-old asymptomatic woman, routine screening examination.

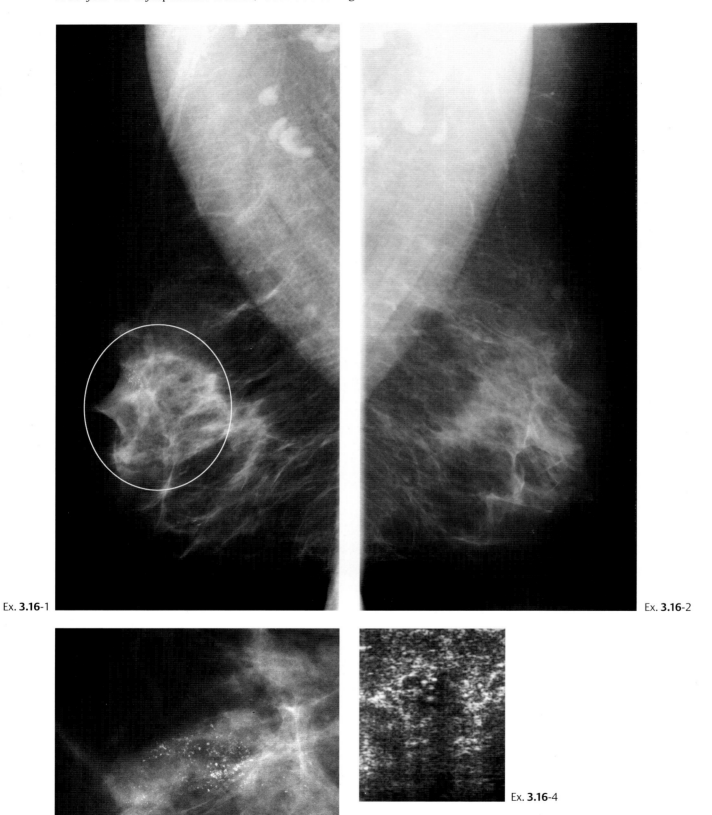

Ex. **3.16**-1

Ex. **3.16**-2

Ex. **3.16**-3

Ex. **3.16**-4

Ex. **3.16**-1 to 4   Screening mammograms (1, 2), right and left MLO projections. A large area with calcifications is seen in the upper portion of the right breast. Microfocus magnification image (3). The calcifications can be better analyzed in the CC projection. Breast ultrasound (4) shows an ill-defined tumor mass containing calcifications.

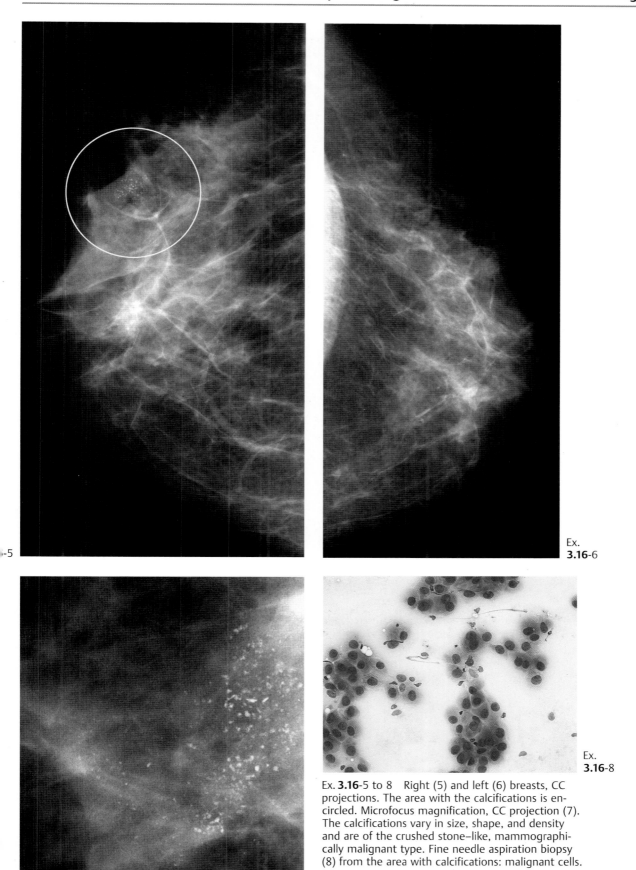

Ex.
3.16-6

Ex.
3.16-8

Ex. **3.16**-5 to 8 Right (5) and left (6) breasts, CC projections. The area with the calcifications is encircled. Microfocus magnification, CC projection (7). The calcifications vary in size, shape, and density and are of the crushed stone–like, mammographically malignant type. Fine needle aspiration biopsy (8) from the area with calcifications: malignant cells.

-5

-7

Example 3.16 continued

Ex. **3.16**-9   Operative specimen radiograph.

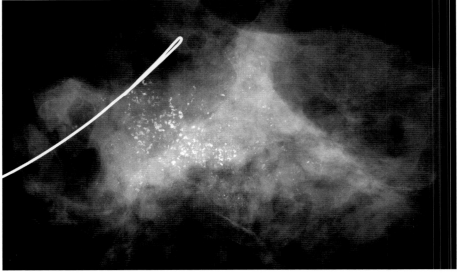

Ex. 3.

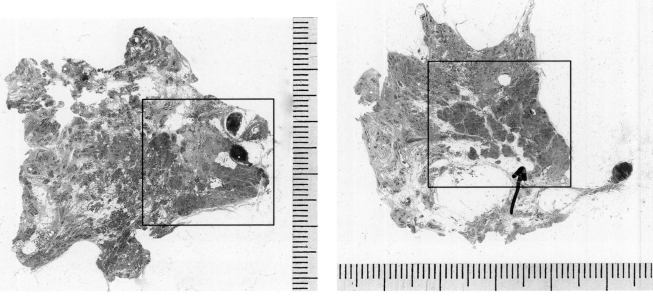

Ex.
3.16-10

Ex. 3.

Ex. **3.16**-10 & 11   Large-section histology slices. The cancerous areas are marked with rectangles. The overall extent of the Grade 2 and 3 in situ carcinoma is 35 mm × 35 mm. The specimen margin is involved. There were no signs of metastases in three intramammary lymph nodes.

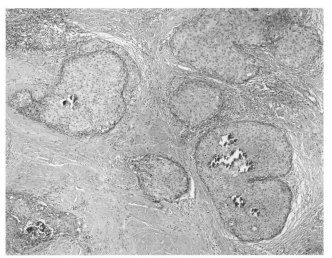

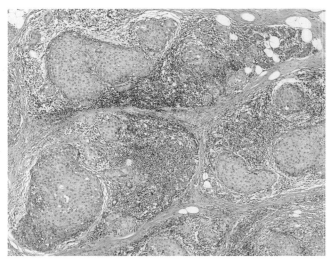

Ex.
3.16-12

Ex. 3.

Ex. **3.16**-12 & 13   Medium-power histological images (H & E). The ducts and acini distended by cancer cells are closely spaced and surrounded by extensive periductal lymphocytic infiltration.

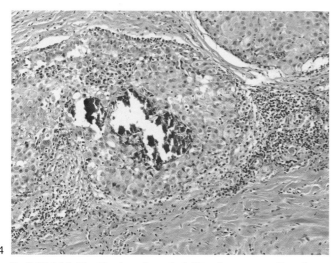

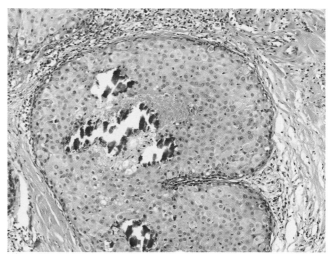

14

Ex. **3.16**-14 & 15   The lymphocytic infiltration surrounding the cancerous ducts raises the suspicion of neoductgenesis. The basement membrane is intact.

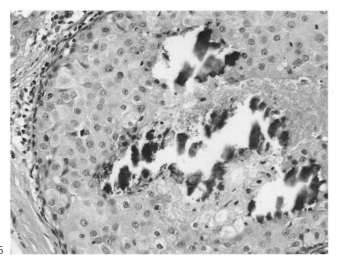

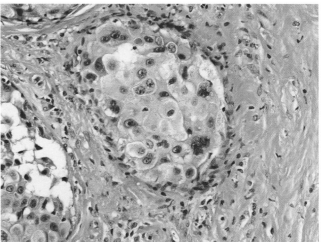

»16

Ex.
3.16-17

Ex. **3.16**-16 & 17   Higher-power histological images: polymorphic carcinoma cells associated with necrosis and amorphous calcifications.

Comment
In this case the malignant type, crushed stone–like calcifications were observed over a large area on the mammograms. The histological features of neoductgenesis and the presence of vascular invasion are at odds with the diagnosis of in situ carcinoma.

Treatment and outcome: Mastectomy. There was no evidence of recurrence at the most recent follow-up examination 7 years after surgery.

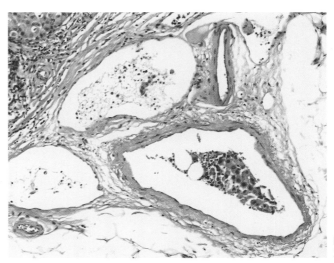

Ex.
3.16-18

Ex. **3.16**-18   Cancer cells were found within a large vessel, demonstrating vascular invasion.

Example 3.17

A 53-year-old asymptomatic woman, called back from mammography screening for assessment of the calcifications detected in the lower-inner quadrant of her right breast. Her most recent mammograms taken 5 years earlier showed no abnormality.

Ex. **3.17**-1 & 2   Right breast, detail of the MLO projection, contact and microfocus magnification images. Multiple clusters of crushed stone–like calcifications are surrounded by a soft-tissue density.

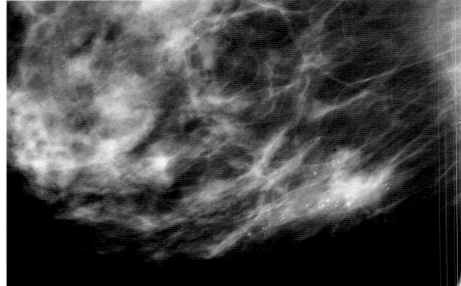

Ex.
3.1

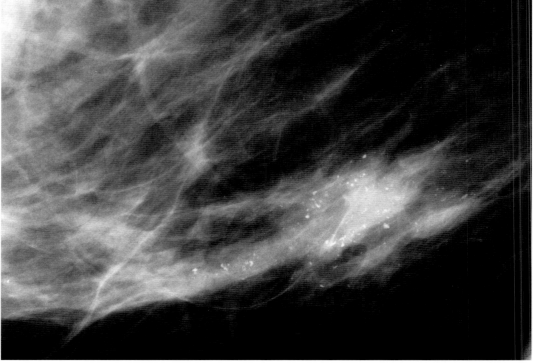

Ex.
3.1

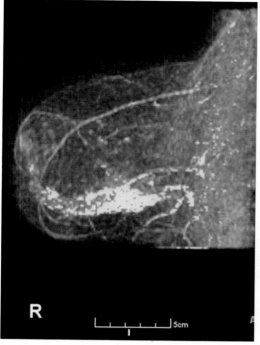

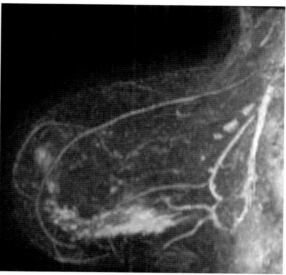

7-3

Ex. 3.17-4

Ex. **3.17**-3 & 4   Right breast, MRI examination, sagittal view: corresponding to the mammographically detected abnormality, there is a similarly shaped density contrast enhancement suggesting malignancy.

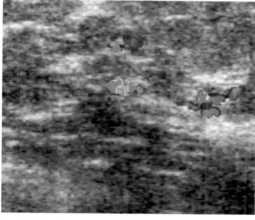

7-5

Ex. **3.17**-5   Breast ultrasound demonstrates greatly increased vascularity, suggesting neoangiogenesis in the region with the malignant type calcifications.

Example 3.17 continued

Ex. **3.17**-6 & 7   Right breast, detail of the CC projection, contact and microfocus magnification images.

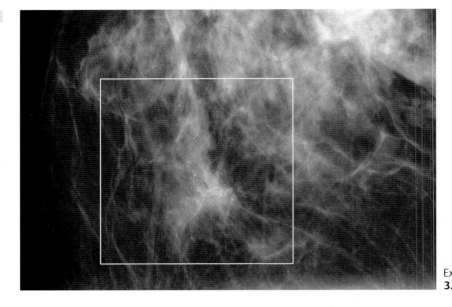

Ex. 3.1

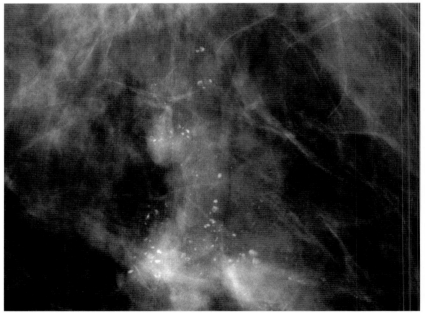

Ex. 3.1

Ex. **3.17**-8   MRI, axial plane. Contrast enhancement outlines the wedge-shaped abnormality in the right breast.

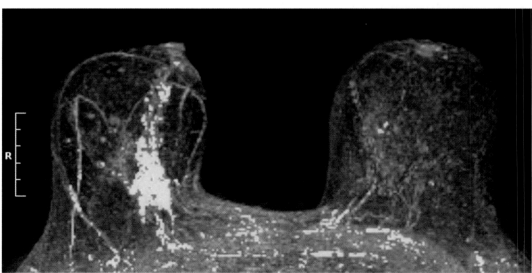

Ex. 3.1

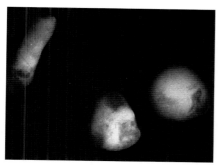

Ex. **3.17**-9

Ex. **3.17**-9   Radiograph of the 14-gauge core specimen.

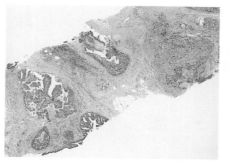

Ex. **3.17**-10

Ex. **3.17**-10   Histological image of the 14-gauge core specimen: in situ carcinoma.

Ex. **3.17**-11   Preoperative localization using the bracketing technique.

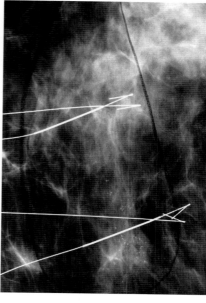

Ex. **3.17**-11

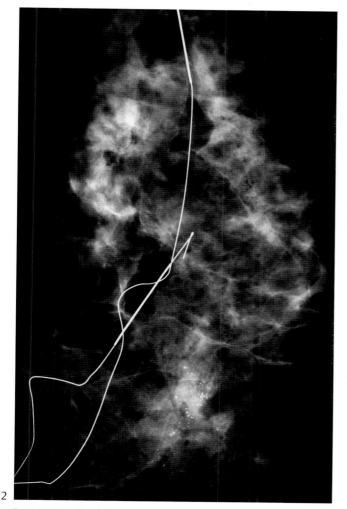

12

Ex. **3.17**-12   Operative specimen radiograph.

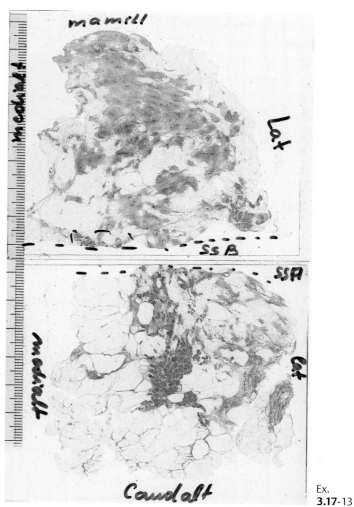

Ex. **3.17**-13

Ex. **3.17**-13   Collage of two large-section histology slices. Grade 1-2-3 in situ carcinoma was demonstrated over an area measuring 70 mm × 30 mm. The circumferential margins were free of tumor.

Example 3.17 continued

Ex. **3.17**-14   Detail image of the operative specimen radiograph demonstrating the calcifications and the associated soft-tissue density.

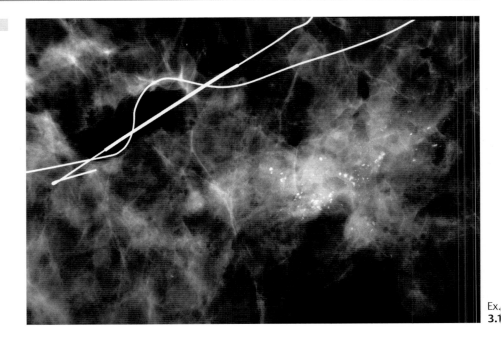

Ex.
3.1

Ex. **3.17**-15   Radiograph of one of the operative specimen slices.

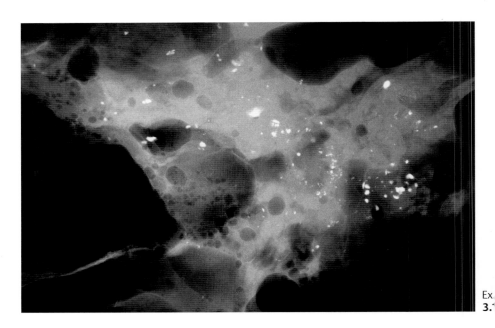

Ex.
3.1

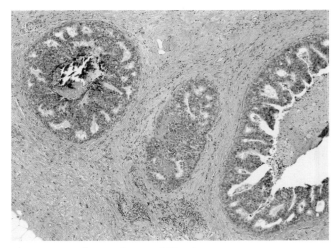

Ex.
3.17-16

Ex.
3.

Ex. **3.17**-16 & 17   Histological images of in situ carcinoma with central necrosis and amorphous calcification.

Treatment and outcome: Sector resection and postoperative irradiation, a very recent case.

3D Image

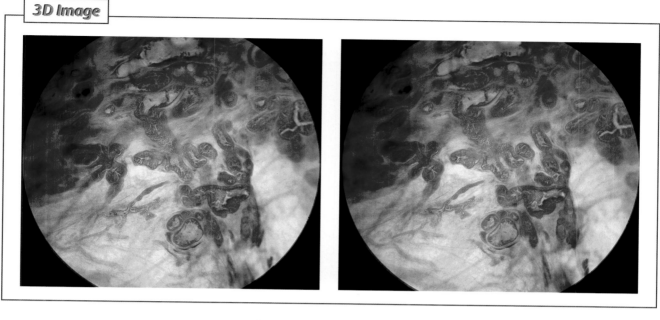

Ex. 3.17-18   Ex. **3.17**-19

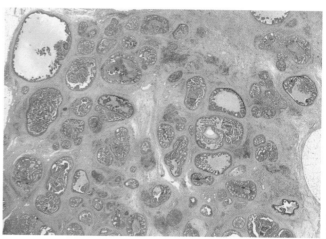

Ex. **3.17**-20

3D Image

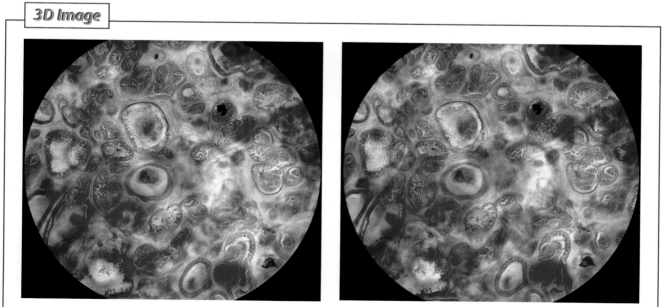

Ex. 3.17-21   Ex. **3.17**-22

Ex. **3.17**-18 to 22   Comparative subgross, thick-section (3D) and conventional histological images demonstrating a large area with non-calcified in situ carcinoma, in addition to those containing amorphous calcifications.

Example 3.18

A 65-year-old asymptomatic woman, called back from mammography screening for assessment of the calcifica- tions detected in the lower-inner quadrant of her left breast. Her most recent mammograms taken 3 years earlier showed no abnormality.

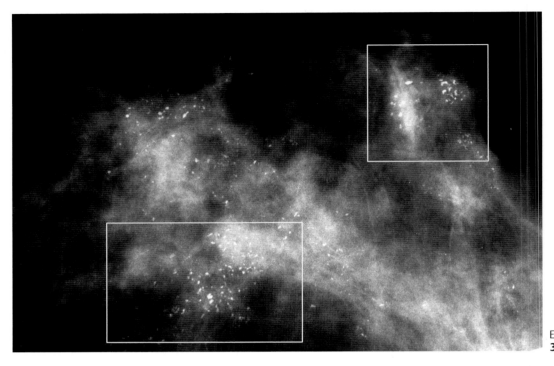

Ex
3.1

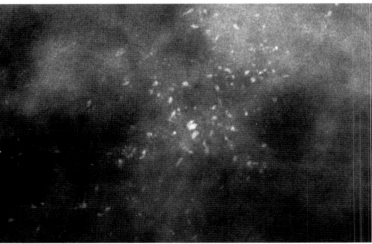

Ex.
3.1

Ex. **3.18**-1 to 3   Left breast, detail of the CC projection (1). Many clusters of calcifications are seen over the entire lateral portion and also in the medial half of the breast. Microfocus magnification images of the clusters (2 & 3) within the rectangles demonstrate the broken needle tip–like/crushed stone–like calcifications that are mammo- graphically malignant.

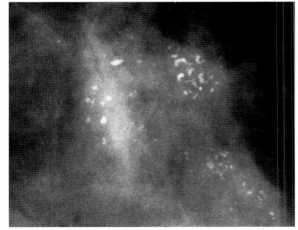

Ex
3.

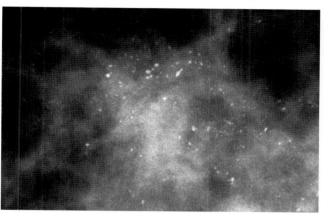

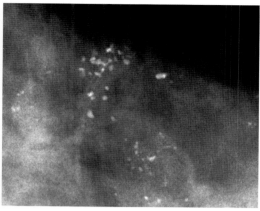

Ex. **3.18**-4 & 5   Further examples of the magnified calcification clusters.

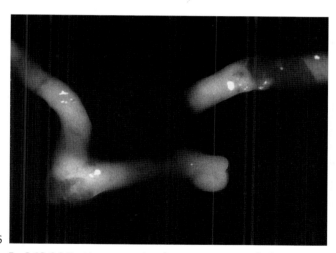

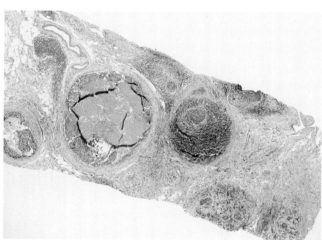

Ex. **3.18**-6 & 7   Vacuum-assisted preoperative needle biopsy. Radiographs of the core needle biopsy specimen (6) and low-power magnification of an histological image of one of the specimen samples (7).

Histology: Multiple foci of in situ carcinoma.

Example 3.18 continued

Ex. **3.18**-8   Detail of the left CC projection for comparison with the large-section histological image (Ex. **3.18**-9).

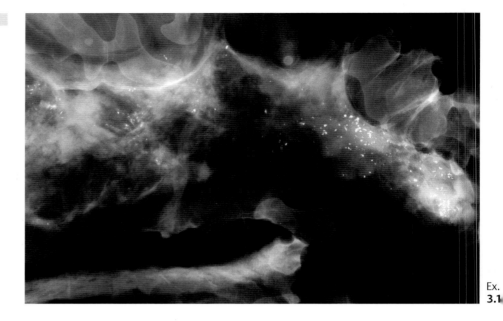

Ex.
3.1

Ex. **3.18**-9   One of the large-section histology slices. The pathologist's marks indicate that the entire section is involved with the disease.

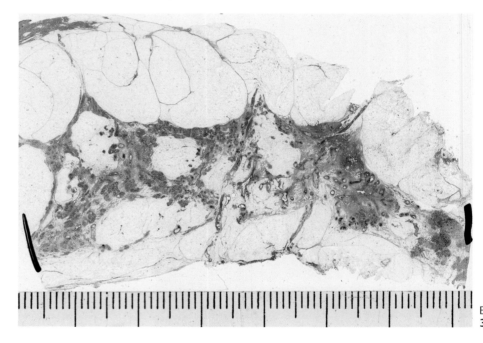

Ex.
3.1

Ex.
3.18-10

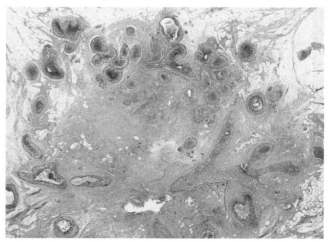

Ex.
3.1

Ex. **3.18**-10 & 11   Medium- and high-power magnification images of this in situ carcinoma with several closely spaced ductlike structures. The higher magnification shows intraluminal calcification.

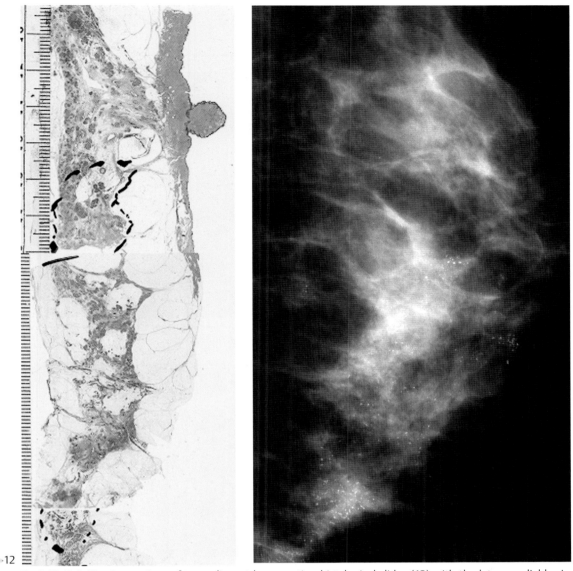

Ex. **3.18**-13

Ex. **3.18**-12 & 13   Comparison of two adjacent large-section histological slides (12) with the lateromedial horizontal mammogram (13). The areas marked by the pathologist contain cancer foci.

3D Image

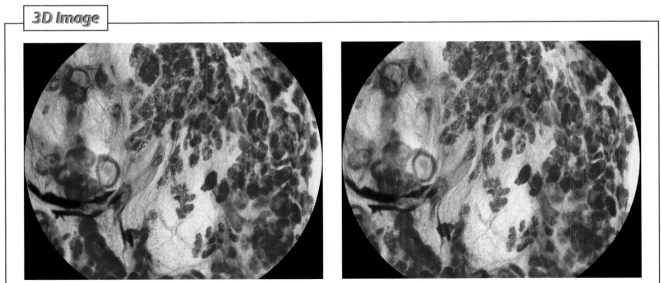

Ex. **3.18**-15

Ex. **3.18**-14 & 15   Subgross, thick-section 3D image pair of cancer-filled, ductlike structures and blood vessels (left side of the image) compared with entirely normal TDLUs (right side of the image).

Example 3.18 continued

3D Image

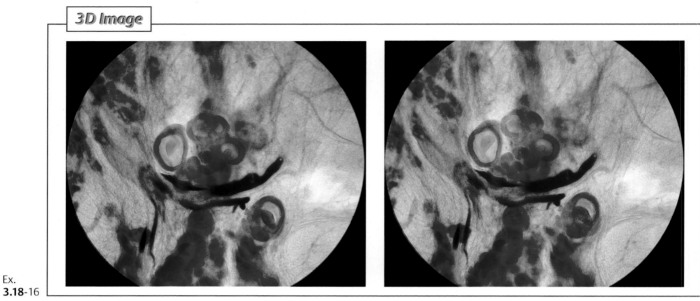

Ex.
3.18-16

Ex.
3.1

Ex. **3.18**-16 & 17   Subgross, thick-section 3D image pair of cancer-filled, ductlike structures and blood vessels.

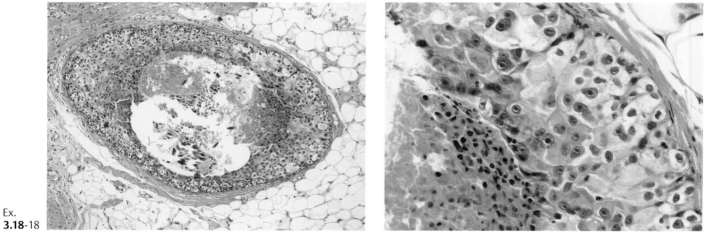

Ex.
3.18-18

Ex.
3.1

Ex. **3.18**-18 & 19   Medium- and high-power magnification histological images. The ductlike structure is distended by high grade in situ carcinoma associated with central necrosis.

3D Image

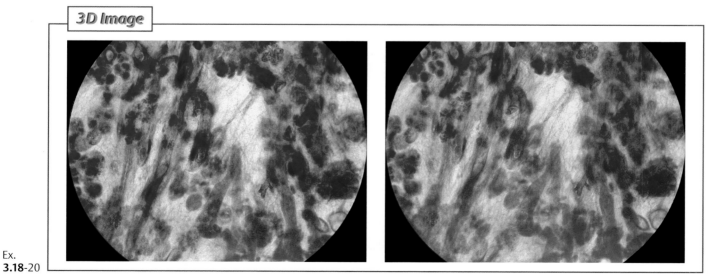

Ex.
3.18-20

Ex.
3.1

Ex. **3.18**-20 & 21   Subgross, thick-section 3D image pair. There are an unnaturally large number of cancer-filled, ductlike structures closely spaced within a limited area.

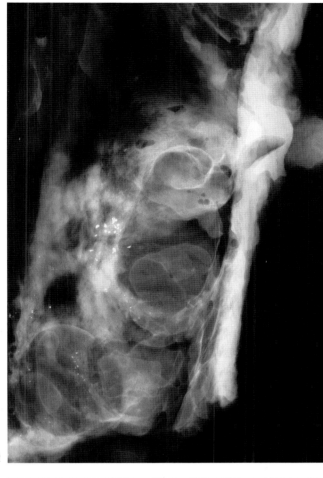

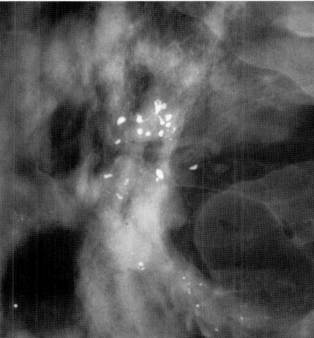

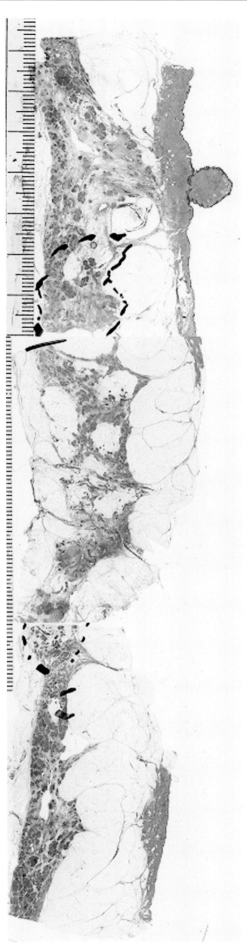

Ex. **3.18**-22 to 24   Operative specimen-slice radiograph containing the crushed stone–like calcifications (22) and a magnified view of the area with the calcifications (23). The mammographic findings can be compared directly with the collage of three large-section histological slides (24).

Ex.
3.18-24

Example 3.18 continued

Ex. **3.18**-25   Large-section histological image. The area with in situ carcinoma has been marked by the pathologist.

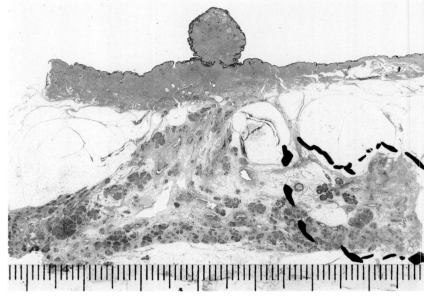

Ex. **3.1**

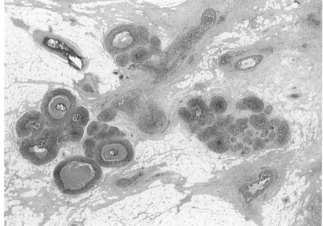

Ex. **3.18**-26

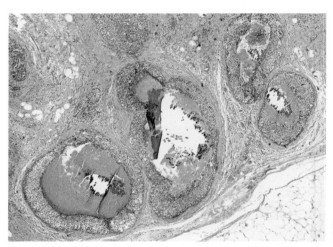

Ex. **3.1**

Ex. **3.18**-26 & 27   Low- and medium-power histological images. The cancer cells distend the individual acini within the TDLU and also fill some of the ducts.

Ex. **3.18**-28   Radiograph of one of the specimen slices (photographic and microfocus magnification make the individual calcification particles easier to analyze).

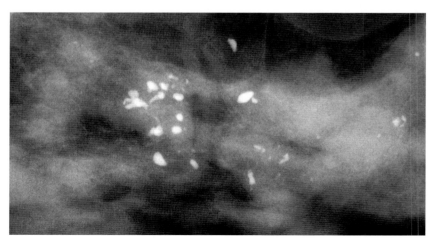

Ex. **3.1**

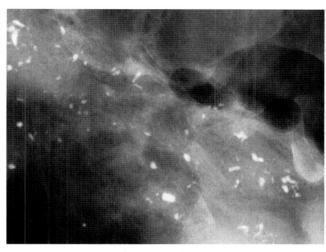
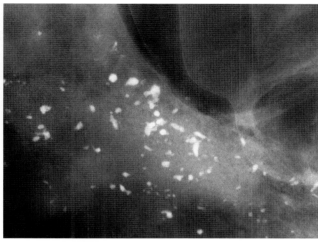

Ex. **3.18**-29 & 30   Microfocus magnification images of two different regions in the specimen slice radiographs containing larger clusters of crushed stone–like calcifications.

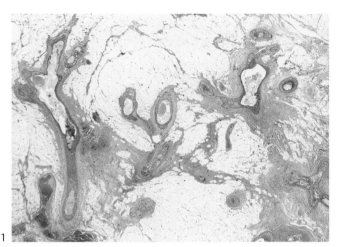
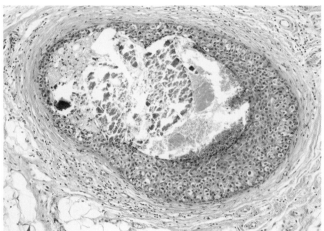

Ex. **3.18**-31 & 32   Low- and medium-power histological images (H & E). Longitudinal and cross sections of numerous ductlike structures distended by carcinoma cells and surrounded by desmoplastic reaction and lymphocytic infiltration, both of which are indicators of neo-ductgenesis.

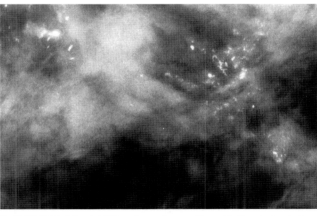
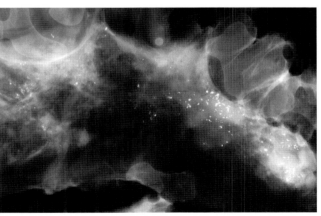

Ex. **3.18**-33 & 34   Additional specimen slices. Both crushed stone–like and casting type calcifications are present, although the pleo-morphic calcifications dominate the mammograms.

Treatment and outcome: Mastectomy. The patient had no signs of recurrence at the first follow-up examination after operation.

Example 3.19

This 67-year-old asymptomatic woman attended mammography screening and no abnormalities were perceived.

Ex. **3.19**-1 to 3   Retrospective analysis of the right CC projection (contact and photographic magnification) reveals two small clusters of calcifications (ovals) and two additional, rodlike calcifications (rectangles).

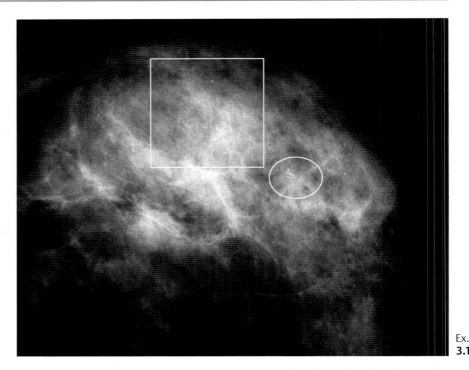

Ex.
3.1

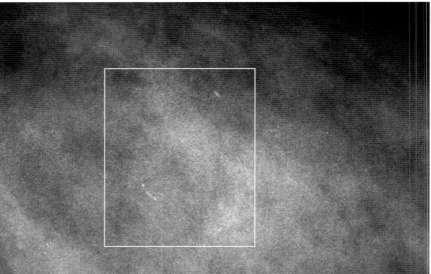

Ex.
3.1

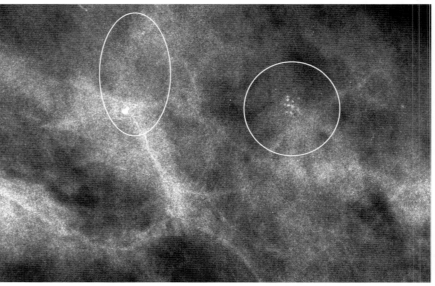

Ex.
3.1

Ex. **3.19**-4 to 6: Three years later, at age 70 years and still asymptomatic, she again attended screening. There is now a large number of crushed stone–like and casting type, mam- mographically malignant type calcifications throughout most of the breast.

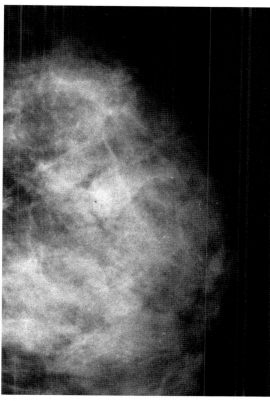

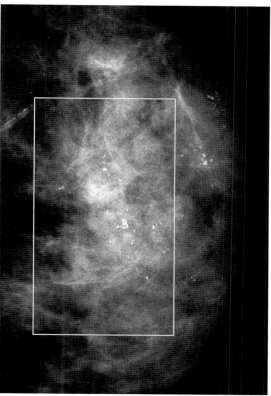

Ex. **3.19**-5

Ex. **3.19**-4   Left breast, MLO projection, first examination. Subtle clusters of calcifications are scattered in the dense tissue.

Ex. **3.19**-5   Left breast, MLO projection, second examination. A large number of clusters of crushed stone–like and casting type calcifications are seen with no associated tumor mass.

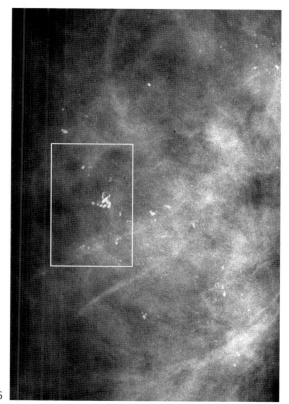

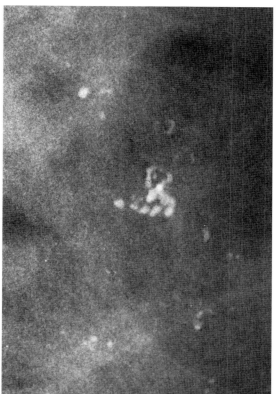

Ex. **3.19**-7

Ex. **3.19**-6   Microfocus magnification of the area within the rectangle in Ex. **3.19**-5.

Ex. **3.19**-7   Further magnification of the area within the rectangle in Ex. 3.**19**-6.

Example 3.19
continued

Ex. **3.19**-8   Left breast, CC projection, second examination. The malignant type calcifications are demonstrable throughout most of the breast.

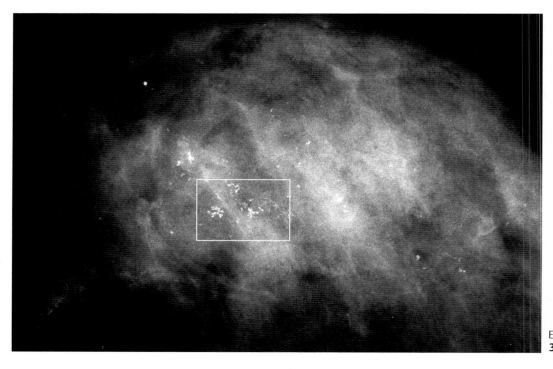

Ex.
3.1

Ex. **3.19**-9   Microfocus magnification image of the area within the rectangle on Ex. **3.19**-8. Numerous crushed stone–like and casting type calcifications have developed since the previous examination.

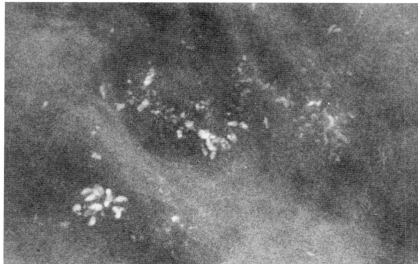

Ex.
3.1

Ex. **3.19**-10   Breast ultrasound. Neoductgenesis often results in an irregular, hypoechogenic image at ultrasound examination.

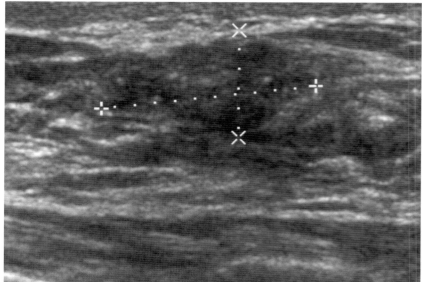

Ex.
3.19

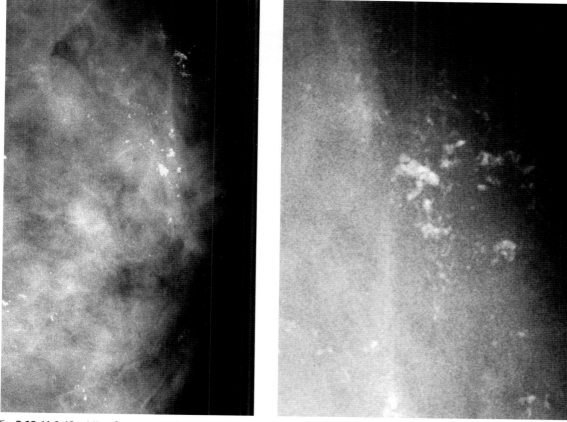

9-11

Ex.
3.19-12

Ex. **3.19**-11 & 12   Microfocus magnification images from the upper portion of the left breast, second examination.

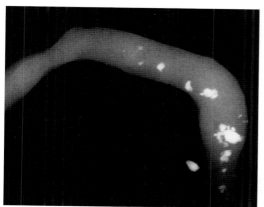

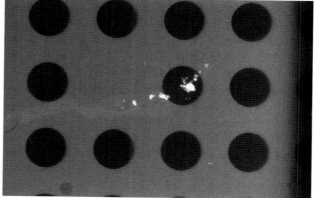

-13

Ex.
3.19-14

Ex. **3.19**-13 & 14   Microfocus magnification images of the vacuum-assisted biopsy specimen containing the calcifications.

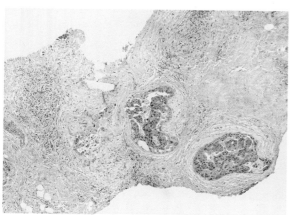

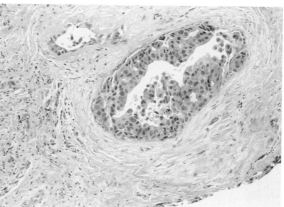

15

Ex.
3.19-16

Ex. **3.19**-15 & 16   Histology of the preoperative biopsy specimen: multiple foci of in situ carcinoma.

Example 3.19 continued

Ex. **3.19**-17   Radiograph of the surgical specimen.

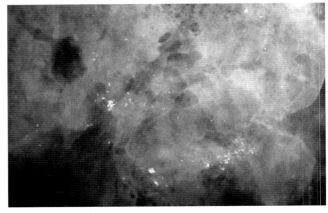

Ex.
3.1

Ex. **3.19**-18   Large-section histological image. The pathologist has outlined the boundaries of the area with in situ carcinoma.

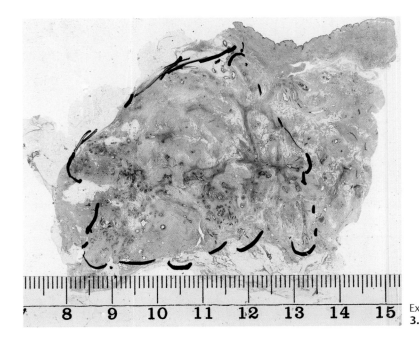

Ex.
3.

3D Image

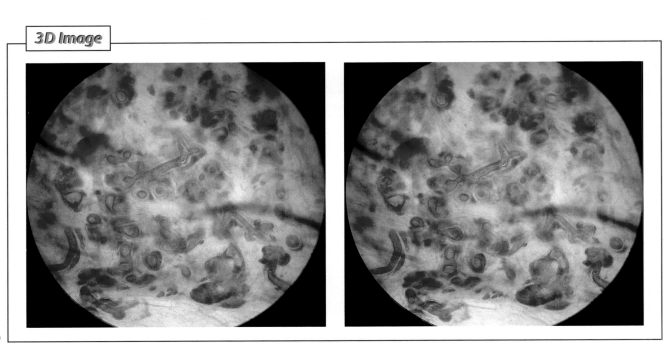

Ex.
3.19-19

Ex.
3.

Ex. **3.19**-19 & 20   Stereoscopic image pair. The cancer-filled ductlike structures are closely spaced.

Ex. **3.19**-21 to 24   Mammographic-histological correlation of neoducts containing cancer cells, necrosis, and amorphous calcifications. Periductal desmoplastic reaction and lymphocytic infiltration can be seen on Ex. **3.19**-22.

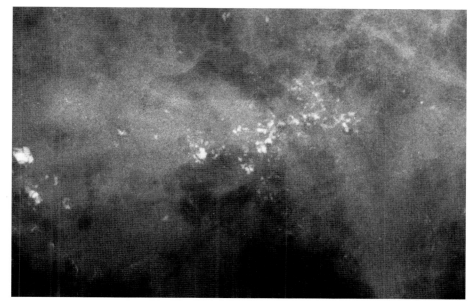

Ex.
3.19-21

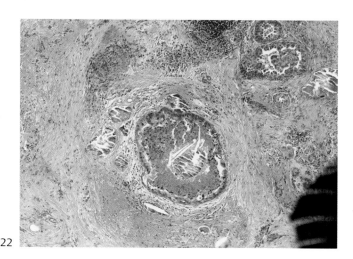

-22

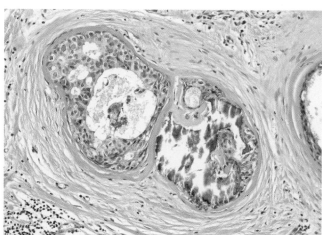

Ex.
3.19-23

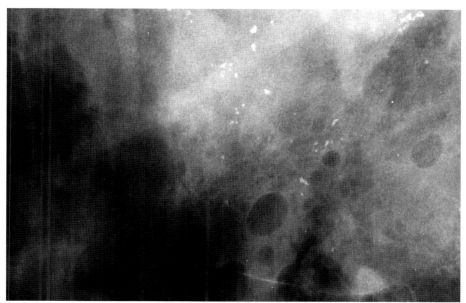

Ex.
3.19-24

Example 3.19 continued

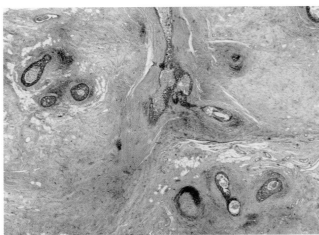

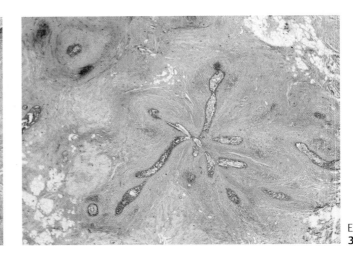

Ex.
3.19-25

Ex.
3.1

3D Image

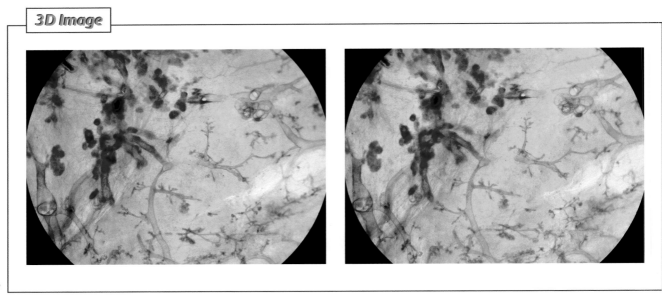

Ex.
3.19-27

Ex.
3.1

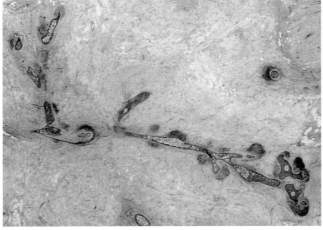

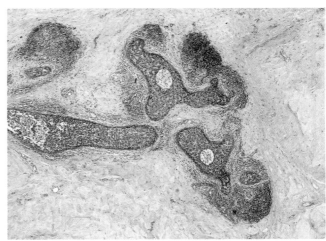

Ex.
3.19-29

Ex.
3.1

Ex. **3.19**-25 to 30   Stereoscopic image pair (27 & 28) of neoducts compared with the conventional histological images of newly formed ducts surrounded by lymphocytic infiltration.

Ex. **3.19**-31   The conglomerate of ductlike structures seen on Ex. **3.19**-32 & 33 is reflected in the ultrasound image.

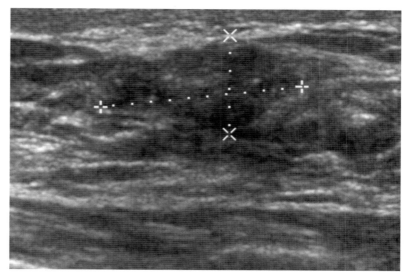

Ex. **3.19**-31

3D Image

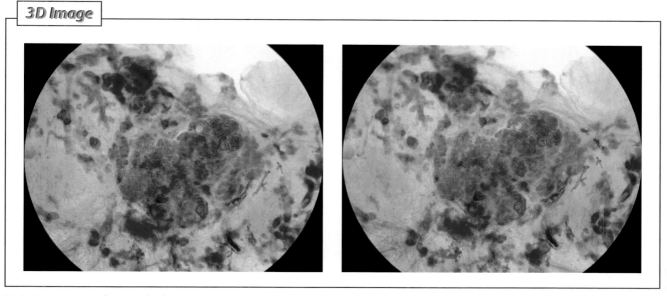

32

Ex. **3.19**-33

Ex. **3.19**-32 & 33   Subgross, thick-section (3D) histological image pair. The newly formed ducts are cramped together in a tumorlike conglomerate.

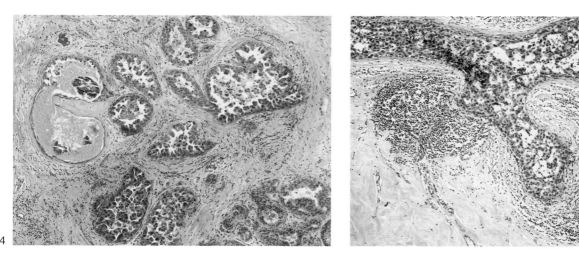

34

Ex. **3.19**-35

Ex. **3.19**-34 & 35   The tightly packed ductlike structures are associated with periductal desmoplastic reaction and lymphocytic infiltration, suggesting neoductgenesis.

Example 3.19 continued

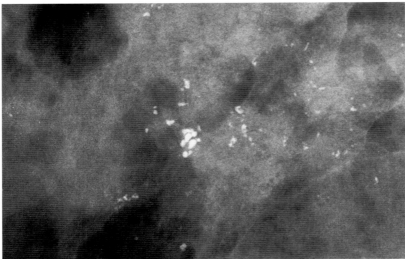

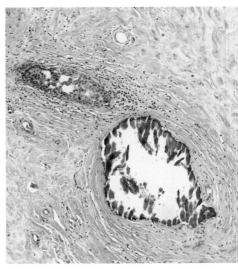

Ex.
3.19-36

Ex.
3.1

Ex. **3.19**-36 & 37   Radiograph of one of the specimen slices (36). The large, smooth-contoured amorphous calcification is surrounded by dense fibrous tissue (lower right); viable cancer cells are seen nearby (upper left) (37).

Ex. **3.19**-38   Detail of a large-section histological image of this extensive cancerous process hidden in the dense fibrous tissue. Numerous budlike protrusions are surrounded by lymphocytic infiltration (sites of neoductgenesis). Note that these neoducts have no associated TDLUs.

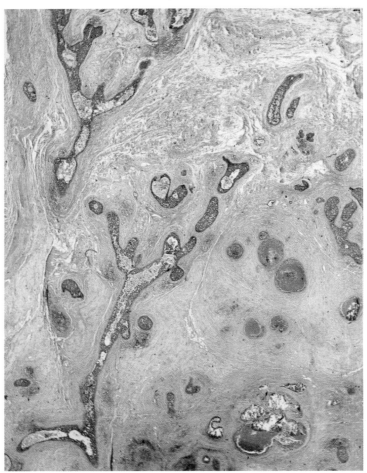

Ex.
3.1

Histology: 75 mm × 55 mm in situ carcinoma, Grades 1 to 3 associated with a 4 mm × 3 mm Grade 3 invasive carcinoma.

Treatment and outcome: Mastectomy. During the first year of follow-up the patient was diagnosed with a malignant lung tumor. It is extremely difficult to distinguish between a possible breast cancer metastasis and a primary lung cancer.

Comment
Unfortunately, distinction between multiple clusters of crushed stone–like calcifications in Group 2A and 2B cases cannot be made solely on the basis of mammography. Breast MRI can be of great help in distinguishing between the two groups.

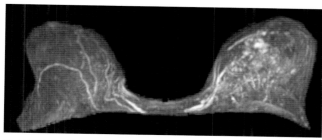

Ex. **3.19**-39   Breast MRI shows contrast enhancement over most of the left breast, confirming the presence of an extensive malignant process.

Ex. **3.19**-40   Histology of one long ductlike structure distended by cancer cells. There are numerous short neoducts with an associated lymphocytic reaction.

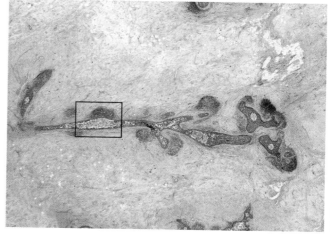

Ex. **3.19**-40

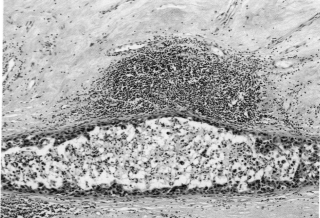

Ex. **3.19**-41   Magnification of the area within the rectangle on Ex. **3.19**-40.

Ex. **3.19**-41

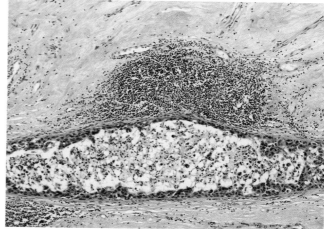

Ex. **3.19**-42   Radiograph of one of the operative specimen slices.

Ex. **3.19**-42

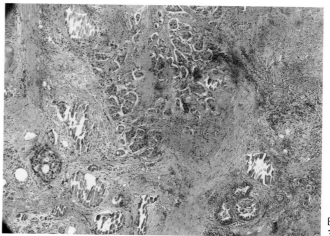

Ex. **3.19**-43   A tiny invasive micropapillary carcinoma is associated with the extensive in situ process.

Ex. **3.19**-43

Chapter 4 Differential Diagnosis of Breast Diseases Producing Clustered, Discernible Calcifications

Clustered, discernible calcifications with a crushed stone–like appearance may be associated with both malignant and benign processes in the breast. Crushed stone–like calcifications are the most frequent among the malignant type calcifications. The most frequent benign, hyperplastic breast changes that may be associated with discernable crushed stone–like calcifications are fibrocystic change, fibroadenoma, and papilloma, all of which may cause considerable differential diagnostic problems (see Fig. **4.2**).

A better understanding of these underlying benign and malignant pathophysiological processes can be gained through the study of subgross, 3D histological images. This understanding will greatly assist in the interpretation of the images and in determining the most likely etiology of the calcifications.

Introduction

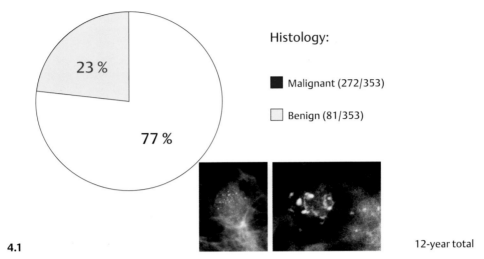

4.1   12-year total

Fig. **4.1**   After thorough preoperative mammographic work-up and the frequent use of percutaneous needle biopsy, one out of four cases of discernible crushed stone–like calcifications sent to surgery was benign in our 12-year, prospective and consecutive patient material (from the Department of Mammography, Falun, Sweden). The indications for surgery also included patient preference.

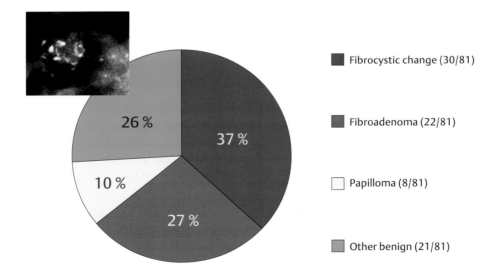

4.2   12-year total

Fig. **4.2**   The most frequent benign, hyperplastic breast changes with associated crushed stone–like calcifications sent to surgery after careful preoperative work-up were **fibrocystic change**, **fibroadenoma** and **papilloma**. One benign, non-hyperplastic process results in **involutional calcifications**, which are discernible and therefore a frequent diagnostic problem.

Fibrocystic Change: Pathophysiology, Imaging, and Differential Diagnosis

Fibrocystic change is a clinically and radiologically detectable form of ANDIs (**A**berrations of **N**ormal **D**evelopment and **I**nvolution[1]), which includes apocrine metaplasia, cysts, ductectasia, and fibrosis. The apocrine metaplastic cells produce a proteinaceous fluid which dilates the TDLUs and the adjoining ducts, most often producing cysts. This excess fluid may result in spontaneous nipple discharge through multiple duct openings in the nipple, often bilaterally. The high protein content and cellular debris give the fluid a cloudy, turbid appearance in varying shades of green, gray, yellow, or milky. Calcified crystals (so-called psammoma bodies) may precipitate in the dilated acini and may occasionally be detectable on the mammogram.

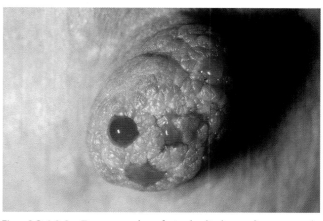

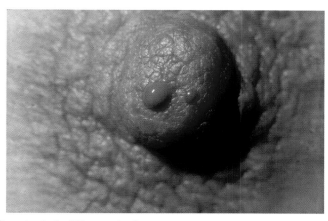

4.3-1　　　　4.3-2

Figs. **4.3**-1 & 2　Two examples of nipple discharge from several orifices, typical of fibrocystic change.

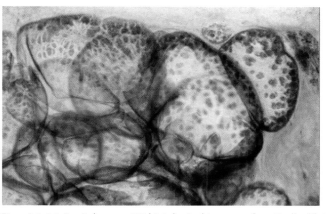

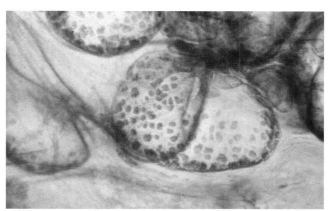

4.4-1　　　　4.4-2

Figs. **4.4**-1 & 2　Subgross, 3D histological images of cystically dilated acini. The apocrine metaplastic cells form micropapillary clusters along the internal surface of the acini.

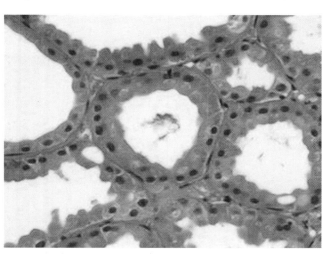

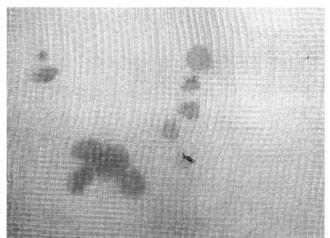

4.5-1　　　　4.5-2

Figs. **4.5**-1 & 2　The long, cylindrical, apocrine metaplastic cells produce fluid in excess. The color of the fluid can be best determined on a white compress pad.

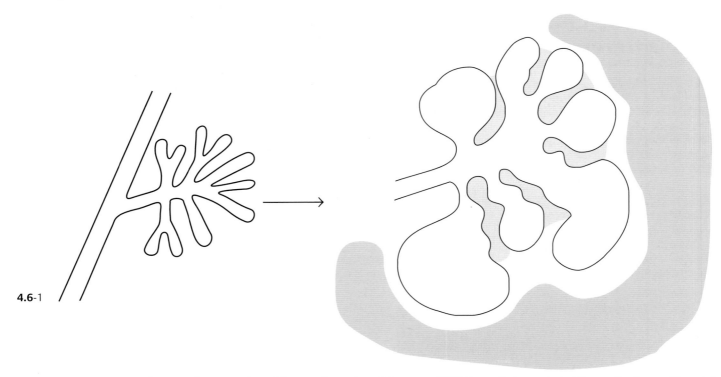

4.6-1

4

Figs. **4.6**-1 & 2   Schematic demonstration of the transformation of the normal TDLU to cystic hyperplasia / fibrocystic change. The acini become cystically dilated and the interlobular connective tissue proliferates as well. The degree of acinar distention can vary considerably within a single TDLU.

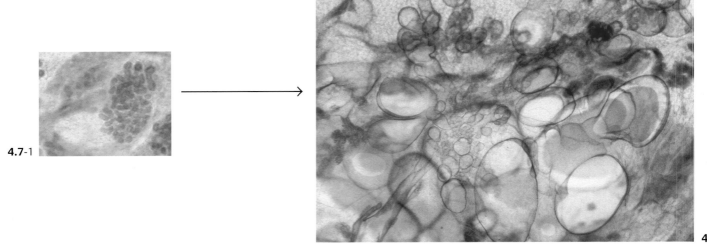

4.7-1

4.7

Figs. **4.7**-1 & 2   Subgross, 3D histological demonstration of a normal TDLU and one with cystic hyperplasia.

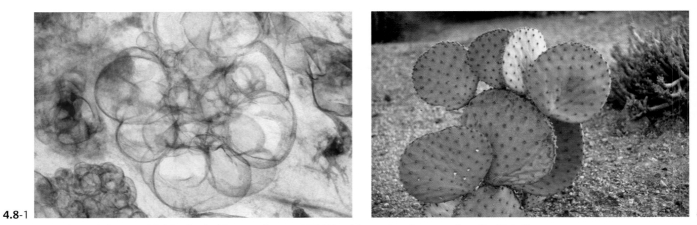

4.8-1

4.8

Figs. **4.8**-1   Subgross, 3D histological image of several TDLUs with varying degrees of cystic dilatation.

3D Image

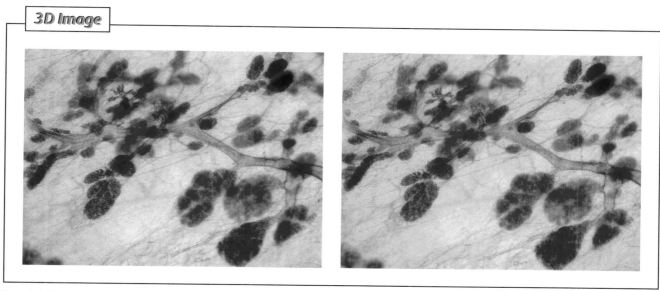

.9-1

4.9-2

Figs. **4.9**-1 & 2   Stereoscopic image pair of normal TDLUs.

3D Image

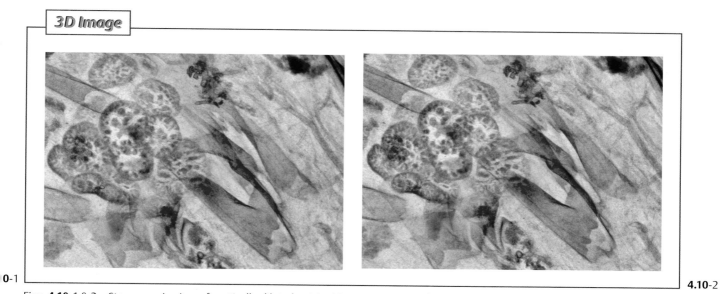

0-1

4.10-2

Figs. **4.10**-1 & 2   Stereoscopic view of cystically dilated acini with apocrine metaplasia and adjoining, distended ducts.

3D Image

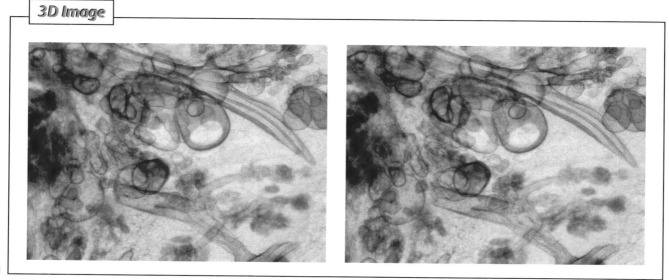

1-1

4.11-2

Figs. **4.11**-1 & 2   Stereoscopic images of ducts and TDLUs with varying degrees of cystic dilatation.

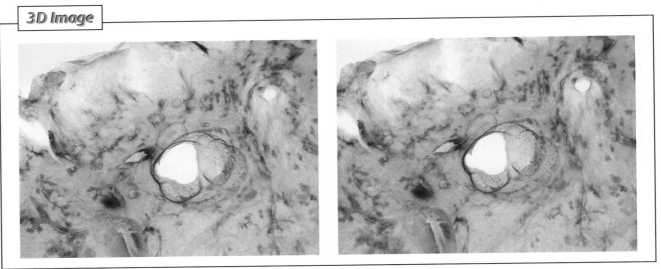

4.12-1   4.12

Figs. **4.12**-1 & 2   Stereoscopic histological images of a solitary, cystically dilated TDLU. The tiny micropapillary growths on the inner wall of the cyst represent apocrine metaplasia. Fibrosis and normal-sized TDLUs and ducts are seen in the surrounding tissue.

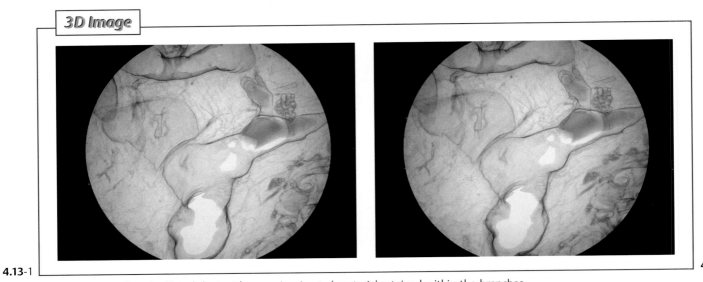

4.13-1   4.1

Figs. **4.13**-1 & 2   Grossly dilated duct with some inspissated material retained within the branches.

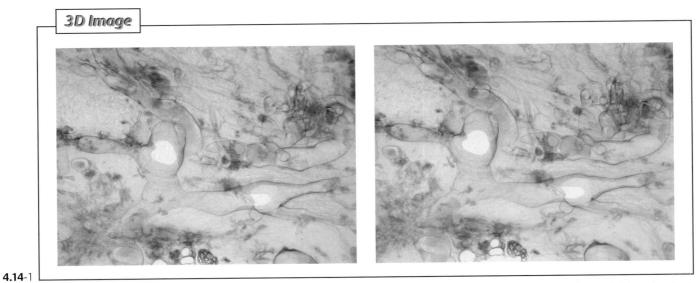

4.14-1   4.1

Figs. **4.14**-1 & 2   The fluid overproduction causes distention of the duct system, making ductectasia an integral part of this pathophysiological process.

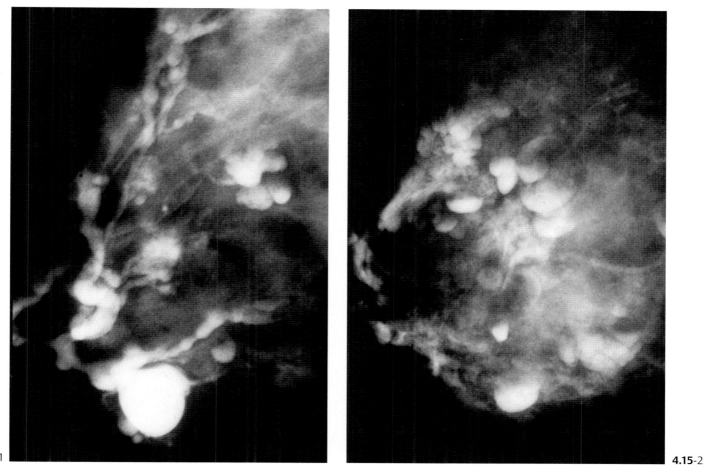

Figs. **4.15**-1 & 2   Galactography of the right breast, MLO (1) and horizontal beam lateromedial (2) projections. There are numerous cystically dilated TDLUs and distended ducts surrounded by fibrosis. These images provide a comprehensive illustration of fibrocystic change. The contrast medium tends to settle in the dependent portion of the cystic cavities. When present, the psammoma body–like calcifications will also settle in a similar manner, producing the characteristic "teacup–like" calcifications.

3D Image

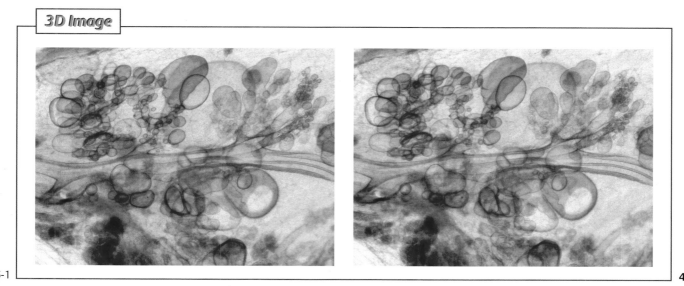

Figs. **4.16**-1 & 2   Stereoscopic, subgross, 3D histological images of several cystically dilated TDLUs having a highly variable degree of acinar dilatation.

Explanatory Illustration of the Pathophysiological Process Leading to the Formation of Teacup–like Calcifications in Fibrocystic Change

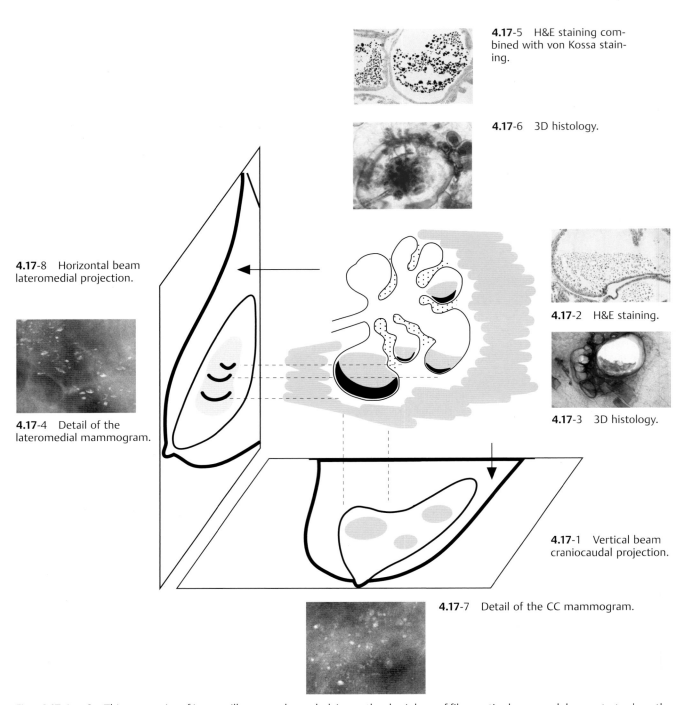

4.17-5   H&E staining combined with von Kossa staining.

4.17-6   3D histology.

4.17-8   Horizontal beam lateromedial projection.

4.17-4   Detail of the lateromedial mammogram.

4.17-2   H&E staining.

4.17-3   3D histology.

4.17-1   Vertical beam craniocaudal projection.

4.17-7   Detail of the CC mammogram.

Figs. **4.17**-1 to 8   This composite of images illustrates the underlying pathophysiology of fibrocystic change and demonstrates how the characteristic mammographic image of the "teacup–like" calcifications is formed in the two orthogonal projections.[2, 3] When viewing calcifications on the mammogram, the most helpful approach is first to imagine their anatomical location in terms of the 3D subgross images and then to attempt to determine the pathological process that has formed them. This stepwise analytical process, which combines the mammogram first with subgross, 3D pathology and then with conventional, 2D pathology, will enable the radiologist to achieve a more specific differential diagnosis.

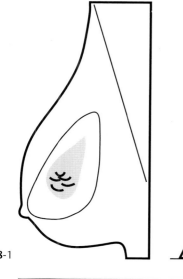

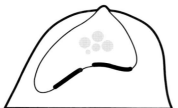

8-1

4.18-2

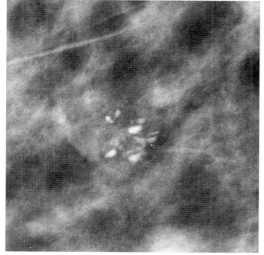

3-3

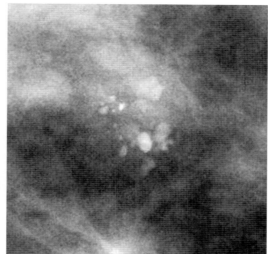

4.18-4

Figs. **4.18**-1 to 5   Sedimentation of the psammoma body–like calcifications in the cystically dilated acini is demonstrated on schematic drawings (1 & 2) and on mammograms taken in orthogonal projections (3 & 4). A similar image is formed on the galactogram when the contrast medium settles to the dependent portion of the cystically dilated acini (5).

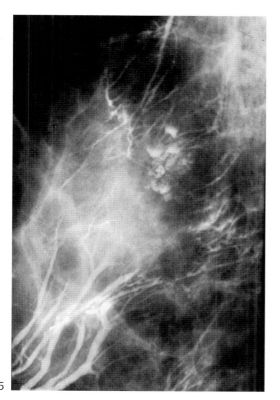

3-5

Comment

When teacup–like calcifications are seen on the mammogram, either as single or multiple clusters or diffusely scattered, the finding indicates fibrocystic change with no mammographic sign of malignancy.

Comparative Mammographic–Histological Demonstration of the Sediment Resulting in Teacup–like Calcifications

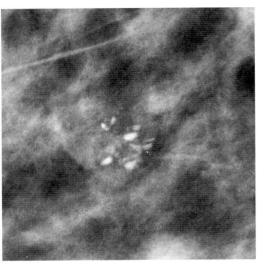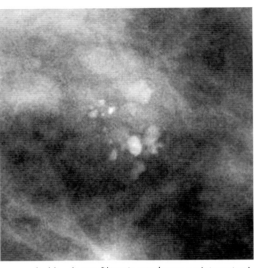

4.19-1   4.19-2

Figs. **4.19**-1 & 2   A cluster of teacup–like calcifications surrounded by dense fibrosis produces a picture typical of fibrocystic change, as demonstrated on the two orthogonal mammographic projections. The histological images below show that each of the individual calcifications on the mammogram is a summation of numerous microscopic psammoma body–like calcifications.

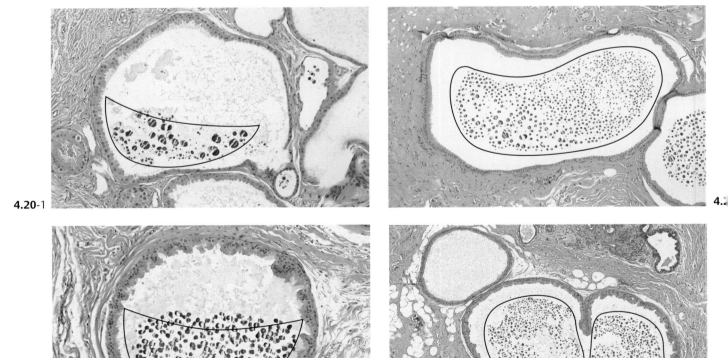

4.20-1   4.2

4.20-3   4.2

Figs. **4.20**-1 to 4   Medium-power histological images show the apocrine metaplastic cell layer lining the cystically dilated acini, which are filled with fluid containing numerous psammoma body–like calcifications. The appearance of the calcifications on the mammogram will depend on the shape of the summation of the calcified particles in the cystically dilated acini. When the shape happens to be teacup–like, the diagnosis of fibrocystic change can be made with confidence. A differential diagnostic problem arises when summation of the calcium particles produces mammographic images resembling crushed stone–like calcifications.

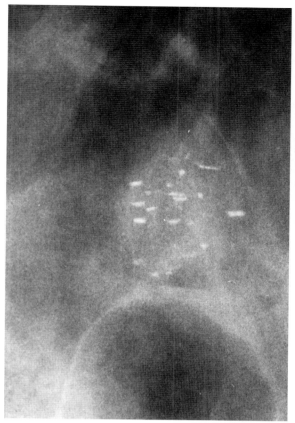

4.21-1

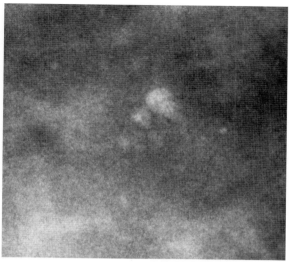

4.21-2

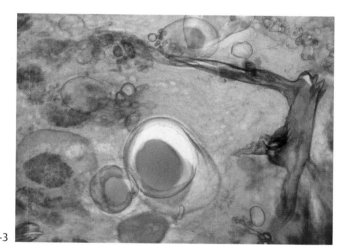

21-3

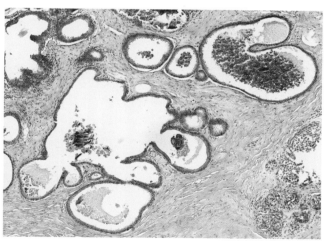

4.21-4

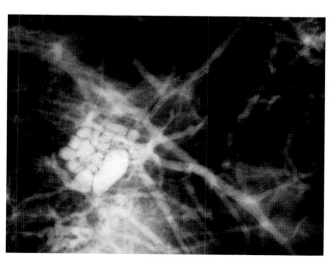

1-5

Figs. **4.21**-1 to 5   Fibrocystic change demonstrated by different methods. Solitary (or multiple) cluster(s) of teacup–like calcifications are the most characteristic features on the mammograms (1 & 2). Galactography is able to show the dilated ducts and acini (5). Subgross, thick-section histological image shows the alterations of ducts and TDLUs caused by the accumulation of excess fluid (3). Conventional histology (4) can show both the structural changes (distention of the TDLUs and ducts) and the cellular details.

Comparative Galactographic–Subgross 3D Histological Demonstration of Fibrocystic Change

The resolving power of mammography and galactography allows visualization of structural changes such as distention and distortion of ducts and TDLUs by pathological processes. Subgross, 3D histology visualizes the same structural changes. This makes it a more useful teaching aid for the imager than is conventional histology, which demonstrates cellular details but is less effective at illustrating the three-dimensional aspects.

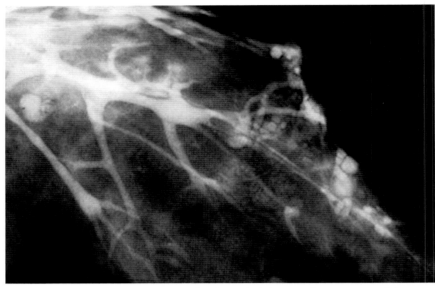

4.2

Figs. **4.22**-1 & 4   A galactogram outlining distended ducts and TDLUs in one lobe.

3D Image

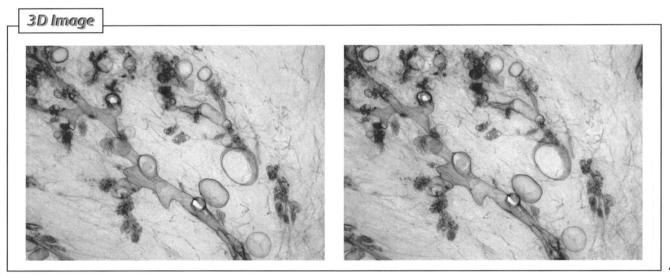

4.22-2

4.2

Figs. **4.22**-2 & 3 Stereoscopic subgross, 3D histological images showing distended ducts and TDLUs.

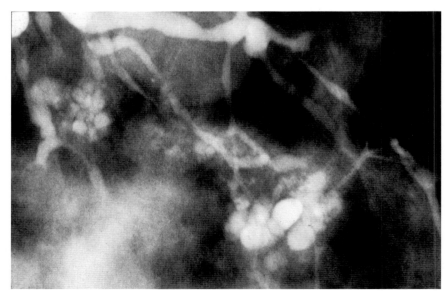

4.2

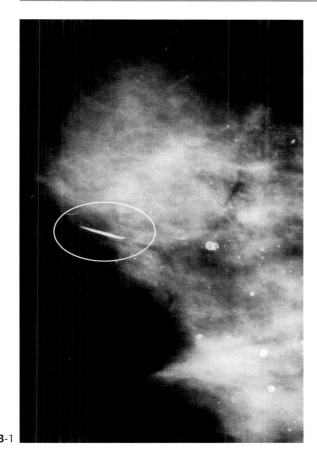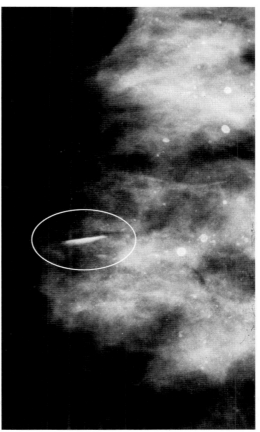

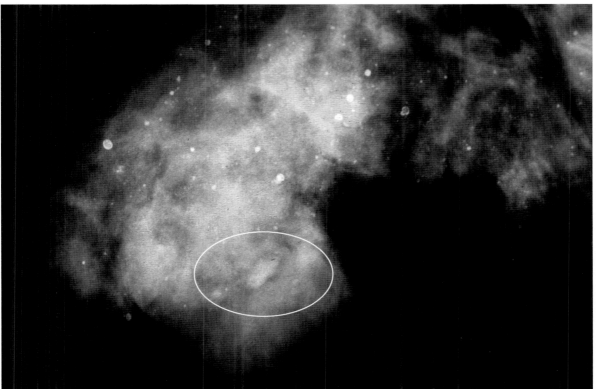

Figs. **4.23**-1 to 3   Right breast MLO (1), horizontal beam lateromedial (2), and CC (3) projections. In addition to numerous, hollow, benign-type calcifications (calcified hematomas) on the mammograms, there is an unusually large "teacup–like" calcification in the dependent portion of a large cyst. Characteristically, it has a high density when viewed from the side and a much lower density on the CC projection, fading into the surrounding fibrosis.

Demonstration of the Natural History of Focal Fibrocystic Change with Calcifications

When the mammographic finding is only a cluster of teacup–like calcifications, the diagnosis of benign fibrocystic change can be made with confidence. The number and density of these benign-type calcifications may increase, decrease, or remain unchanged at serial mammographic examinations. Since malignant-type calcifications may also either increase or decrease in number and density, or even remain unchanged for years, the differential diagnostic value of such changes over time is unreliable. Numerous supporting examples appear in this book (Examples 1.1, p. 10; 2.2, p. 28; 2.7, p. 43; 2.14, p. 77; 2.15, p. 84; 2.16, p. 90); in *Breast Cancer: The Art and Science of Early Detection with*

Mammography. Perception, Interpretation, Histopathological Correlation (Figures 6.51, p. 214; 6.52, p. 215; 6.61, pp. 228–9) and in *Breast Cancer: Early Detection with Mammography. Casting Type Calcifications: Sign of a Subtype with Deceptive Features* (Examples 2.2, p. 80; 2.3, p. 86; 2.4, p. 90; 2.10, p. 118; 2.11, p. 124; 4.4, p. 206; 5.2, p. 238).

> **Conclusion:** Changes in the appearance of calcifications at follow-up mammography do not constitute a reliable diagnostic criterion for the exclusion of malignancy.

The following two examples demonstrate temporal changes in the mammographic appearance of calcifications associated with fibrocystic change.

Example 4.1

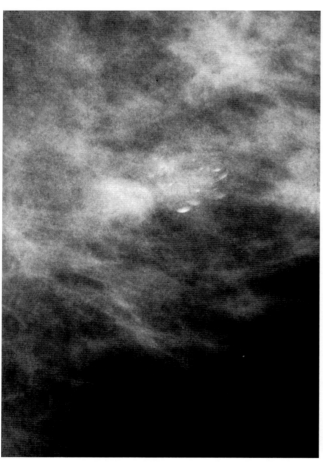 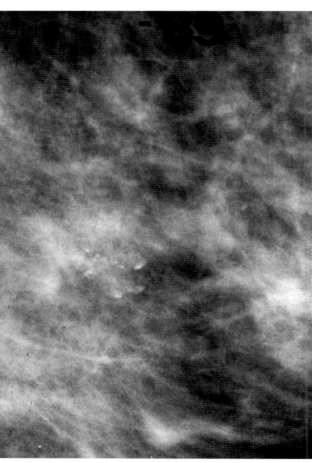

Ex. **4.1**-1

Ex. 4

Ex. **4.1**-1 & 2   Detail of the left MLO projection on two consecutive examinations. This woman had a cluster of teacup–like calcifications on her first screening mammogram at age 41 years (1). The calcifications appear to decrease in density at the next examination 2 years later (2).

Example 4.2

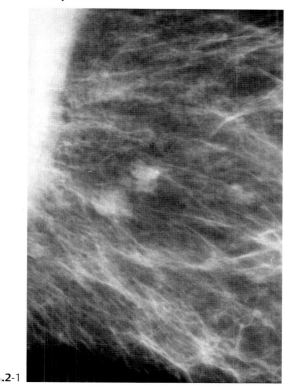

.2-1

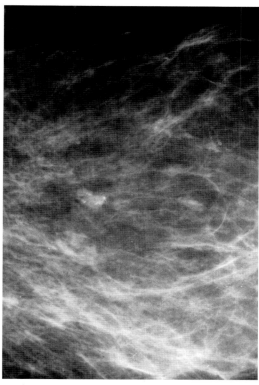

Ex. **4.2**-2

Ex. **4.2**-1   Left MLO projection. Multiple oval-shaped, low-density lesions suggesting cyst(s). One of them contains a solitary calcification.

Ex. **4.2**-2   MLO projection 2 years later. More calcifications have appeared after a 2-year interval.

Ex. **4.2**-4

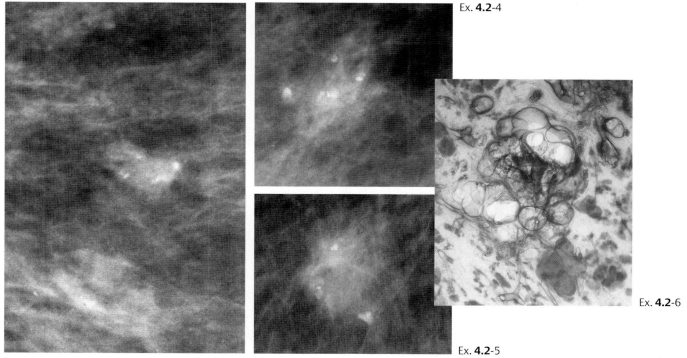

Ex. **4.2**-6

2-3

Ex. **4.2**-5

Ex. **4.2**-3 to 5   Microfocus magnification images demonstrate the individual, de-novo, irregular calcifications within cystically dilated acini. As illustrated on the 3D histological image (Ex. **4.2**-6), the calcifications fill in the unevenly distended acini.

Comment

Fibrocystic change with or without associated calcifications is the most frequently occurring hyperplastic breast change and the most frequent cause of call-backs from screening. When the mammographic signs are unequivocal, it is safe to return these women to regular screening. If doubt exists, large-bore percutaneous needle biopsy is the procedure of choice. Short-term follow-up does not solve the diagnostic problem.

Demonstration of the Bilateral, Extensive Fibrocystic Change with Calcifications

When the mammographic finding consists of bilateral, multiple clusters of teacup–like calcifications that give the impression of being diffusely scattered, the most probable diagnosis is benign fibrocystic change. However, when there are large variations in the size, density, and shape of the calcifications associated with fibrocystic change, percutaneous or surgical biopsy is indicated.

Example 4.3

A 54-year-old woman, screening examination.

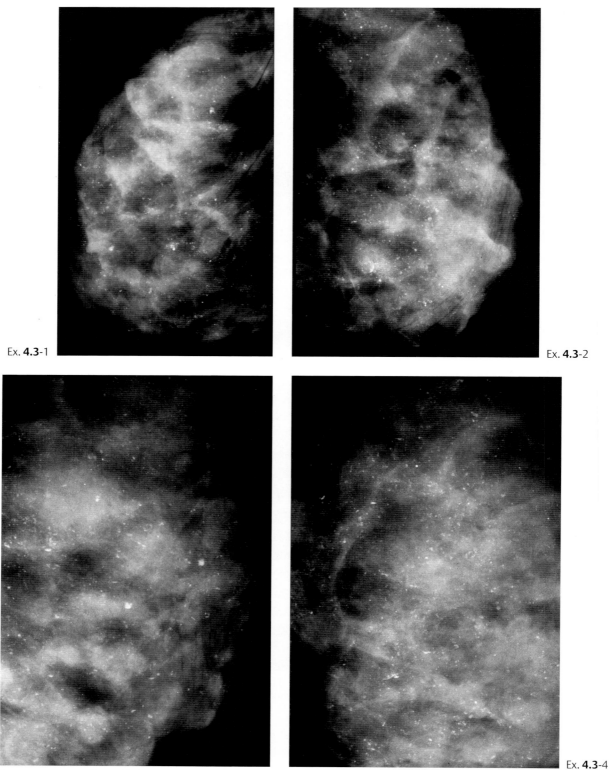

Ex. **4.3**-1

Ex. **4.3**-2

Ex. **4.3**-3

Ex. **4.3**-4

Ex. **4.3**-1 to 4   Right and left MLO (1 & 2) and lateromedial horizontal projections (3 & 4). Innumerable teacup–like calcifications are seen against a background of fibrosis.

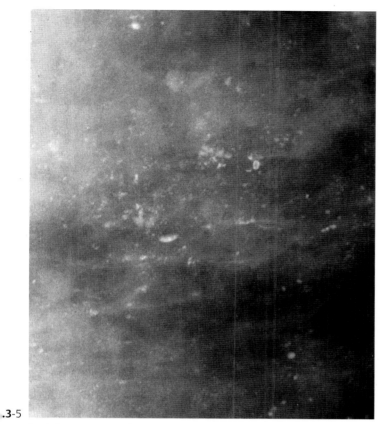

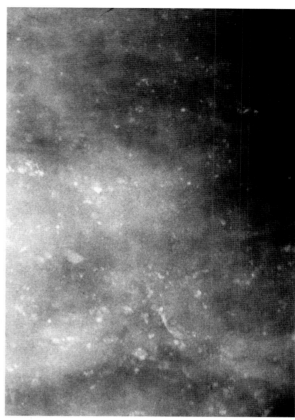

.3-5

Ex. **4.3**-6

Ex. **4.3**-5 & 6 Microfocus magnification images of the right and left breasts of the same patient, lateromedial horizontal projections. In addition to the teacup–like calcifications, circular masses of varying size are seen, suggesting cysts. There are also clusters where the individual calcifications vary in size and shape; this prompted further examination.

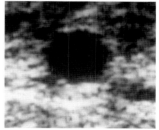

Ex. **4.3**-7

Ex. **4.3**-7 Breast ultrasound: one of the many simple cysts.

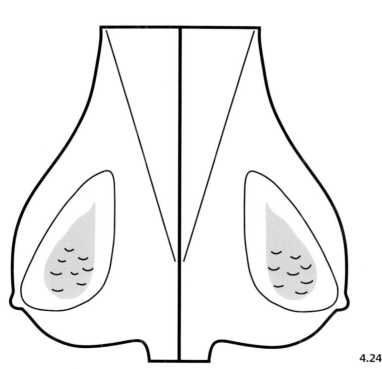

4.24

Fig. **4.24** Schematic drawing of bilateral fibrocystic change with scattered teacup–like calcifications.

Example 4.3 continued

Fig. **4.25** Schematic drawing of bilateral fibrocystic change with teacup–like calcifications on the CC projection.

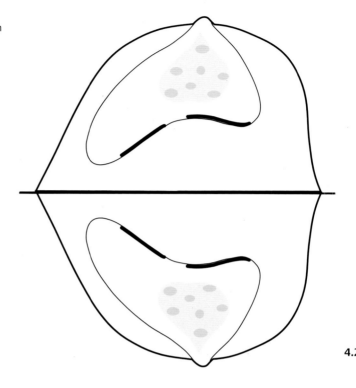

4.2

Ex.

Ex. **4.3**-8 Detail image of the right CC microfocus magnification mammogram showing the numerous teacup–like calcifications against the dense fibrous background.

Demonstration of the Bilateral, Extensive Fibrocystic Change with Calcifications

Ex. **4.3**-9 to 11   Three microfocus magnification images of the right and left CC projections. The shape of the sedimented calcifications in the dependent portion of the tiny cystic cavities resembles teacups or saucers seen from above.

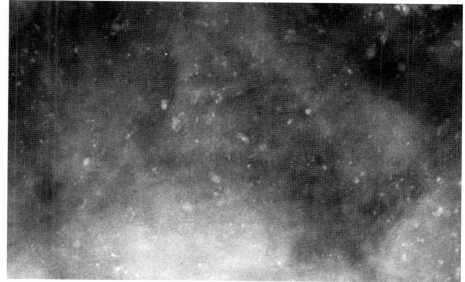

Ex. **4.3**-9

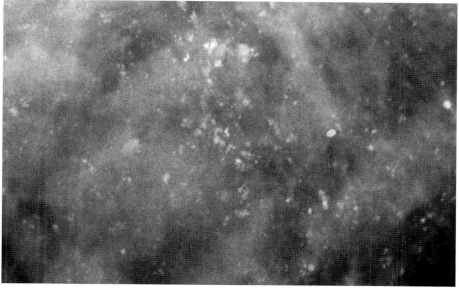

Ex. **4.3**-10

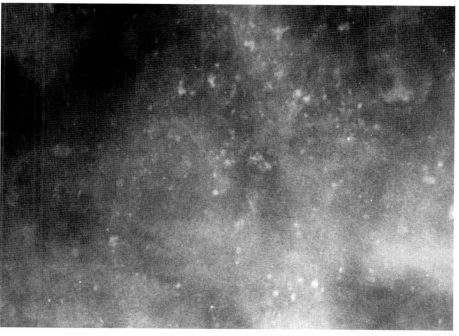

Ex. **4.3**-11

Example 4.3 continued

Ex. **4.3**-12   Specimen radiograph from the left breast shows a large number of calcifications.

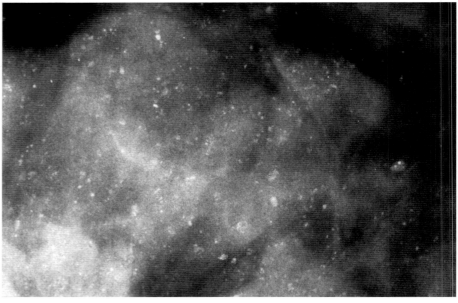

Ex. **4.3**

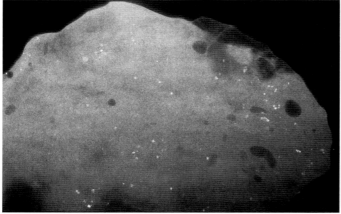

Ex. **4.3**-13

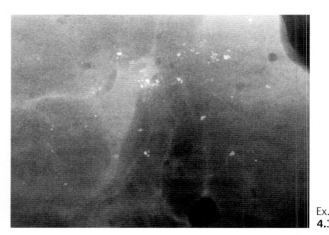

Ex. **4.3**

Ex. **4.3**-13 & 14   Sliced specimen radiographs.

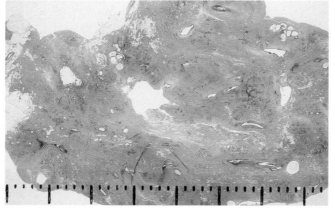

Ex. **4.3**-15

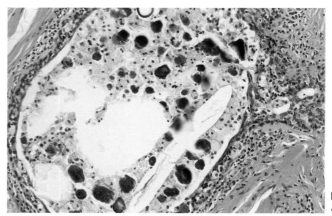

Ex. **4.3**

Ex. **4.3**-15 & 16   Large-section (15) and medium-power histological images (16) demonstrating fibrocystic change with psammoma body–like calcifications.

Demonstration of the Bilateral, Extensive Fibrocystic Change with Calcifications

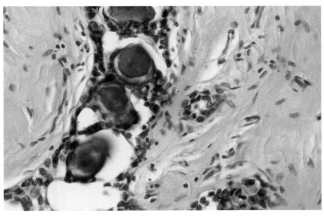

Ex. **4.3**-17

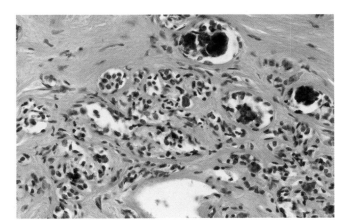

Ex. **4.3**-18

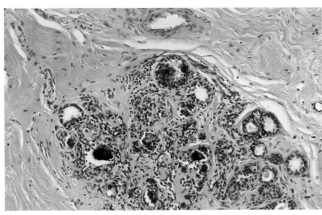

Ex. **4.3**-19

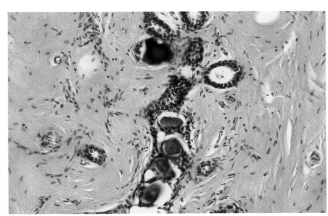

Ex. **4.3**-20

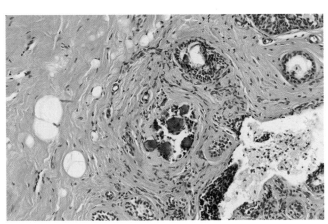

Ex. **4.3**-21

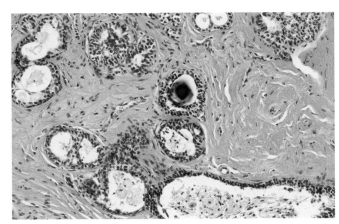

Ex. **4.3**-22

Ex. **4.3**-17 to 22   A series of low- and medium-power histological images showing involutional changes associated with psammoma body–like calcifications. No histological signs of malignancy were found. Ex. **4.3**-15 & 16 are tissue samples from the **right** breast; Ex. **4.3**-17 to 22 are tissue samples from the **left** breast.

Demonstration of the Three Types of Calcifications Occurring in Fibrocystic Change

Example 4.4

A 44-year-old woman presented with greenish discharge from the left nipple. Following the mammographic work-up, galactography was performed to elucidate the cause of the discharge.

Ex. **4.4**-1 & 2   Left breast, MLO projection and microfocus magnification. The calcifications outlined by the rectangle have the typical appearance of milk of calcium sediment within small cysts.

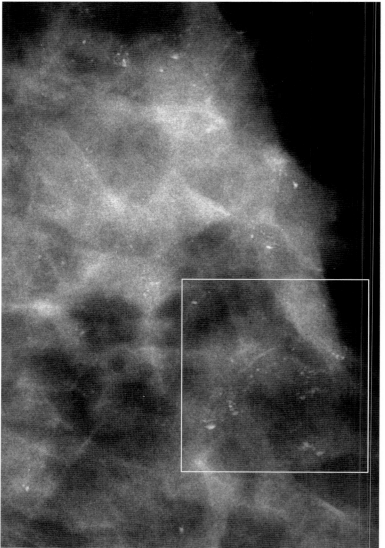

Ex.

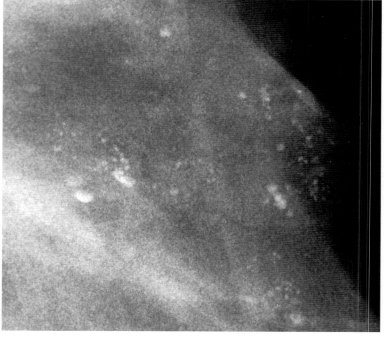

Ex.

Ex. **4.4**-3 Detail image of the galactogram. The contrast medium settles in the dependent portions of some of the cysts, filling others entirely, mimicking the calcifications seen on the mammogram.

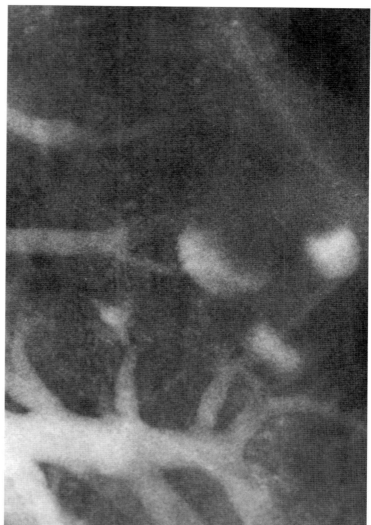

Ex. **4.4**-3

3D Image

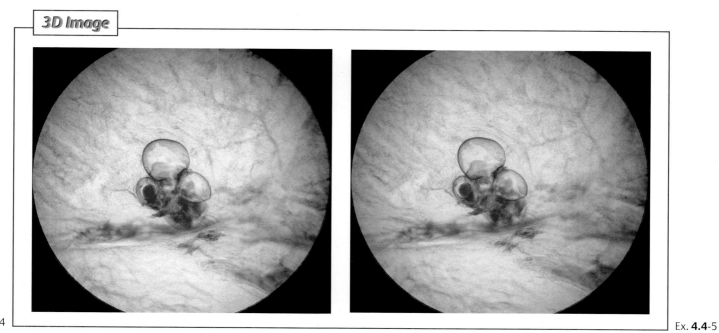

4-4

Ex. **4.4**-5

Ex. **4.4**-4 & 5 Subgross, thick-section (3D) histology. The single, cystically dilated TDLU containing milk of calcium sediment illustrates the underlying cause of the galactographic and mammographic findings.

Example 4.4 continued

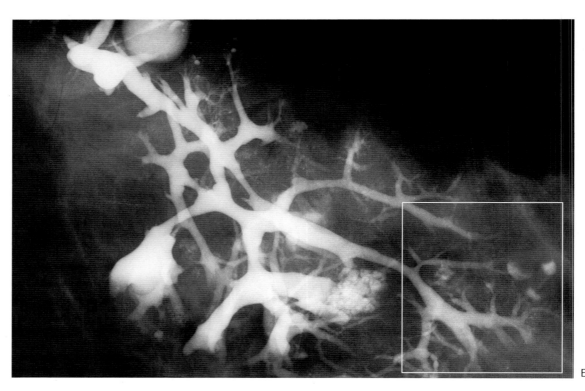

Ex.

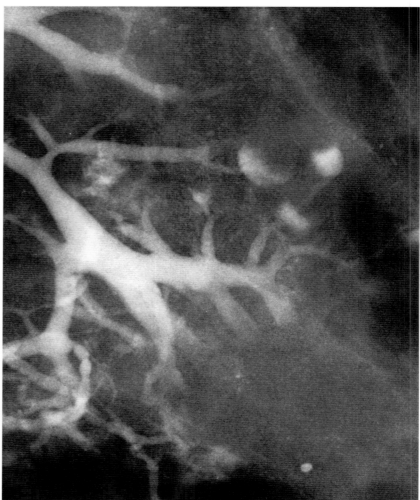

Ex. **4.4**-6 & 7   The galactogram outlines the entire lobe with its dilated ducts. Some of the TDLUs are also cystically dilated.

Ex.

Demonstration of the Three Types of Calcifications Occurring in Fibrocystic Change

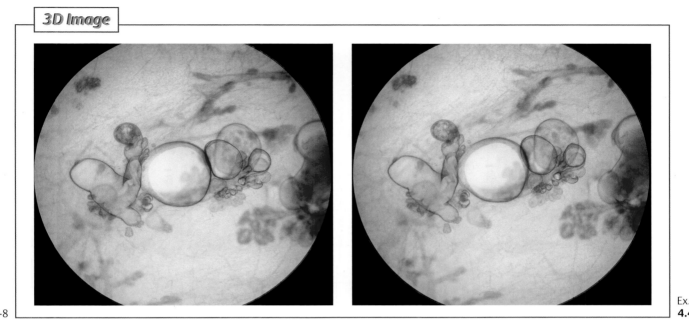

Ex. **4.4**-8

Ex. **4.4**-9

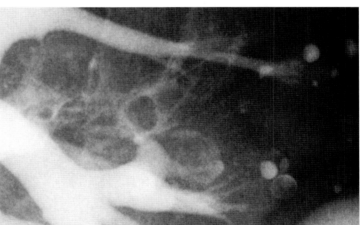

Ex. **4.4**-10

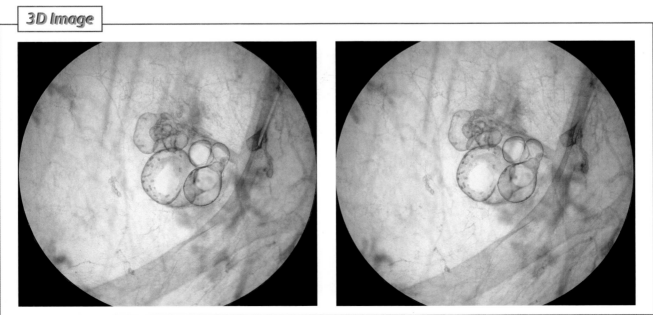

Ex. **4.4**-11

Ex. **4.4**-12

Ex. **4.4**-8 to 12   Galactographic–subgross histological illustration of tiny cystically dilated acini.

Example 4.4 continued

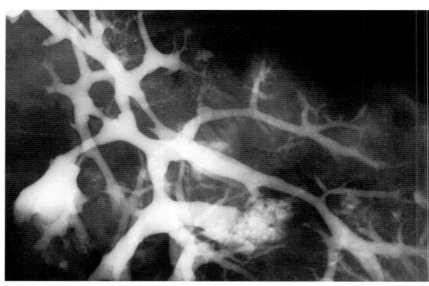

Ex.
4.4

3D Image

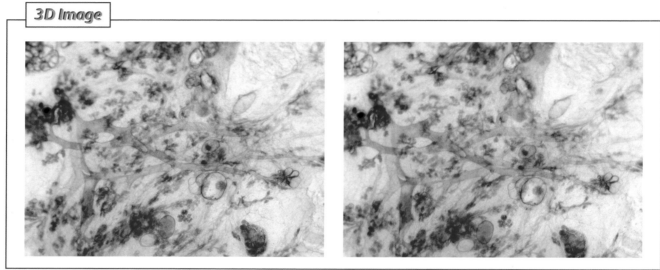

Ex.
4.4-14

Ex.
4.4

3D Image

Ex.
4.4-16

Ex.
4.4

Ex. **4.4**-13 to 17   Galactographic/3D histological correlation of fibrocystic change with ductectasia, multiple cystically dilated TDLUs and associated fibrosis.

**Demonstration of the Three Types of
Calcifications Occurring in Fibrocystic Change**

Ex. **4.4**-18   The contrast medium outlines
the dilated subsegmental and terminal ducts
and fills a cystically dilated TDLU on this galactogram.

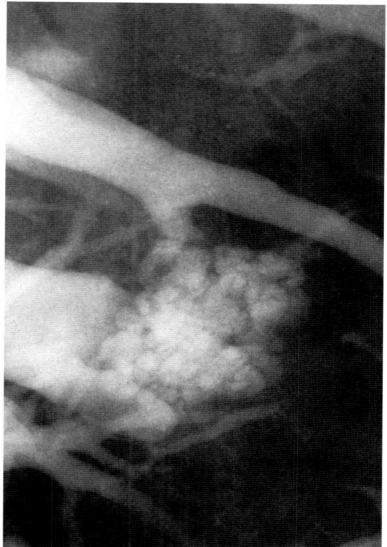

Ex.
4.4-18

3D Image

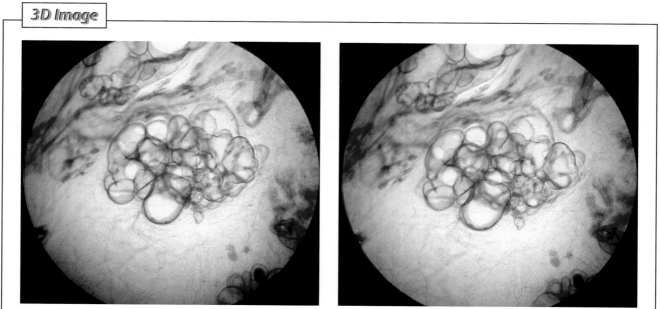

-19

Ex.
4.4-20

Ex. **4.4**-19 & 20   A cystically dilated TDLU is illustrated on this stereoscopic, subgross, thick-section histology slide.

Example 4.4 continued

Three types of calcifications may be associated with fibrocystic change: **psammoma body–like calcifications, amorphous calcifications,** and **calcium oxalate (weddellite) crystals**.

The most frequently occurring is the **psammoma body–like calcification**. Their summation appears on the mammogram as sediments, teacup–like or rounded/oval calcifications, causing minimal differential diagnostic problems (Ex. **4.4**-21 to 24).

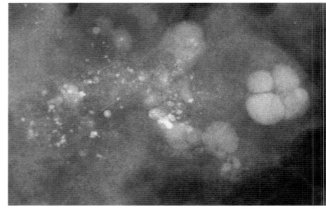

Ex.
4.

3D Image

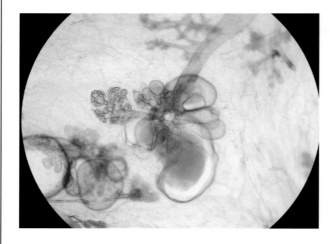

Ex.
4.4-22

Ex.
4.

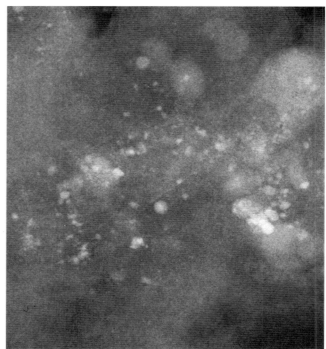

Ex. **4.4**-21 to 24   Specimen radiographs and correlative subgross, thick-section (3D) histology show several cystically dilated TDLUs. Some of these are filled with contrast medium, while others are made visible by the presence of milk of calcium.

Ex.
4.4

Demonstration of the Three Types of Calcifications Occurring in Fibrocystic Change

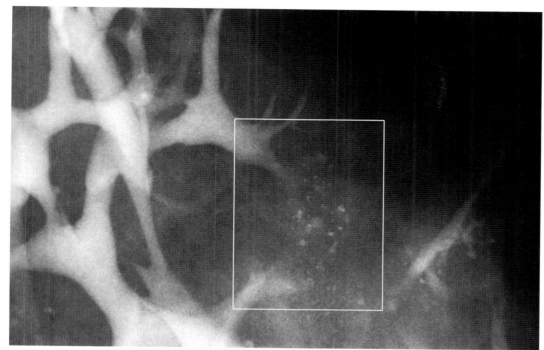

Ex. **4.4**-25

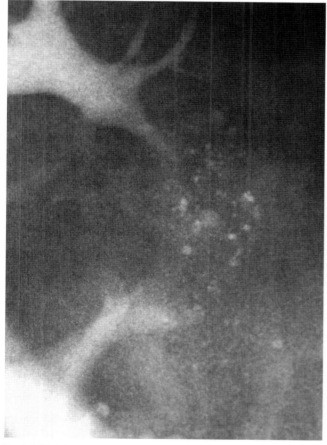

-26

Ex. **4.4**-25 & 26   Some of the cystically dilated TDLUs containing milk of calcium are not filled by contrast medium.

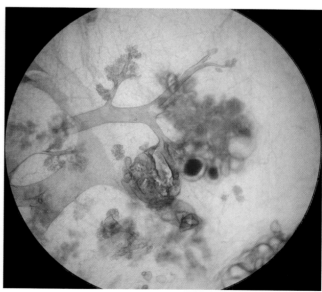

Ex. **4.4**-27

Ex. **4.4**-27   Subgross, 3D histological image of the distended TDLU, corresponding to the TDLU shown in Ex. **4.4**-8 & 9. Some of the acini are fluid-filled; others contain cell proliferation, preventing the contrast medium from filling the TDLU.

Example 4.4 continued

Whenever **amorphous calcifications** (see p. 17) are formed in the breast tissue, their mammographic image may resemble the crushed stone–like calcifications associated with malignant processes. In these cases biopsy becomes necessary for the correct diagnosis (Ex. **4.4**-28 to 34).

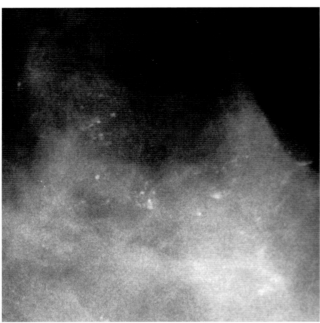

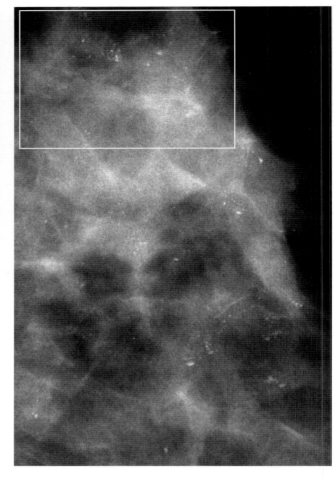

Ex.
4.4-28

Ex. **4.4**-28 & 29   In addition to the diagnostically characteristic teacup–like calcifications discussed above, there are several clusters of calcifications in the axillary tail of the left breast which resemble crushed stone–like calcifications, posing a differential diagnostic problem.

Ex.
4.4

Ex. **4.4**-30   Specimen radiograph. The suspicious clusters of calcifications have been surgically removed. Microfocus magnification images of the clusters within the rectangles are correlated with histological images in Ex. **4.4**-32 & 33.

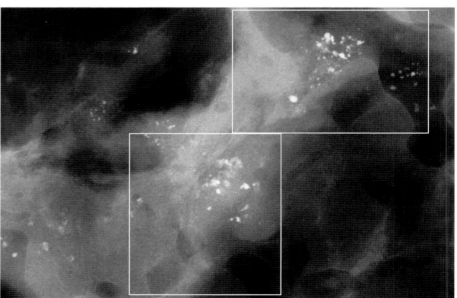

Ex.
4.4

Demonstration of the Three Types of Calcifications Occurring in Fibrocystic Change

Ex. **4.4**-31 to 34   Magnified views of the areas outlined by rectangles in Ex. **4.4**-30. Surprisingly, amorphous calcifications were found within the cyst fluid at histology (32, 33) (ovals), which explains the presence of crushed stone–like calcifications on the mammograms.

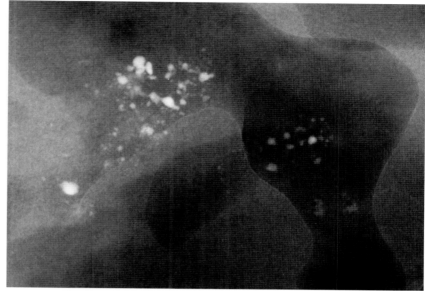

Ex. **4.4**-31

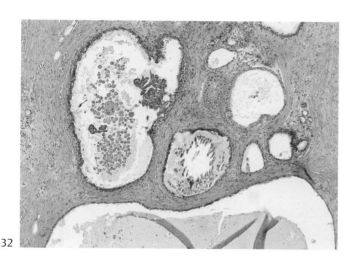

4-32

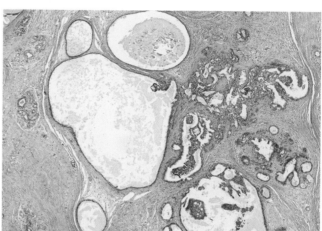

Ex. **4.4**-33

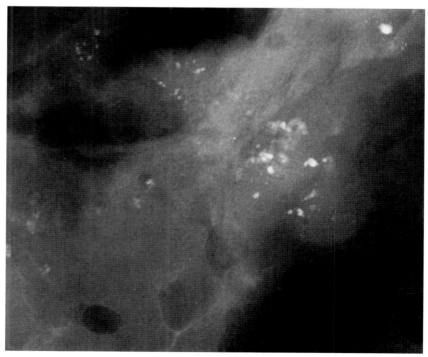

Ex. **4.4**-34

Example 4.4 continued

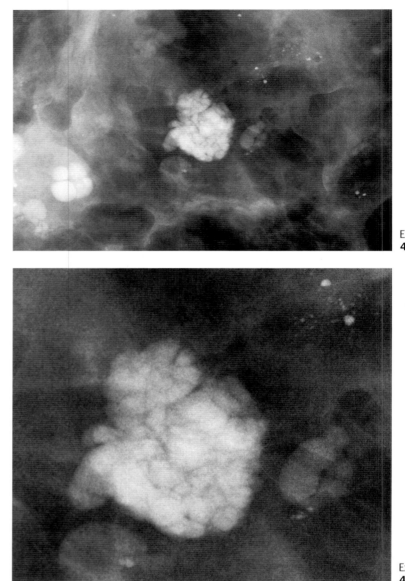

Ex.
4.4

Ex.
4.4

3D Image

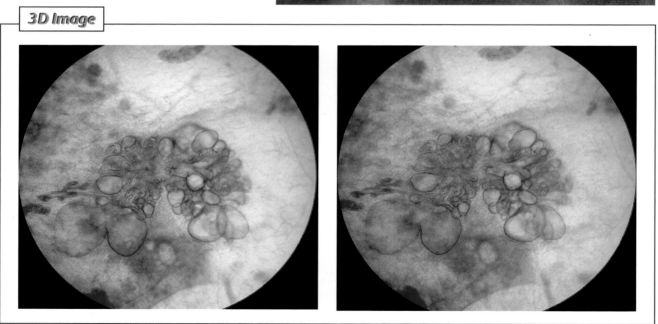

Ex.
4.4-37

Ex.
4.4

Ex. **4.4**-35 to 38   Specimen radiographs show several cystically dilated TDLUs, some of which are filled with contrast media. The sub-gross, thick-section (3D) histology illustrates the unevenly distended acini within a TDLU.

Demonstration of the Three Types of Calcifications Occurring in Fibrocystic Change

The third type of calcification associated with benign fibrocystic change, which may be confused with the crushed stone–like calcifications, are those caused by **calcium oxalate crystals.** These may cause differential diagnostic problems.

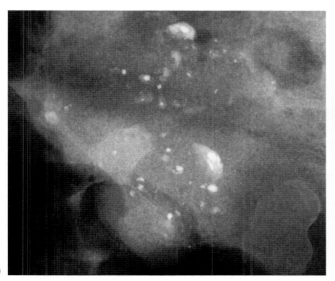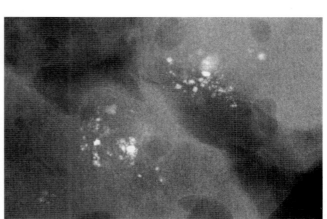

Ex. **4.4**-39 & 40   Details of specimen radiographs. There is a mixture of circular-oval and irregular, discernible calcifications, not characteristic of the crushed stone–like calcifications.

3D Image

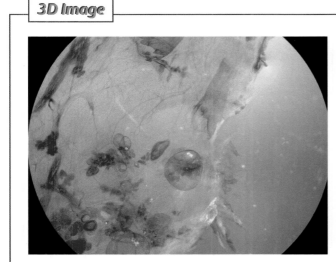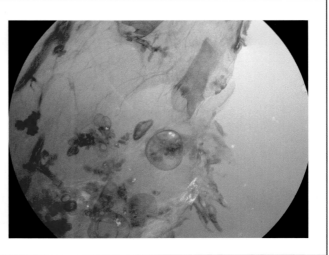

Ex. **4.4**-41 & 42   Subgross, thick-section (3D) histological image pair demonstrating spherical/oval cystic cavities within which the calcifications are formed.

Example 4.4 continued

Ex. **4.4**-43   Specimen slice radiograph containing octahedron-shaped calcium oxalate crystals, termed weddellite (ovals). Some of these crystals have an irregular form and are difficult to distinguish from crushed stone–like calcifications.[4, 5]

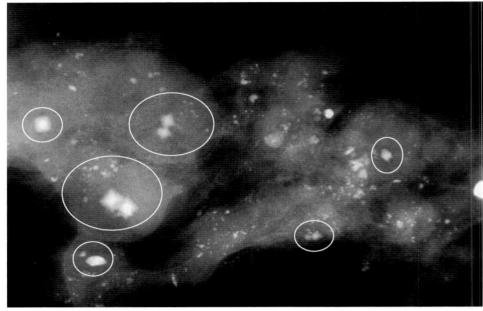

Ex. **4.4**

3D Image

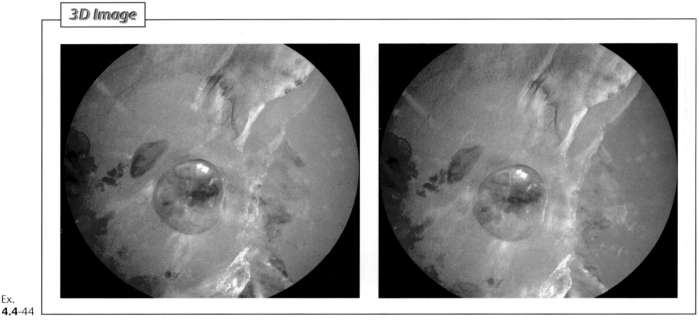

Ex. **4.4**-44

Ex. **4.4**

Ex. **4.4**-44 & 45   Subgross, thick-section (3D) histology of a cyst containing two adjacent calcium oxalate (weddellite) crystals illuminated with reflected light.

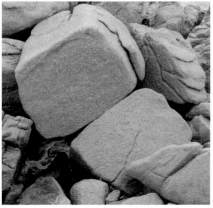

Ex. **4.4**

Demonstration of the Three Types of Calcifications Occurring in Fibrocystic Change

3D Image

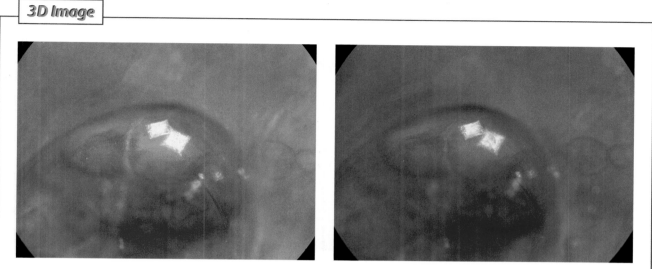

Ex. 4.4-46

Ex. **4.4**-47

Ex. **4.4**-46 to 48   Subgross histological–mammographic correlation of calcium oxalate (weddellite) crystals at higher magnification.

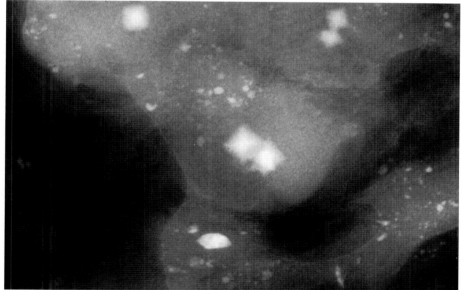

Ex. **4.4**-48

The name "**weddellite**" originates from calcium oxalate crystals discovered in sediment samples from the Weddell Sea in Antarctica.[4] The sea was named after the British explorer and seal hunter James Weddell (1787–1834), who explored the southern seas on the brigantine *Jane* (Christophe Frouge, M.D., personal communication). Weddellite crystals in breast tissue were first described in a biopsy specimen[5] and subsequently on mammograms[6]. The crystals are birefringent and easily detectable with polarized light at microscopy, but are otherwise often overlooked. This explains the discrepancy that occurs when the calcifications are ob-

vious on the specimen radiograph but are either not seen or not appreciated at microscopic examination. These crystals are more easily perceived with digital mammography, since the pixellated structure of the images emphasizes their sharp corners. Although the basic crystalline structure is an octahedron, they are often elongated and irregular in shape, causing differential diagnostic problems. Reliable diagnosis can be best achieved with thorough histological–mammographic correlation employing specimen radiography and adequate communication.

Another Case Demonstrating Weddellite Crystals

Example 4.5

A 45-year-old asymptomatic woman, screening examination. The clinical breast examination was normal.

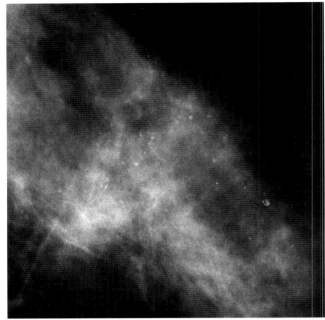

Ex. **4.5**-1 & 2   Left breast, detail of the CC projection (1) and microfocus magnification (2). There are clusters of calcifications against the background of extensive fibrosis. No tumor mass is demonstrable.

Ex.

Ex.

Ex. **4.5**-3   Breast ultrasound: the fluid-filled, dilated ducts and cystically dilated TDLUs contain the calcifications.

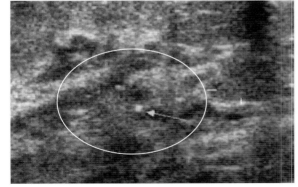

Ex.

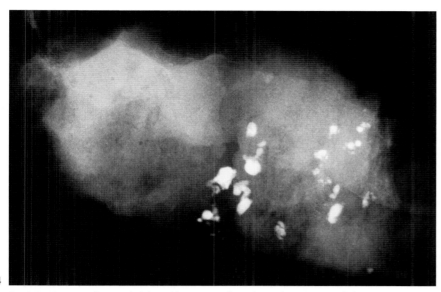

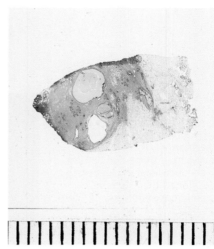

Ex. **4.5**-4 & 5   Radiograph (4) and low power histological image (5) of the preoperative 15-mm diameter (RF-assisted) biopsy specimen. Some of the large calcifications are squared, others are bullet–like.

Ex. **4.5**-5

Ex. **4.5**-6 & 7   Histological examination using polarized light demonstrates calcium oxalate crystals (weddellite) in small, fluid-filled cysts. The individual calcium particles have irregular shape on the mammogram and their density varies, making the mammographic differential diagnosis very difficult, if not impossible. No signs of atypia or malignancy were found at histology.

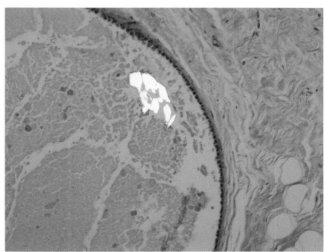

Ex. **4.5**-6

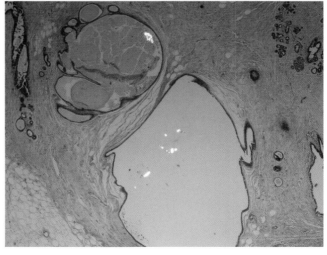

Ex. **4.5**-7

Another Case Demonstrating Different Types of Calcifications Occurring in Fibrocystic Change

Example 4.6

A 49-year-old asymptomatic woman, screening examination. Clinical breast examination was normal. She was called back to the assessment center for further work-up of the calcifications detected in her right breast.

Ex. **4.6**-1   Right breast, detail of the CC projection. The dense fibrous tissue contains several clusters of discernible calcifications. It is difficult to analyze the shape and density of the individual calcium particles due to the extensive, superimposed fibrosis.

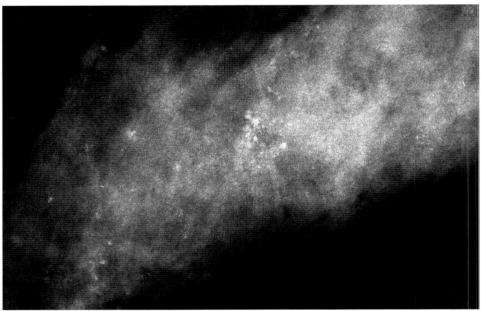

Ex.

Ex. **4.6**-2   Right breast, detail of the microfocus magnification, MLO projection. The microcalcifications in the different clusters vary greatly in shape and density.

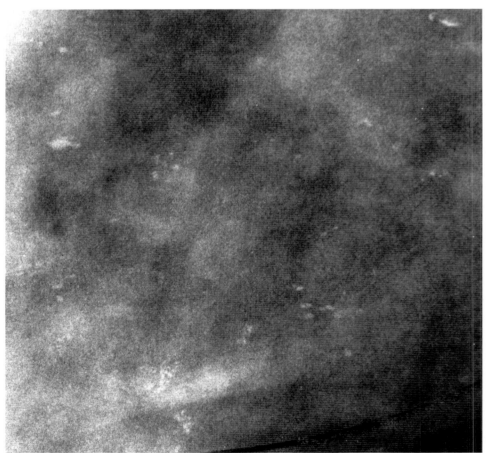

Ex.

Ex. **4.6**-3 & 4   Microfocus magnification radiographs of two specimen slices showing the different clusters of calcifications. No tumor mass is demonstrable.

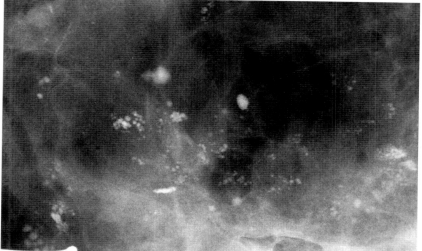

Ex. **4.6**-3

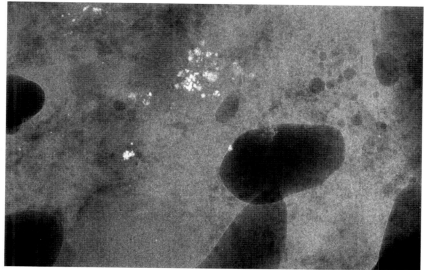

Ex. **4.6**-4

Ex. **4.6**-5   One of the large-section histological slices. A group of calcifications has been encircled by the pathologist.

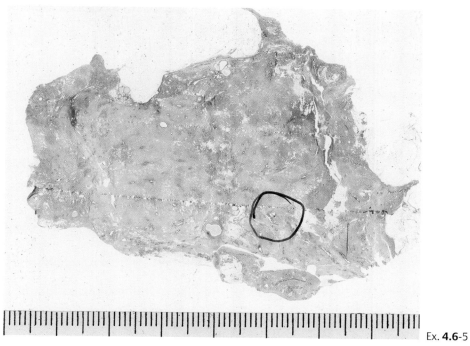

Ex. **4.6**-5

Example 4.6 continued

Ex. **4.6**-6 & 7   Radiographs of two additional specimen slices. The round calcifications (within rectangles) correspond to psammoma body–like calcifications at histology (Ex. **4.6**-8), while the calcifications within the ovals are weddellites (Ex. **4.6**-10 & 11).

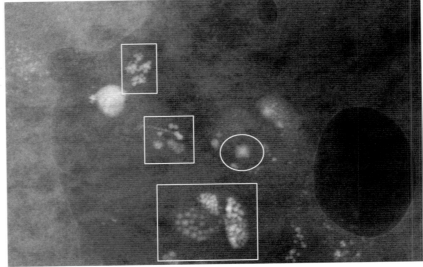

Ex. **4**

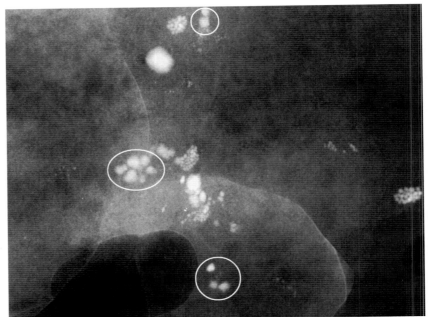

Ex.

Ex. **4.6**-8   Medium-power histological image of two cystically dilated acini lined by apocrine metaplastic cells. There are numerous psammoma body–like calcifications within the cyst fluid.

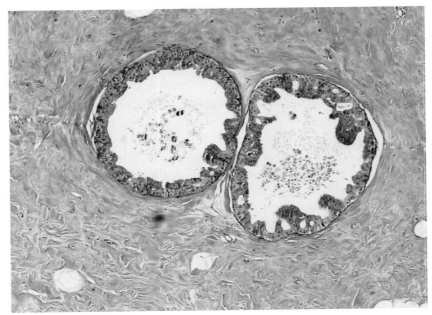

Ex.

Ex. **4.6**-9 Radiograph of a specimen slice containing both clusters of psammoma body–like calcifications (rectangles) and calcium oxalate crystals, weddellites (oval).

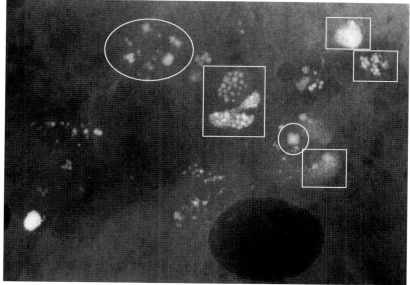

Ex. **4.6**-9

Ex. **4.6**-10 & 11 Conventional histological image (H&E) (10) and a histological image using polarized light (11) demonstrate the calcium oxalate crystals within the cystic cavities.

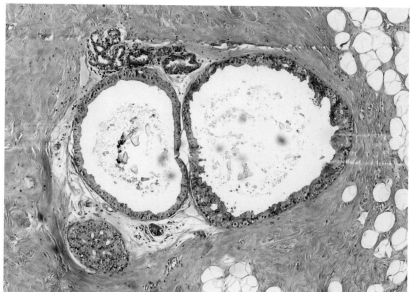

Ex. **4.6**-10

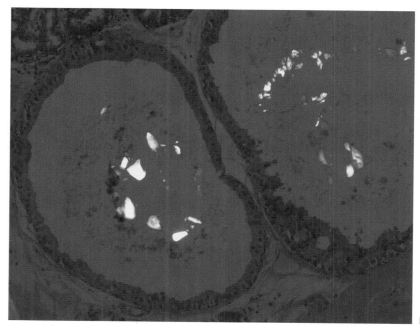

Ex. **4.6**-11

Example 4.6 continued

Ex. **4.6**-12   Radiograph of one of the specimen slices with clusters of calcifications against a fibrous background.

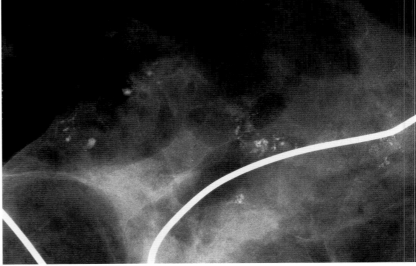

Ex.
4.6

Ex. **4.6**-13 & 14   Low- and medium-power histological images (H&E). The histological examination revealed atypical ductal hyperplasia (ADH) and lobular carcinoma in situ (2 mm × 3 mm LCIS) unrelated to the mammographically demonstrable calcifications.

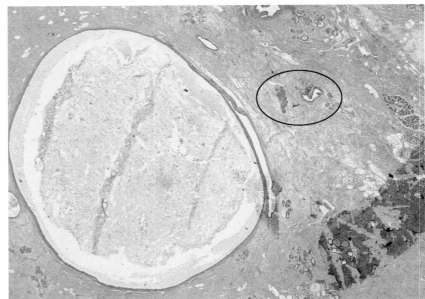

Ex.
4.

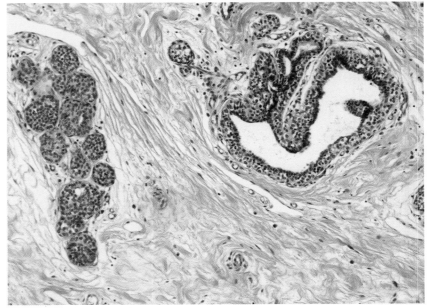

Ex.
4.

Mammographic and ultrasound examination of the **left breast** 4 years after surgery of the **right breast.**

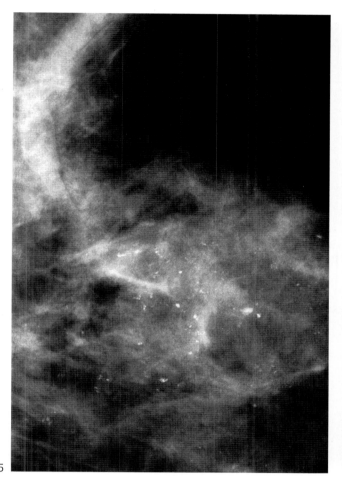

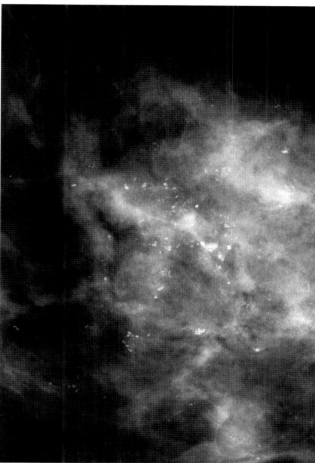

Ex. **4.6**-15

Ex. **4.6**-16

Ex. **4.6**-15 & 16   Detail of the left MLO projection (15), showing a large number of calcifications with no associated tumor mass. Microfocus magnification (16): the individual calcifications show great variation in form, density, and size. No tumor mass is demonstrable on the mammograms.

Ex. **4.6**-17   Microfocus magnification of the lateral portion of the left CC projection. There are a large number of calcifications with no associated tumor mass. The individual calcifications show great variation in form, size, and density, but they appear to be diffusely scattered rather than clustered.

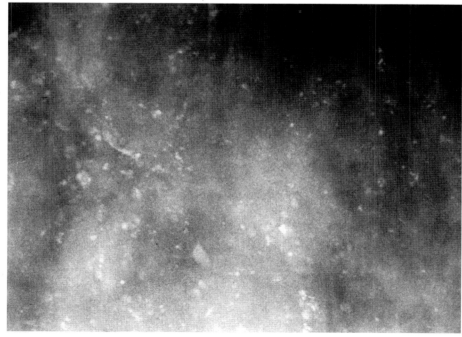

Ex. **4.6**-17

Example 4.6 continued

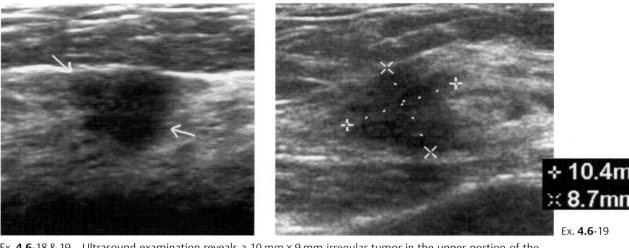

Ex. **4.6**-18

Ex. **4.6**-19

Ex. **4.6**-18 & 19   Ultrasound examination reveals a 10 mm × 9 mm irregular tumor in the upper portion of the **left breast.** The lesion has the ultrasound features of a malignant tumor.

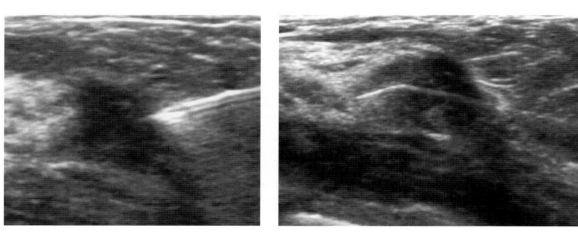

Ex. **4.6**-20

Ex. **4.6**-21

Ex. **4.6**-20 & 21   Preoperative 14-g needle biopsy.

Ex. **4.6**-22   Histology of the 14-g needle biopsy specimen: invasive cribriform carcinoma.

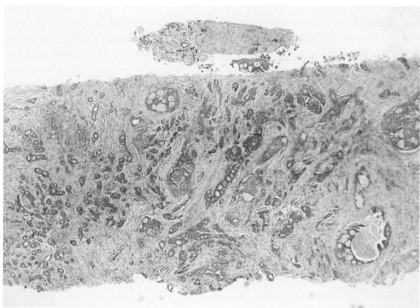

Ex. **4.6**-22

Ex. **4.6**-23 Radiograph of the operative specimen. The architectural distortion corresponds to the ultrasound finding and invasive carcinoma.

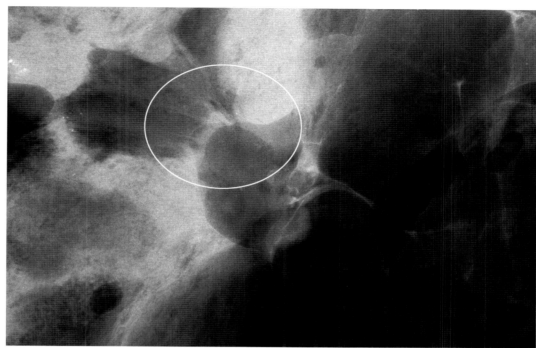

Ex. **4.6**-23

Ex. **4.6**-24 Large-section histology. The invasive carcinoma is encircled. Additional in situ carcinoma foci have been marked by the pathologist.

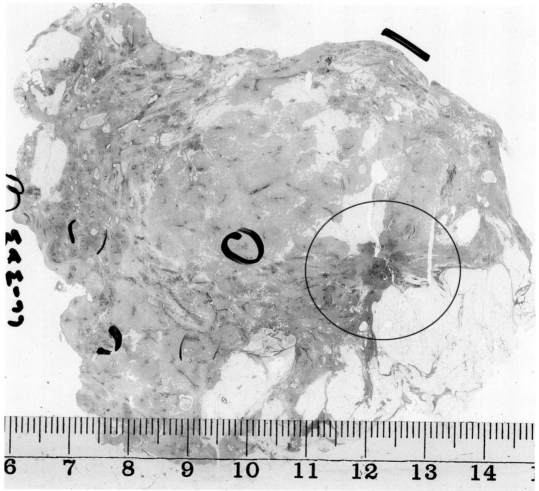

Ex. **4.6**-24

Example 4.6 continued

Ex. **4.6**-25 to 27　Low- and medium-power magnification of the 10 mm × 9 mm invasive cribriform carcinoma (25 & 26). There are in situ cribriform carcinoma foci within the invasive tumor (27).

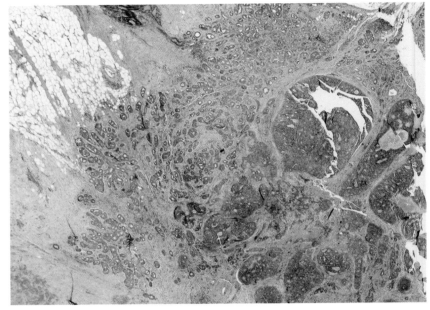

Ex. **4.6**-

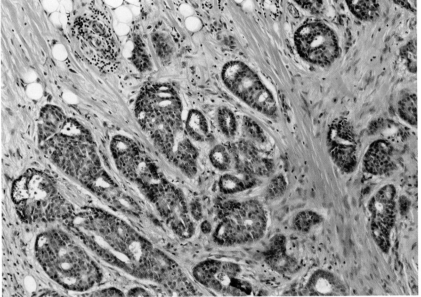

Ex. **4.6**-

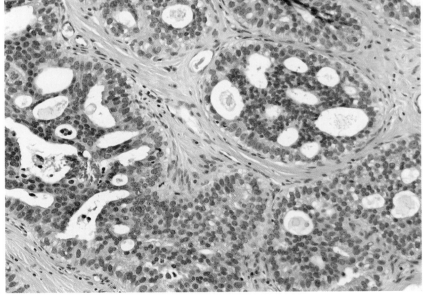

Ex. **4.6**-

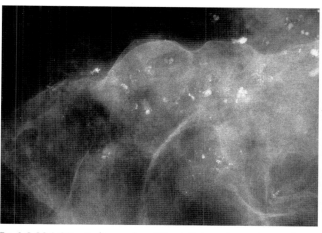

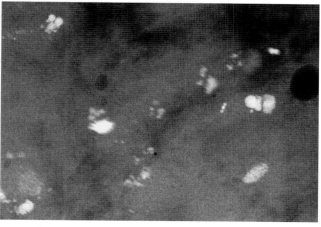

6-28   Ex. **4.6**-29

Ex. **4.6**-28 & 29   Radiographs of the left breast specimen slices containing clusters of tiny, dotlike calcifications.

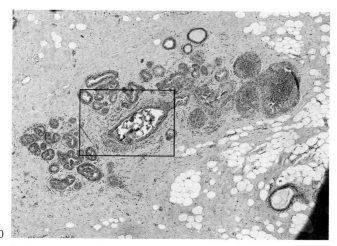

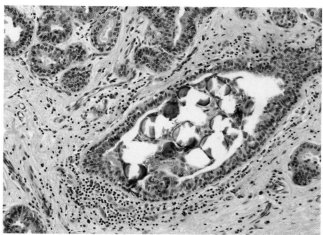

6-30   Ex. **4.6**-31

Ex. **4.6**-30 & 31   The tiny calcifications seen within the clusters of calcifications on images Ex. **4.6**-28 & 29 correspond to psammoma body–like calcifications at histological examination.

Example 4.6 continued

Ex. **4.6**-32 & 33   Detail of the region with calcifications in the left breast. MLO contact (32) and microfocus magnification (33).

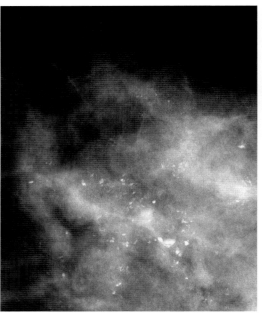

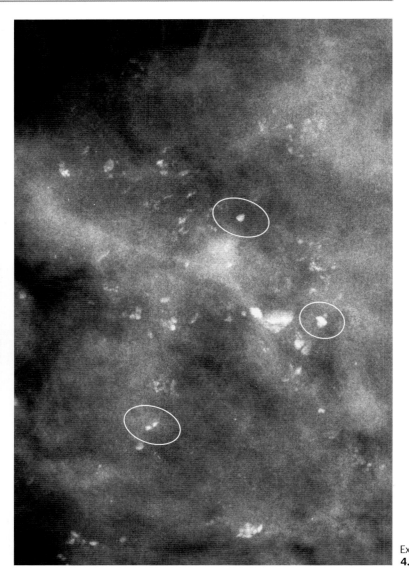

Ex.
4.6-32

Ex.
4.6

Ex. **4.6**-34   Histological examination shows large, **amorphous calcifications** corresponding to the high-density, irregular calcifications encircled on the mammographic image Ex. **4.6**-33. These are localized within involuted breast tissue. There is no evidence of malignancy.

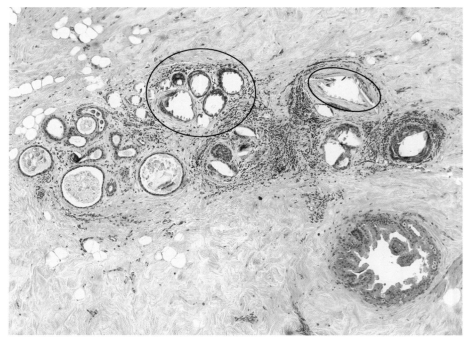

Ex.
4.6

Ex. **4.6**-35 Radiograph of an additional slice also contains squared calcifications (rectangle) in addition to the rounded, obviously benign type calcifications.

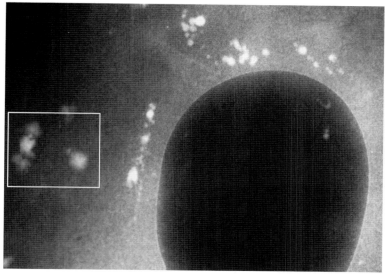

Ex. **4.6**-35

Ex. **4.6**-36 & 37 Histological examination using polarized light reveals the nature of the calcifications within the rectangle on Ex. **4.6**-35: **calcium oxalate,** so-called "**weddellites**," within cystic cavities. No sign of malignancy.

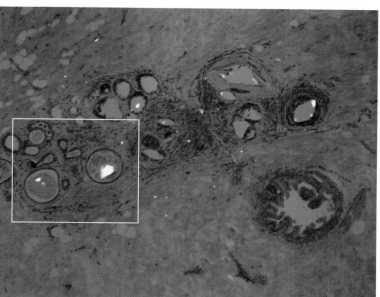

Ex. **4.6**-36

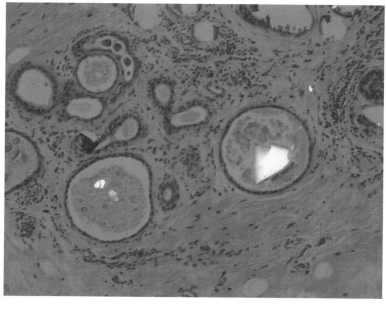

Ex. **4.6**-37

A Case Demonstrating the Differential Diagnostic Problem Caused by the Occurrence of Clustered Crushed Stone–like Calcifications in a Breast with Fibrocystic Change

Example 4.7

A 39-year-old woman with greenish discharge from the right nipple. Galactography shows changes corresponding to fibrocystic changes, including cystic dilatation of several TDLUs and ductectasia. Following galactography, there was cessation of her spontaneous discharge, which recurred 3 years later.

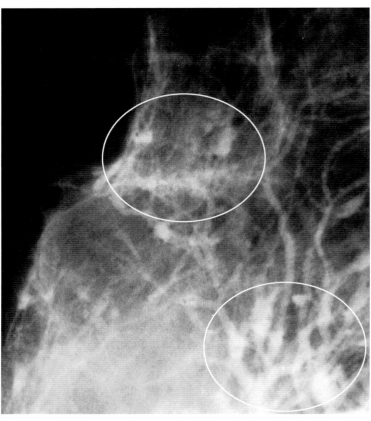

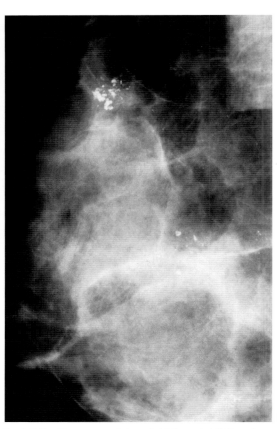

Ex. **4.7**-1

Ex. ⬤

Ex. **4.7**-1   Right breast galactography, MLO projection, detail of the axillary tail. The contrast-filled dilated ducts and their branches drain the cystically dilated TDLUs.

Ex. **4.7**-2   Three years later: right breast, MLO projection, detail of the axillary tail. Multiple clusters of crushed stone–like calcifications are seen with no associated tumor mass.

Ex. **4.7**-3 Microfocus magnification, MLO projection, detail of the right the axillary tail. The pleomorphic calcifications are in close proximity to each other, are irregular in size and density, and are of the mammographically malignant type.

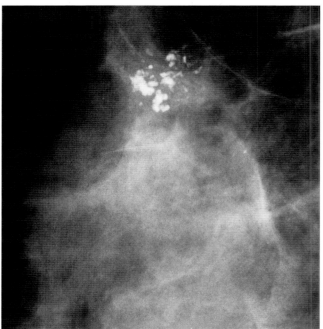

Ex.

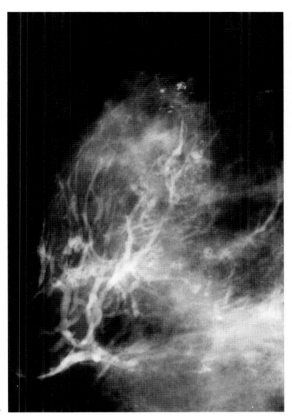

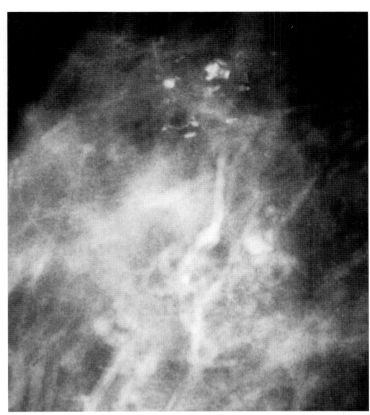

7-4

Ex. **4.7**-5

Ex. **4.7**-4 & 5   Repeat galactography: the distended, contrast-filled ducts and their branches can be followed to the area with the clusters of calcifications, suggesting that the irregular calcifications might be caused by fibrocystic change.

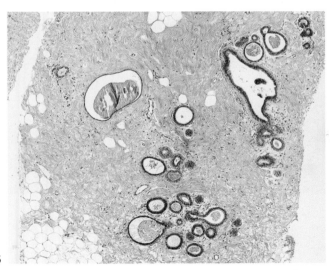

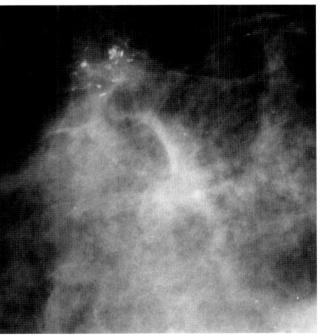

7-6

Ex. **4.6**-6   Histological diagnosis of the 14-gauge core biopsy samples: fibrocystic change without signs of malignancy.

Ex. **4.7**-7

Ex. **4.7**-7   Post-biopsy mammogram: the number of calcifications has decreased considerably compared with the prebiopsy mammogram (Ex. **4.7**-7 vs. **4.7**-3).

Treatment and follow-up: The patient declined surgical biopsy and no longer attended mammography screening. However, according to the Cancer and Population Registries, she was still alive and did not have breast cancer 14 years after the biopsy.

Involutional Type Calcifications: Pathophysiology, Imaging, and Differential Diagnosis

Screening of asymptomatic women brings to light many calcifications of benign origin. **Involutional type calcifications** produce typical findings that may, in some cases, cause differential diagnostic problems, making interventional procedures necessary. The **underlying pathophysiology** may follow one of two pathways:

(1) During involution of the fibroglandular tissue the acini within the individual TDLUs gradually decrease in number and the remaining acini may contain secretions, some of which will calcify. These remaining acini may become some-

what distended as they tend to fill the space vacated by the involuting TDLU. The lobule does not increase in overall size, so these slightly distended acini are not considered to be cysts. Within the alkaline, proteinaceous fluid the precipitating calcification(s) generally assume a spherical shape, which is very distinctive on high-resolution specimen radiography. The glandular tissue may eventually undergo complete involution, leaving behind the calcifications embedded in the adipose or fibrous connective tissue (Fig. **4.26**-2).

Fig. **4.26**-1 Subgross, thick-section (3D) histological image. The round, tiny, dotlike calcifications are localized within involuting acini that are cystically dilated.

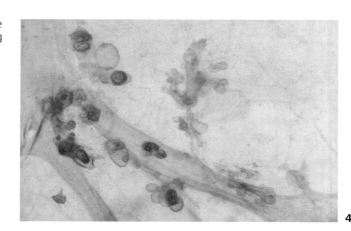

4.2●

Fig. **4.26**-2 Illustration of the development of involutional type calcifications. The remainder of the involuting acini become somewhat distended by secretions (left). Rounded calcifications may be formed within the retained secretions (center). Following complete involution (right), only the high-density, rounded/oval, dotlike calcifications are seen on the mammogram.

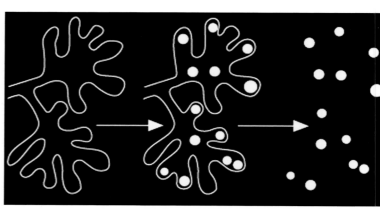

4.26

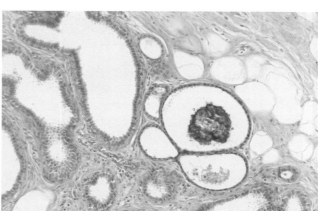

4.26-3

4.26

Figs. **4.26**-3 & 4   Subgross, thick-section (3D) (3) and conventional (4) histological images of large, spherical calcifications within distended acini. These are seen on the mammogram as round, high-density calcifications that are easy to perceive.

(2) An even more frequently occurring pathway leading to the formation of involutional type calcifications occurs when small areas within the involuting stroma become hy-alinized and may gradually calcify (Figs. **4.26**-5 & 6 and Examples 4.8 to 4.14).

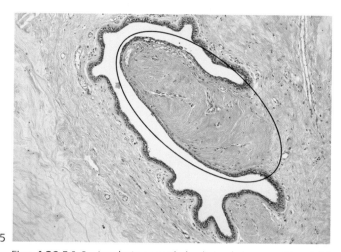
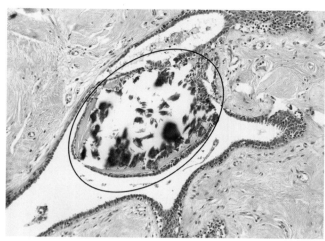

26-5   4.26-6

Figs. **4.26**-5 & 6   Involuting, partly hyalinized stroma without (5) and with "involutional type calcification" (6).

In most cases the involutional type calcifications can be un-equivocally diagnosed because of their **characteristic mammographic appearance**:

1. **Distribution**: Unlike the typically clustered distribution of the malignant type calcifications, the involutional type calcifications are **scattered** and may be present within a part of a lobe, in most of the breast, and are often bilateral (Example 4.11).
2. **Shape** and **density** of the calcifications: (a) Since the fluid distends the acinus to a tiny spherical cavity with a smooth inner wall, and the involutional type calcifications fill all or most of this cavity and assume its shape, the resulting calcified crystalline balls will appear as small, very dense spheres. (b) The more frequently occurring option is that the tiny hyalinized areas in the stroma protrude into a smaller duct or a spherical cavity, assuming a regular, round or oval shape. On the two-dimensional mammogram (best seen on the microfocus magnification images or on magnified specimen radiographs)

the involutional type calcifications resemble tiny dots with high opacity. The term "punctate" or dotlike calcifications is appropriate, as these are analogous to **a series of dots made by the point of a pen or pencil.** Understandably, dots of equal size will have an essentially identical appearance.

The underlying pathophysiological processes producing these calcifications are radically different from the processes producing the various types of malignant type calcifications. For this reason, the typical distribution and shape of the involutional type calcifications differs considerably from that of malignant type calcifications formed within the TDLUs. Summation of innumerable involutional type calcifications may cause differential diagnostic problems, but these can usually be resolved by thorough mammographic work-up and occasionally by larger-bore needle biopsy.

Unfortunately, there is a tendency to confuse involutional type calcifications with the cotton ball–like / powdery calcifications. The distinction should be fairly straightforward (see Table **4.1**)

Table **4.1**   Mammographic features distinguishing involutional type calcifications from powdery calcifications

	Distribution	Shape
Involutional type calcifications	Diffusely scattered	Dotlike, punctate, individually discernible
Powdery, cotton ball–like calcifications	Multiple clusters, not diffuse	Not individually discernible. Accumulation of many within TDLUs: faint, cotton ball–like

Demonstration of the difference between powdery (Fig. 4.27-1) and involutional type (Fig. 4.27-2) calcifications

Fig. **4.27**-1   Multiple clusters of powdery calcifications: aggregates of large numbers of psammoma body–like calcifications within slightly distended TDLUs, resembling cotton balls.

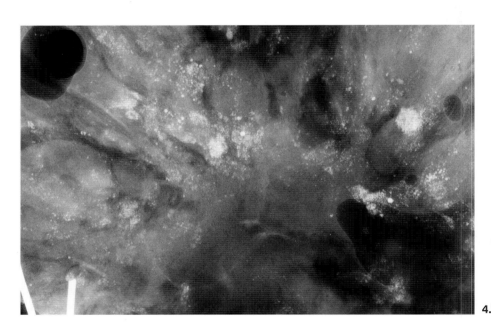

4.2

Fig. **4.27**-2   Diffusely scattered, dotlike, punctate, involutional type calcifications.

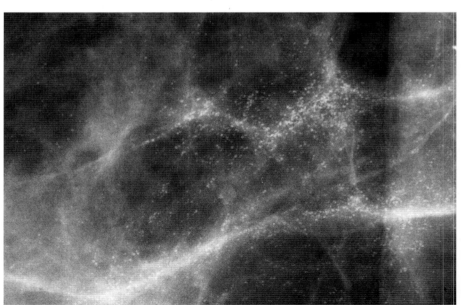

4.2

Examples 4.8 to 4.14 are illustrative examples of involutional type calcifications confirmed by either biopsy or long-term follow-up. Each case is from routine screening before the advent of large-bore needle biopsy.

Example 4.8

A 49-year-old asymptomatic woman, called back from screening for assessment of the oval shaped lesion in the upper portion of the right breast and for evaluation of the retroareolar calcifications.

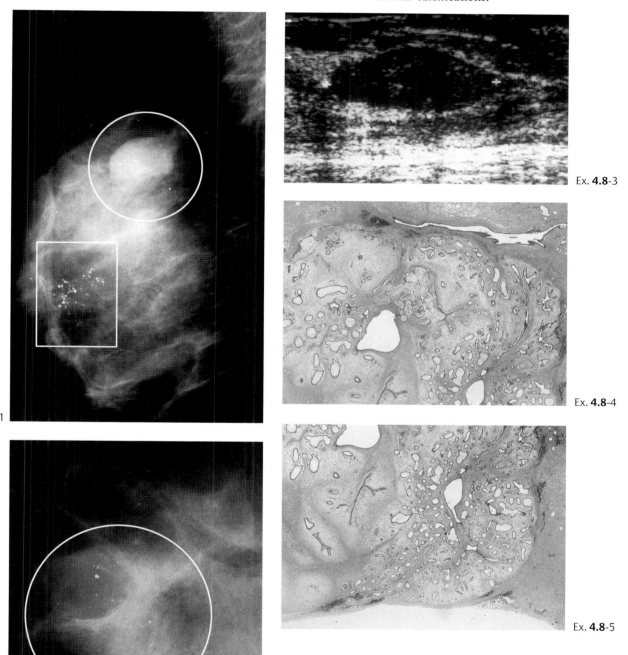

Ex. **4.8**-1

Ex. **4.8**-2

Ex. **4.8**-3

Ex. **4.8**-4

Ex. **4.8**-5

Ex. **4.8**-1 to 5   Right breast, MLO projection (1), micro-focus magnification (2), and breast ultrasound (3) demonstrate a solitary, low-density, oval benign tumor. The calcifications are scattered, high-density, dotlike, mammographically benign type. Histology of the preoperative 14-g biopsy showed a fibroadenoma (4, 5). Surgical removal of both the fibroadenoma and the area with calcifications was performed at the patient's request.

Example 4.8 continued

Ex. **4.8**-6   Radiograph of the specimen containing the calcifications. The individual calcifications have high density and, although their sizes vary, the calcium particles of equal size have an identical, dotlike appearance. The background is homogenous, ground glass–like fibrous tissue.

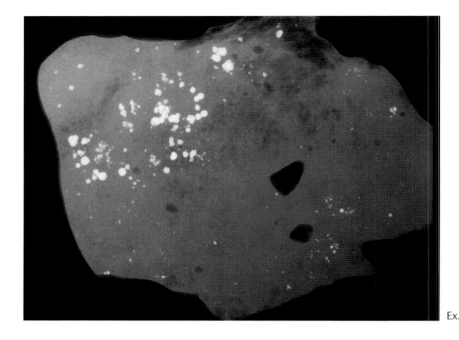

Ex.

Ex. **4.8**-7   Low-power, large-section histological image. Round calcifications are scattered within the stroma, which contains a few atrophic glandular elements.

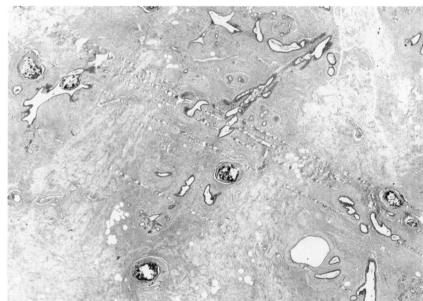

Ex.

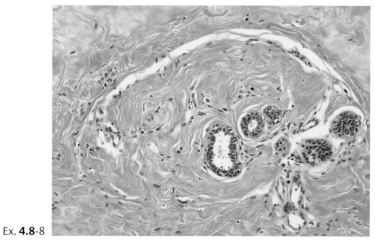

Ex. **4.8**-8

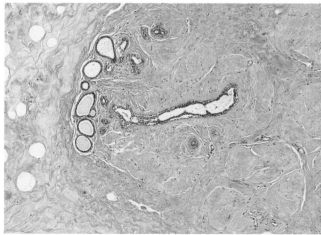

Ex.

Ex. **4.8**-8 & 9   Medium-power histological images of areas of involuting stroma and atrophic glandular tissue.

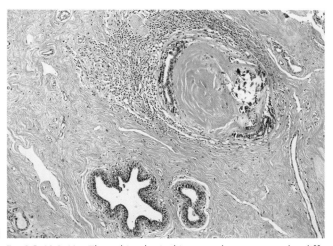

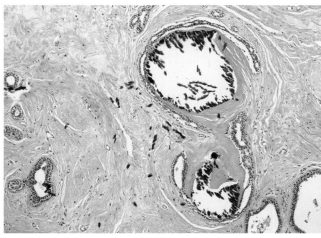

-10

Ex. **4.8**-10 & 11   These histological images demonstrate the different phases of the calcification process within the hyalinized stroma.

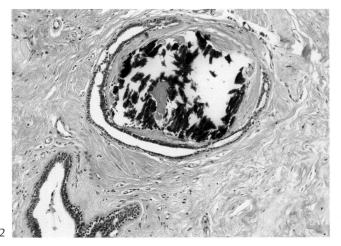

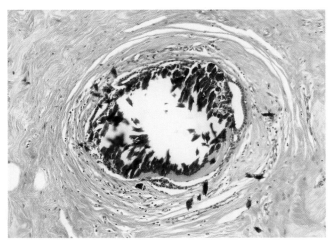

-12

Ex.
4.8-13

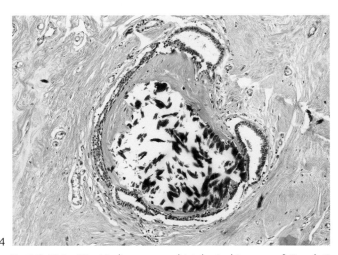

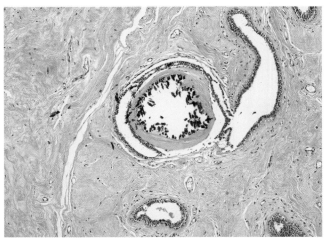

-14

Ex.
4.8-15

Ex. **4.8**-12 to 15   Medium-power histological images of "involutional type" calcifications. These correspond to the high-density, scattered, round calcifications seen on the mammograms.

Example 4.9

A 48-year-old asymptomatic woman. The mammograms of her right breast showed a group of microcalcifications without an associated tumor mass.

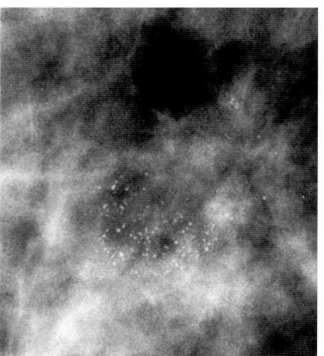

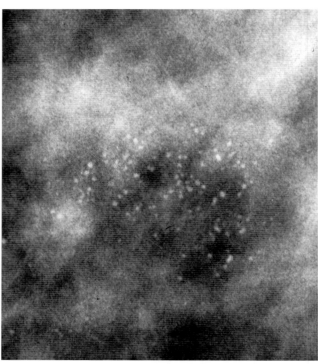

Ex. **4.9**-1

Ex.

Ex. **4.9**-1 & 2   Right breast, detail of the MLO projection (1) and microfocus magnification of the region with microcalcifications (2). Within an area measuring 20 mm × 20 mm, diffusely scattered, discernible calcifications are seen. The slight variations in density and shape of the individual calcifications particles lead to surgical biopsy (this is a case from the era before the introduction of larger-bore needle biopsies).

Ex. **4.9**-3   Radiograph of the surgical specimen. The calcifications have been removed with a good margin.

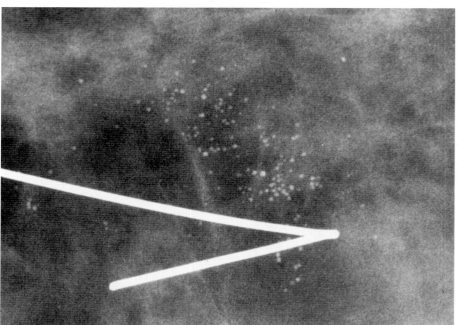

Ex.

Ex. **4.9**-4   Low-power histological image of the large-section. Rounded calcifications are seen scattered within the fibrous tissue.

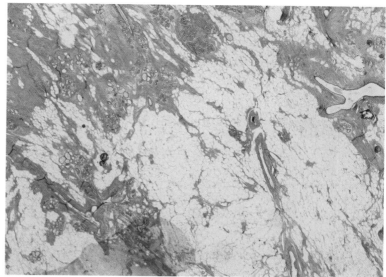

Ex. **4.9**-4

Ex. **4.9**-5   Radiograph of the surgical specimen slice containing the calcifications.

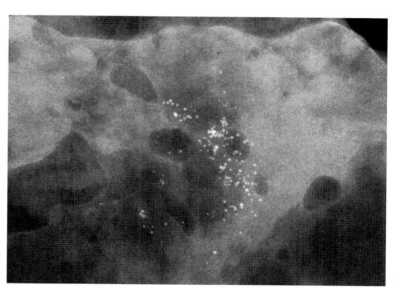

Ex. **4.9**-5

Ex. **4.9**-6   Medium-power histological examination. The spherical calcifications are not localized within the glandular tissue, but are in the stroma.

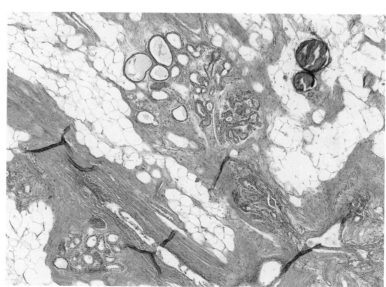

Ex. **4.9**-6

Example 4.9 continued

Ex. **4.9**-7   Radiograph of the paraffin block. The calcifications have the typical feature of involutional type calcifications: the discernible, round calcifications are scattered and have a high and even density. Although the calcified particles cover a range of sizes, any two particles of the same size have an almost identical appearance.

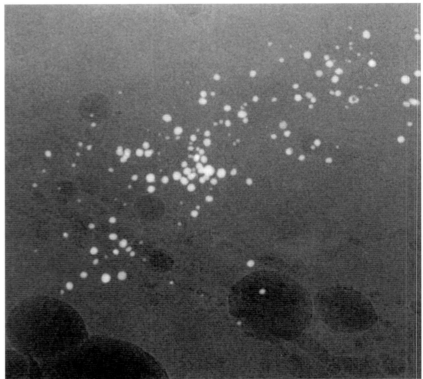

Ex.

Ex. **4.9**-8   Medium-power histological image. The few remaining acini of the involuting TDLU contain secretions. The involutional type calcifications are outside the TDLUs, scattered within the dense fibrous stroma.

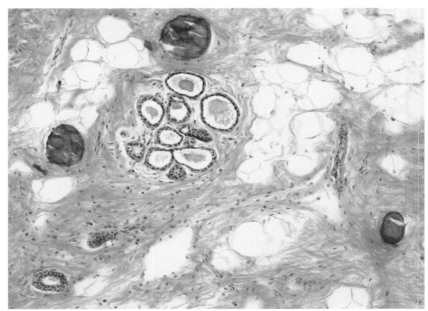

Ex.

Ex. **4.9**-9 & 10   Additional histological slides demonstrating that the spherical calcifications are localized in fibrous tissue. There are no signs of malignancy.

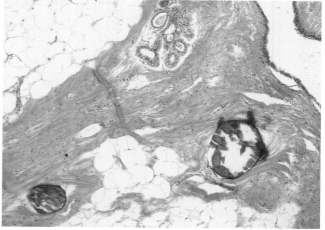

Ex. **4.9**-9

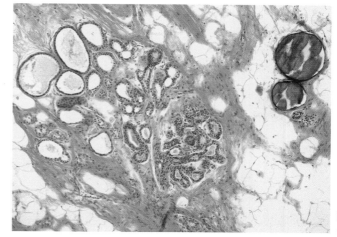

Ex. **4.9**-10

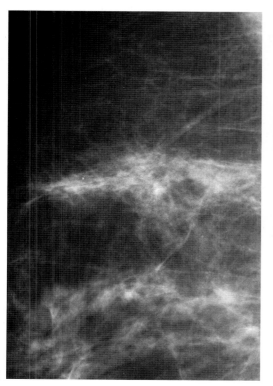

-11

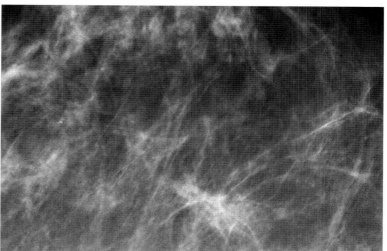

Ex. **4.9**-12

Ex. **4.9**-11 & 12   Details of the right MLO and CC projections 16 years after surgery. A small postoperative scar is seen at the site of the biopsy without any mammographic abnormality.

Example 4.10

A 52-year-old asymptomatic woman. Microcalcifications have been detected in the upper portion of her left mammogram. The clinical breast examination was normal.

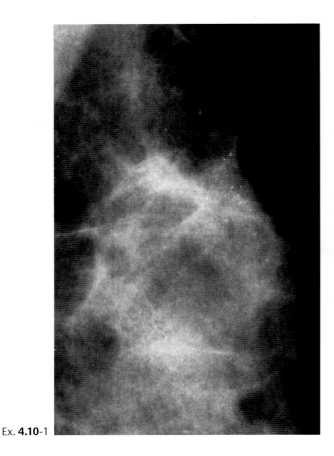

Ex. **4.10**-1

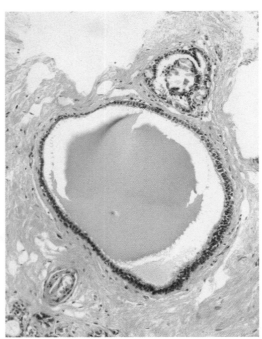

Ex. **4.10**-2

Ex. **4.10**-1 & 2   Left MLO projection at first screening (1). Tiny scattered calcifications are seen in the upper portion of the fibroglandular tissue. Histological examination of the 14-g core biopsy specimen reveals atrophic glandular tissue, occasional cystic dilatations with intraluminal secretion and involutional type calcifications in the stroma (2).

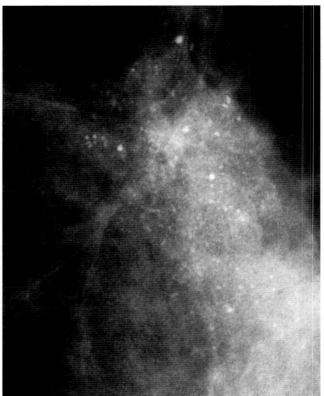

Ex. **4.10**-3   Mammogram 3 years later: microfocus magnification of the region with calcifications. The scattered, round calcifications are seen against a dense, homogeneous, fibrous background.

Ex.
4.1

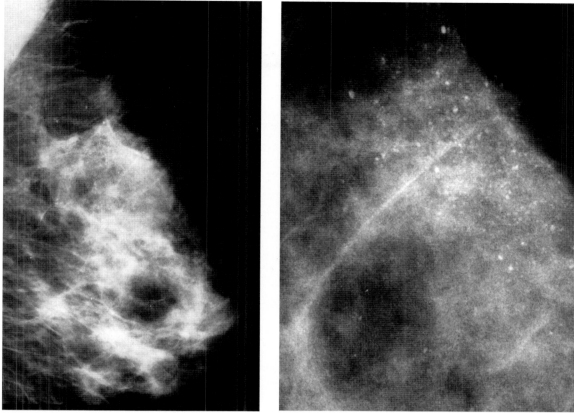

Ex.
4.10-5

Ex. **4.10**-4 & 5   Screening mammogram a further 3 years later: MLO projection (4) and microfocus magnification (5) show no change.

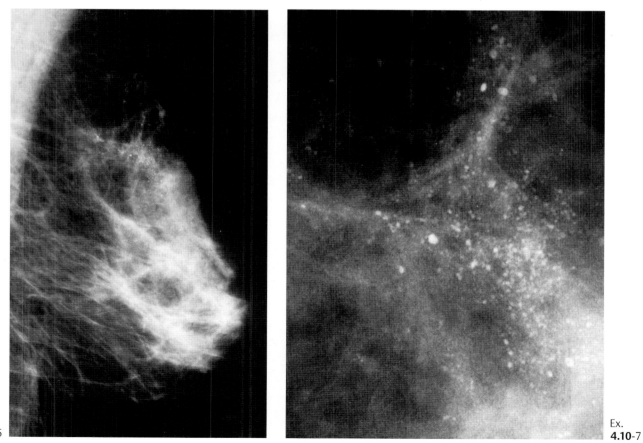

10-6

Ex.
4.10-7

Ex. **4.10**-6 & 7   MLO projection (6) and microfocus magnification (7) a further 2 years later. As the involution progresses, the amount of fibrous tissue decreases and the involutional type calcifications increase, occupying a larger region in the upper portion of the left breast.

Example 4.11

A 44-year-old asymptomatic woman, called back from mammographic screening for assessment of the diffusely scattered, bilateral microcalcifications.

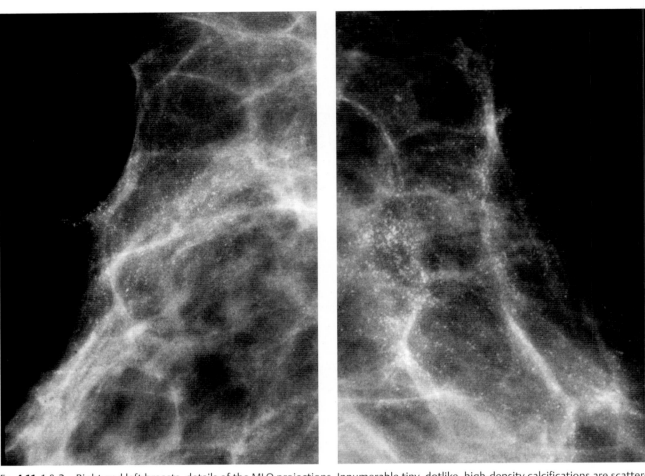

Ex.
4.11-1

Ex.
4.11-

Ex. **4.11**-1 & 2   Right and left breasts, details of the MLO projections. Innumerable tiny, dotlike, high-density calcifications are scattered over the upper portions of both breasts. No tumor mass is seen.

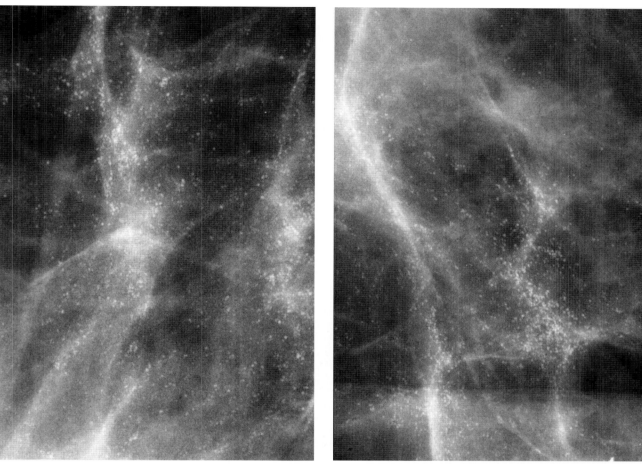

Ex. **11**-3

Ex. **4.11**-4

Ex. **4.11**-3 & 4   Microfocus magnification of the upper regions of the right and left breasts demonstrates the characteristic appearance of involutional type calcifications, an unequivocally benign finding. There is no suspicion of malignancy.

Example 4.12

A 55-year-old asymptomatic woman, screening examination.

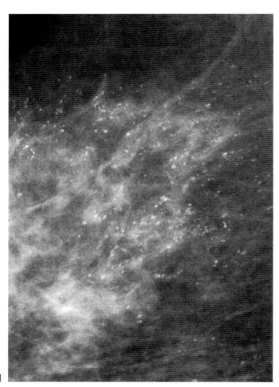

Ex. **4.12**-1

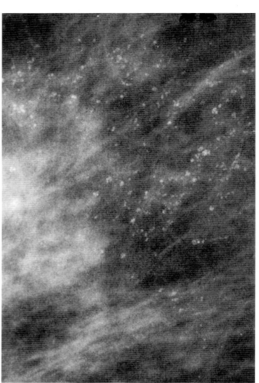

Ex. **4.12**-2

Ex. **4.12**-1   Right breast, detail of the MLO projection. The scattered, dotlike, spherical calcifications have high and even density. The mammographic features are characteristic of involutional type calcifications.

Ex. **4.12**-2   Two years later, at the next mammographic screening examination, the woman is still asymptomatic. The mammographic characteristics of the scattered, dotlike calcifications have not changed.

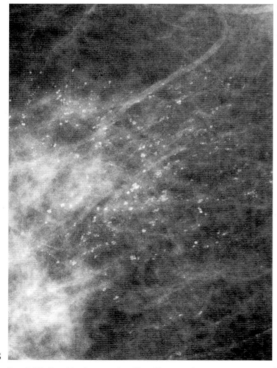

Ex. **4.12**-3

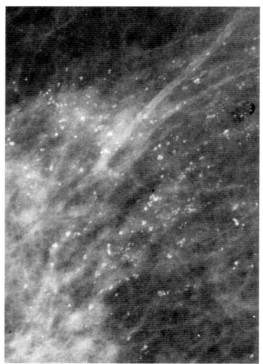

Ex. **4.12**-4

Ex. **4.12**-3   Next examination 3 years later: as expected, the involutional type calcifications show no change.

Ex. **4.12**-4   Ten years after the first examination (1) the mammographic image is unchanged.

Example 4.13

A 53-year-old asymptomatic woman, screening examination.

Ex. **4.13**-1 & 2   Right breast, detail of the MLO projection. Despite the 7-year time interval between the two examinations, the involutional type calcifications in the upper portion of the breast have the same mammographic appearance.

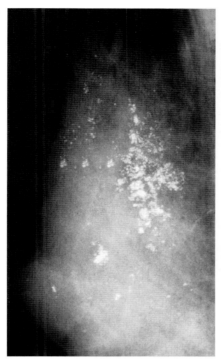
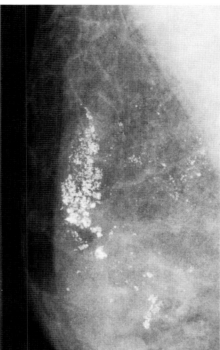

Ex. **4.13**-1

Ex. **4.13**-2

Example 4.14

A 68-year-old asymptomatic woman, screening examination.

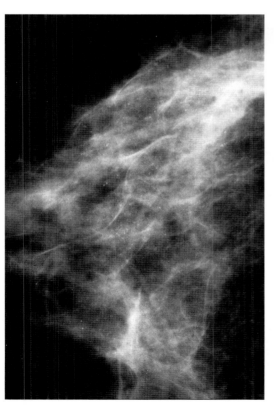
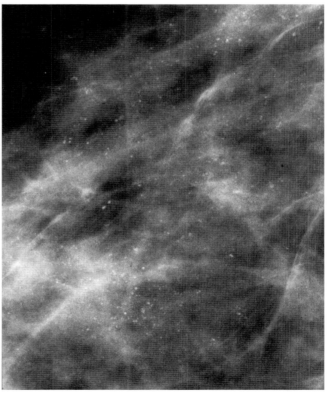

14-1

Ex. 4.14-2

Ex. **4.14**-1 & 2   Right breast, CC projection (1) and microfocus magnification (2). A large number of tiny, dotlike, rounded calcifications are seen scattered in the involuting parenchyma (Pattern I). No mammographic signs of malignancy are demonstrable.

Fibroadenoma

The next benign breast lesion associated with calcifications is the fibroadenoma. The need for surgical biopsy has decreased considerably because of the reliable histological diagnosis obtained by larger-bore needle biopsy.

Fig. **4.28** The second most frequent benign, hyperplastic breast change which may be associated with crushed stone–like calcifications sent to surgery after careful preoperative work-up is the **fibroadenoma.**

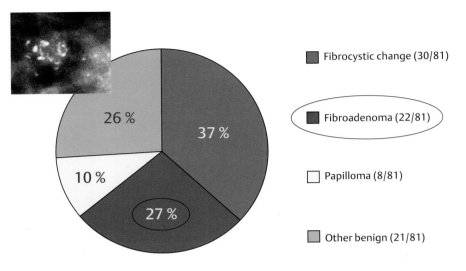

Fibrocystic change (30/81)

Fibroadenoma (22/81)

Papilloma (8/81)

Other benign (21/81)

12-year total **4.28**

Schematic illustration of the natural history of fibroadenomas in relation to the mammographic findings and differential diagnostic problems

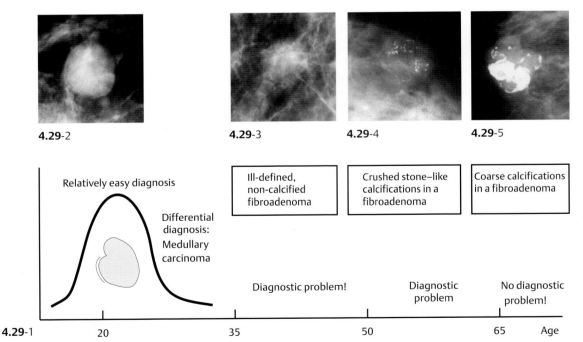

4.29-2   **4.29**-3   **4.29**-4   **4.29**-5

Relatively easy diagnosis

Differential diagnosis: Medullary carcinoma

Ill-defined, non-calcified fibroadenoma

Crushed stone–like calcifications in a fibroadenoma

Coarse calcifications in a fibroadenoma

Diagnostic problem!   Diagnostic problem   No diagnostic problem!

4.29-1   20   35   50   65   Age

Fig. **4.29**-1 to 5   The mammographic appearance of fibroadenomas according to patient age. In its initial phase of development, the fibroadenoma is low-density radiopaque with a partial or extensive halo sign. Its shape is round or oval, and often has a lobulated contour. In young women the rarely occurring medullary carcinoma may have a similar appearance (2). As the woman approaches menopausal age, the fibroadenoma tends to undergo involution, resulting in an ill-defined contour, making mammographic differentiation from invasive breast cancers difficult (3). During this process of involution, calcifications may appear within the fibroadenoma. When the calcifications are crushed stone–like, their mammographic appearance may resemble that of the calcification particles associated with Grade 2 in situ carcinoma (4). Here again, the distinction between benign and malignant type calcifications based only on mammographic appearance may be difficult or impossible. Larger-bore needle biopsy can provide a definite answer. On the other hand, the development of large, coarse, popcorn–like calcifications pathognomic for fibroadenomas (5). Biopsy should not be necessary in these cases.

Fibroadenomas are benign biphasic tumors arising from the epithelium and stroma of the terminal ductal lobular units (TDLUs). The epithelial component usually contains two layers (a layer of epithelial cells and a layer of myoepithelial cells) within glandlike structures and may undergo benign proliferation or, rarely, malignant transformation. The stromal component initially represents overgrowth of the specialized intralobular connective tissue containing large amounts of intercellular mucin. During involution, the amount of the mucin and the cellularity of the stromal component both decrease with the simultaneous formation of collagen fibers. This collagen may lose its fibrillar character and become hyalinized, within which dystrophic calcifications may develop.

Fig. **4.30**-1 & 2   Subgross, thick-section (3D) histological images of a fibroadenoma. The proliferating stroma dominates the image.

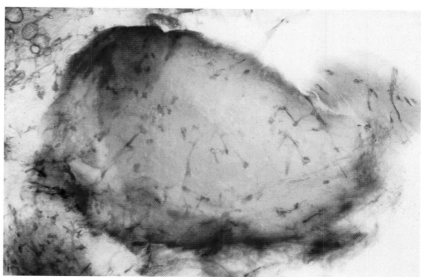

4.30-1

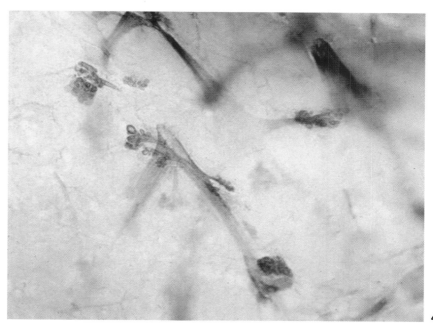

4.30-2

Example 4.15

A 59-year-old asymptomatic woman, screening examination. The mammographically detected microcalcifications in the lateral portion of the left breast were evaluated at the assessment center.

Ex. **4.15**-1 & 2   Left breast, detail of the CC projection (1) and microfocus magnification of the region with calcifications (2). There are numerous clusters of tiny, irregular, discernible calcifications without an associated tumor mass, suggesting malignancy. The calcifications occupy a large area (rectangle), further supporting the suspicion of malignancy.

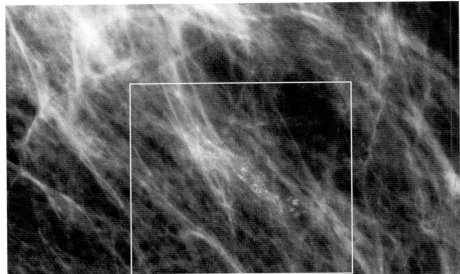

Ex.
4.15-

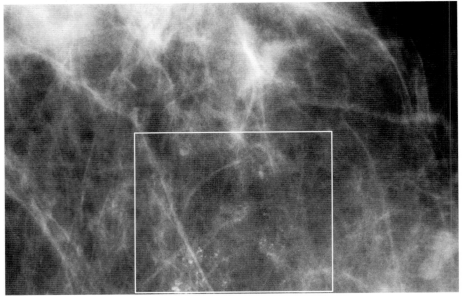

Ex.
4.15

Ex. **4.15**-3   Radiograph of the operative specimen. The multiple clusters of irregular calcifications have been removed.

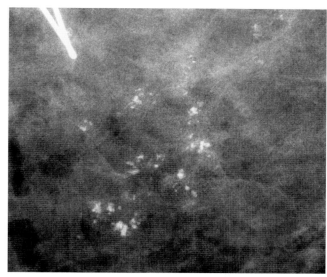

Ex. **4.15**-3

Ex. **4.15**-4   Large-section histology. The low-power magnification shows the calcifications in multiple clusters (oval).

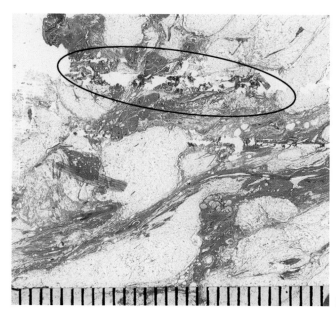

Ex. **4.15**-4

Ex. **4.15**-5   Medium-power histological image. The calcifications are localized within tiny fibroadenomas adjacent to each other.

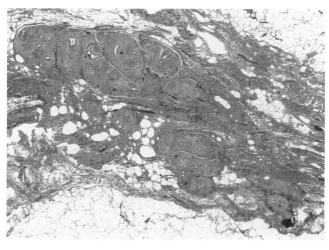

Ex. **4.15**-5

Example 4.15 continued

Ex. **4.15**-6 to 8   Continuing with progressively higher magnification, the histological image demonstrates that the calcifications are situated in the hyalinized fibrous stroma of the fibroadenoma. There are no signs of malignancy.

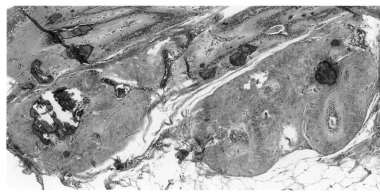

Ex. **4.15**

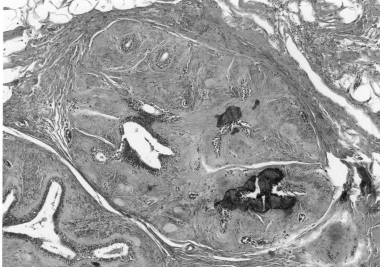

Ex. **4.15**

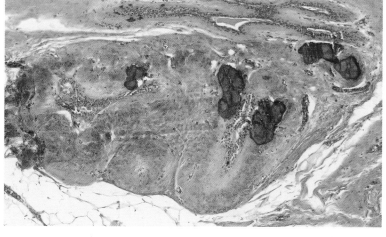

Ex. **4.15**

Ex. **4.15**-9   At still higher magnification, the details of this fibroadenoma can be seen more clearly.

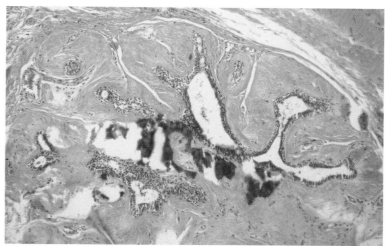

Ex.
4.15-9

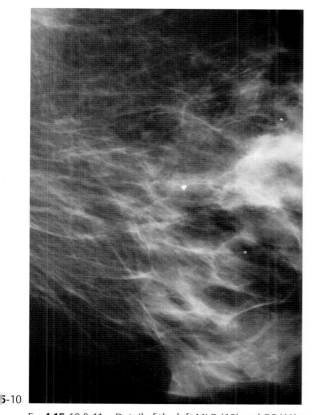

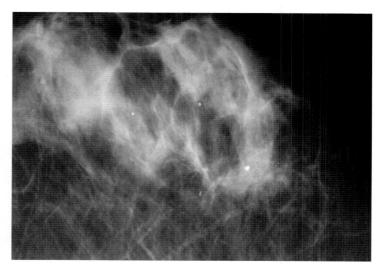

5-10

Ex.
4.15-11

Ex. **4.15**-10 & 11   Detail of the left MLO (10) and CC (11) projections. Fourteen years later, mammographic screening examination shows no abnormality at the site of surgery.

Follow-up: After a diagnostic biopsy of her left breast, the patient participated in regular mammography screening examinations, and no abnormality has been found during the past 14 years of follow-up.

Example 4.16

A 65-year-old asymptomatic woman, screening examination. She was called back for evaluation of the multiple clusters of calcifications in her left breast.

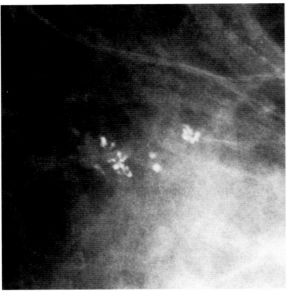

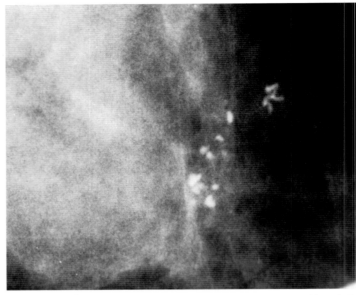

Ex. 4.16-1

Ex. 4.16-2

Ex. **4.16**-1 & 2   Left breast, MLO and CC microfocus magnification images of the region with the clustered, irregular, discernible calcifications without an associated tumor mass. The mammographic analysis suggests malignancy.

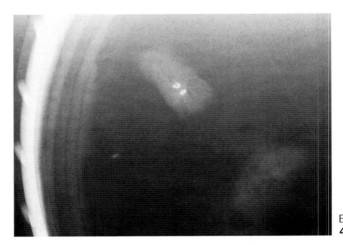

Ex. **4.16**-3   Radiograph of the 14-gauge preoperative needle biopsy specimen containing calcifications.

Ex. 4.16-3

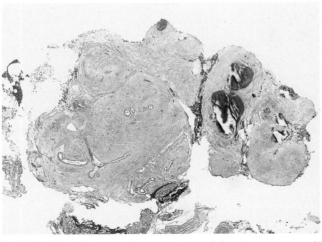

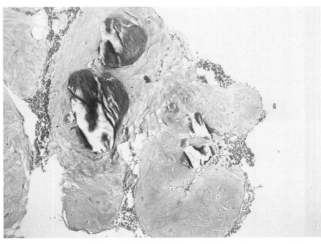

Ex. 4.16-4

Ex. 4.16-5

Ex. **4.16**-4 & 5   Histological examination of the 14-gauge core biopsy specimen: partially calcified, hyalinized fibroadenoma with no signs of malignancy.

Due to the obvious discordance between the mammographic and histological diagnoses, diagnostic surgical biopsy was performed.

Ex. **4.16**-6 to 8 Histological examination of the surgical biopsy specimen confirmed the diagnosis of benign fibroadenomas.

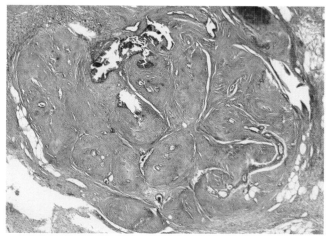

Ex. **4.16**-6

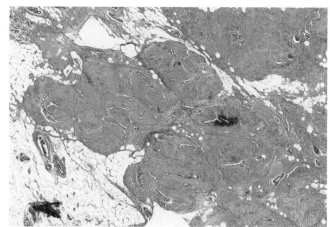

Ex. **4.16**-7

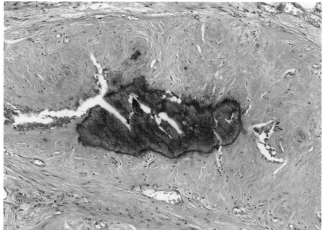

Ex. **4.16**-8

Follow-up: The patient continued with regular mammographic screening examinations. No abnormality was found at the site of biopsy during the next 14 years of follow-up.

Comment and lesson learned
Mammographic analysis of crushed stone–like, discernible calcifications may not allow the distinction between benign and malignant diseases. In such cases, larger-bore needle biopsy becomes necessary to reach the correct diagnosis. Both the malignant (Grade 2 in situ carcinoma) and the benign processes (fibrocystic change, fibroadenoma, papilloma, traumatic fat necrosis) are intimately associated with the calcifications themselves. Consequently, a preoperative percutaneous larger-bore needle biopsy harvesting calcifications from the lesion will provide an unequivocal histological diagnosis, despite the perceived discordance between the mammographic appearance of the calcifications and the benign histological diagnosis.

Example 4.17

A 69-year-old asymptomatic woman, mammographic screening examination. She was called back to the assessment center for further work-up of the de-novo calcifications surrounded by an ill-defined density at the posterior margin of the fibroglandular tissue.

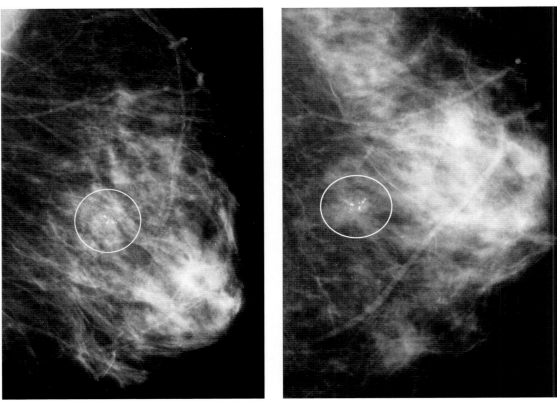

Ex.
4.17-1

Ex.
4.17-

Ex. **4.17**-1 & 2   Left breast, MLO and CC projections. There is a cluster of discrete calcifications in the central portion of the breast, associated with an ill-defined density.

Ex. **4.17**-3 Microfocus magnification view in the CC projection of the region containing the calcifications. The individual calcification particles are discernible and their shape, size, and density are variable as in mammographically malignant type calcifications. These features suggest malignancy.

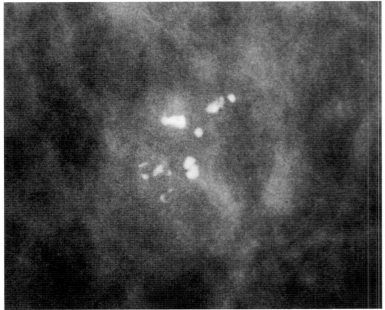

Ex.
4.17

Ex. **4.17**-4 & 5   Histological examination of the 14-gauge core biopsy specimen shows a benign fibroadenoma with amorphous stromal calcifications.

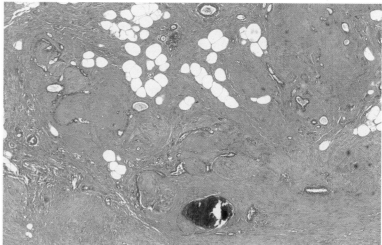

Ex. **4.17**-4

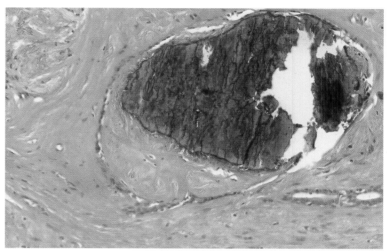

Ex. **4.17**-5

Implications for treatment and follow-up: The individual calcification particles in discernible clusters of calcifications are closely related to the tissue producing them so that larger-bore needle biopsy specimen containing the calcifications will also contain the tissue necessary for reliable histological diagnosis. Further management can then be based on the results of the percutaneous biopsy. When benign, the case is closed and the woman can be returned to regular screening examinations.

Follow-up: In this case, no surgery was performed and her subsequent screening examinations over the next 13 years have shown no evidence of malignancy at the site of the percutaneous biopsy.

Example 4.18

A 40-year-old asymptomatic woman, mammographic screening examination. She was called back to the assess- ment center for evaluation of the partially calcified solitary circular mass in the upper portion of the right breast.

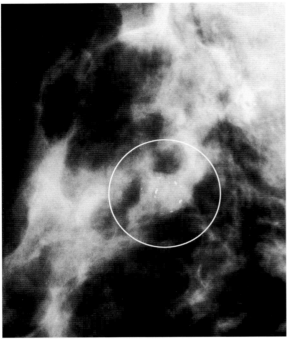

Ex. **4.18**-1

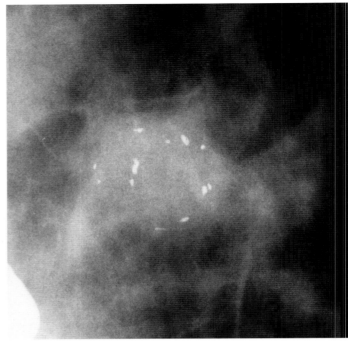

Ex. **4.18**-

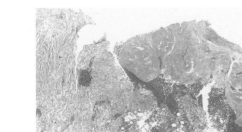

Ex. **4.18**-2

Ex. **4.18**-1 to 5   Right breast, detail of the MLO (1) and CC (2) projections and microfocus magnification (3). There are broken needle tip–like calcifications within an ill-defined circular lesion. The mammographic analysis cannot give a reliable, final diagnosis.
Histology of the ultrasound guided 14-gauge core biopsy (4, 5): benign fibroadenoma.

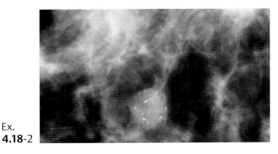

Ex. **4.18**-4

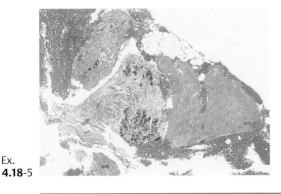

Ex. **4.18**-5

Treatment and follow-up: No surgery was performed. Her subsequent screening mammograms showed a gradual accumulation of a coarse calcification in this shrinking fibroadenoma (Ex. **4.18**-6).

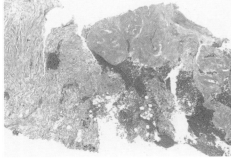

Ex. **4.18**-6   Right breast, screening mammogram 12 years following the percutaneous needle biopsy.

Ex. **4.18**-6

Example 4.19

A 63-year-old asymptomatic woman, mammographic screening examination. Multiple clusters of irregular calcifications are perceived on the mammograms of the right breast.

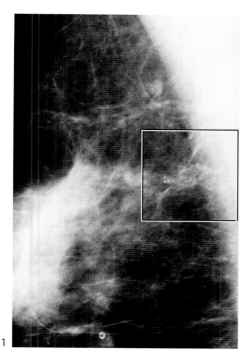

19-1

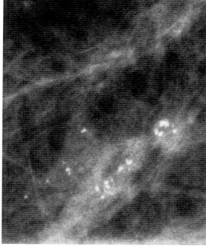

Ex. **4.19**-2

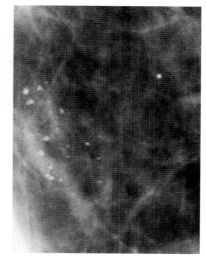

Ex. **4.19**-3

Ex. **4.19**-1 to 3   Right breast, detail of the MLO projection and microfocus magnification images (2, 3). There are multiple clusters of calcifications surrounded by a nonspecific density in the upper portion of the breast, close to the chest wall (rectangle). The shape and density of the individual, discernible calcifications are variable, suggesting malignancy, especially when the ill-defined density is also taken into account.

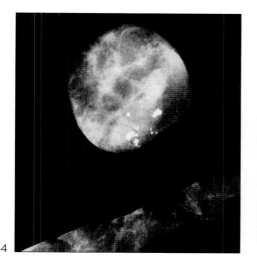

9-4

Follow-up: Because of the reliability of the histological diagnosis, no surgery was performed. She participated in regular mammography screening for the next 9 years and no abnormality has developed.

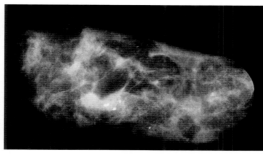

Ex. **4.19**-4 & 5   Microfocus magnification radiographs of the vacuum-assisted needle biopsy specimen. A representative sample of the calcifications has been removed.

Ex.
4.19-5

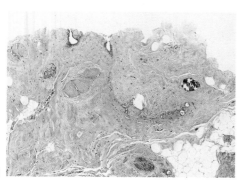

9-6

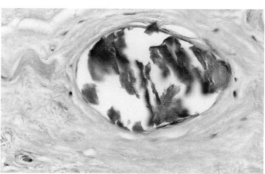

Ex. **4.19**-6 & 7   Low- and higher-power histological images (H&E) demonstrate a benign fibroadenoma with calcification. There are no signs of malignancy.

Ex.
4.19-7

Example 4.20

A 41-year-old asymptomatic woman, mammographic screening examination. She was called back from screening for evaluation of the microcalcifications detected on the mammogram of her left breast.

Ex. **4.20**-1 & 2 Left breast, MLO projection (1) and detail of the CC projection (2). Multiple clusters of discernible calcifications are seen (rectangle) without an associated tumor mass.

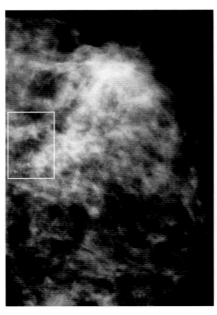

Ex. **4.20**-1

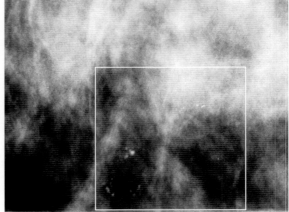

Ex. **4.20**

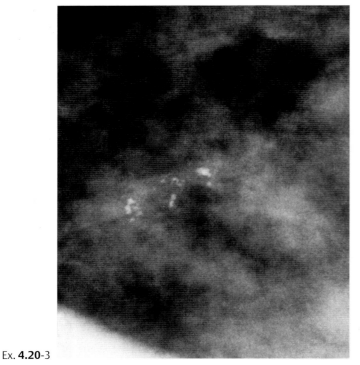

Ex. **4.20**-3

Ex. **4.20**-3 Microfocus magnification and spot compression of the area with the clustered calcifications. Some of the individual calcification particles are broken needle tip–like, and the form and density of the remainder are highly variable, as often seen in malignant type calcifications.

Ex. **4.20**-4

Ex. **4.20**-5

Ex. **4.20**-4 & 5 Low- and intermediate-power histological images (H&E). The histological diagnosis is a partially calcified benign fibroadenoma.

Treatment and follow-up: Following a satisfactory diagnostic work-up, including histology, there is no indication for surgery of this involuting fibroadenoma. Regular screening examinations have shown no evidence of malignancy over the following 12 years.

Example 4.21

A 43-year-old asymptomatic woman, mammographic screening examination. She was called back for further examination of the partially calcified circular, ill-defined tumor that was detected on the mammograms of the right breast. Following mammographic work-up, 14-gauge core biopsy revealed atypical cells, but did not provide a definitive diagnosis. A surgical biopsy was then performed.

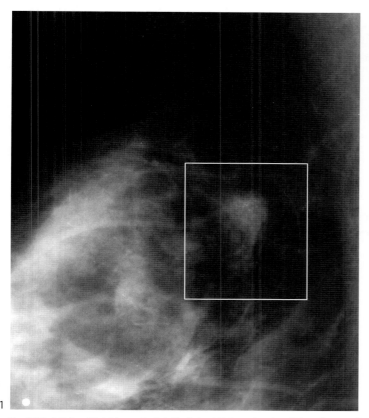

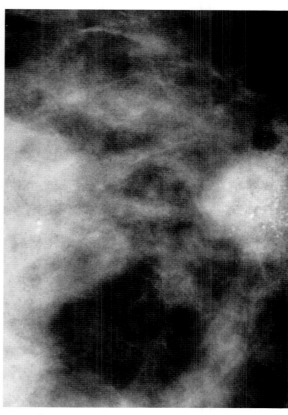

Ex. **4.21**-1 & 2   Right breast, detail of the MLO projection (1) and microfocus magnification (2). There is a high density, ill-defined, lobulated, spherical tumor mass close to the chest wall, containing discrete microcalcifications.

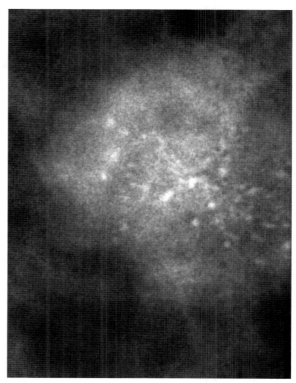

Ex. **4.21**-3   Photographic enlargement of a detail of the microfocus magnification image for better analysis of the microcalcifications. The irregular, crushed stone–like and short branching calcifications are of the mammographically malignant type.

Example 4.21 continued

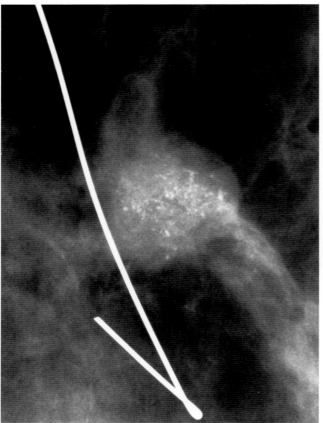

Ex.
4.21-4

Ex. **4.21**-4   Radiograph of the surgical specimen containing the mammographically detected lesion.

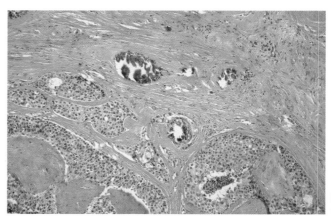

Ex.
4.2

Ex. **4.21**-5   Low-power, large-section histological image shows a fibroadenoma containing in situ carcinoma.

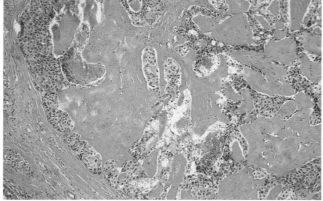

Ex.
4.21-6

Ex.
4.2

Ex. **4.21**-6 & 7   Medium-power histological images demonstrating in situ carcinoma growing within a fibroadenoma. The calcifications are localized within the hyalinized, fibrous tissue, unrelated to the in situ cancer.

Comment
This case demonstrates the value of the percutaneous large-core needle biopsy, which reliably selected the malignant case from among many fibroadenomas containing suspicious calcifications.

Ex. **4.21**-8 & 9   Right breast, detail images of the MLO (1) and CC (2) projections 14 years after surgery. There are no signs of malignancy.

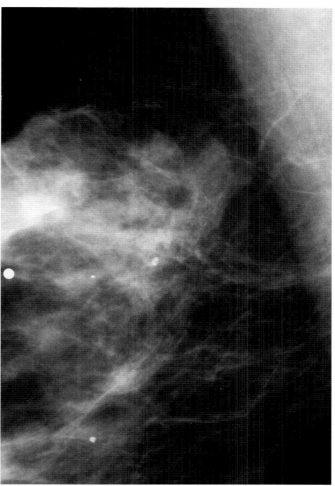

Ex. **4.21**-8

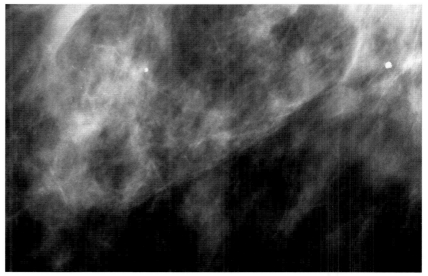

Ex. **4.21**-9

Treatment and follow-up: Surgical biopsy with no adjuvant therapy. There has been no evidence of malignancy during 14 years of follow-up.

Papilloma

Another benign breast lesion associated with calcifications is the **intraductal papilloma**.

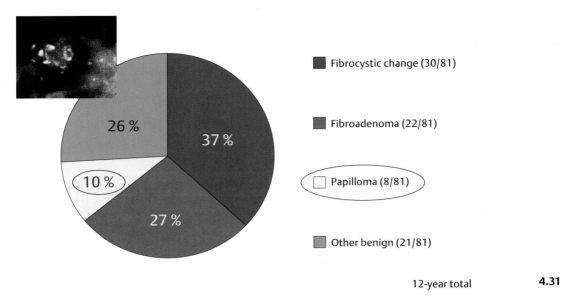

- Fibrocystic change (30/81)
- Fibroadenoma (22/81)
- Papilloma (8/81)
- Other benign (21/81)

37 %

26 %

10 %

27 %

12-year total   **4.31**

Fig **4.31**   One of the benign, hyperplastic breast changes which may be associated with crushed stone–like calcifications the **intraductal papilloma**.

Papillomas are benign tumors of the mammary ductal epithelium. They may be central when arising in a main duct, or peripheral, arising in subsegmental ducts. They may be solitary or multiple as well as intracystic. The basic structures of a papilloma are branching fronds of fibrovascular stroma covered with bi-layered epithelium (a layer of epithelial cells and a layer of myoepithelial cells). The epithelium may proliferate, undergo metaplasia or undergo malignant transformation. The fibrovascular stroma may become hyalinized and calcified. Although calcifications may appear in the lumina of the epithelial proliferations, most of the calcifications within the papillomas are located in the stroma.

3D Image

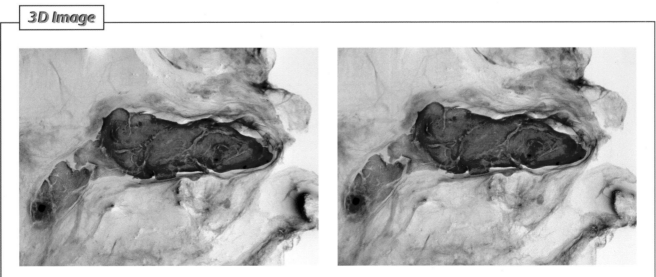

4.32-1   4.32

Figs. **4.32**-1 & 2   Stereoscopic, subgross, thick-section (3D) image pair of a large intraductal papilloma.

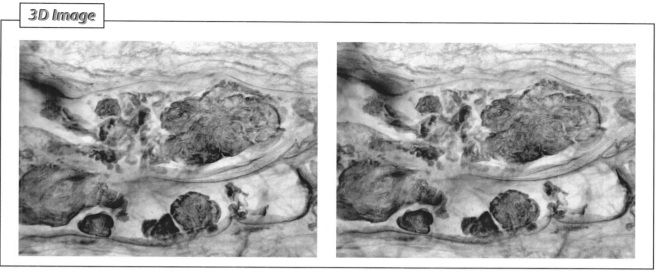

4.33-1   4.33-2

Figs. **4.33**-1 & 2   Stereoscopic, subgross, thick-section (3D) image pair of a two neighboring dilated ducts containing numerous benign papillomas.

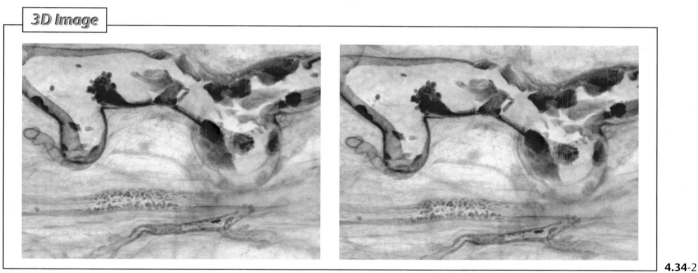

4.34-1   4.34-2

Figs. **4.34**-1 & 2   This 3D image pair shows three ducts: the uppermost is considerably distended and contains numerous benign papillomas; there is micropapillary in situ carcinoma in the two lower ducts.

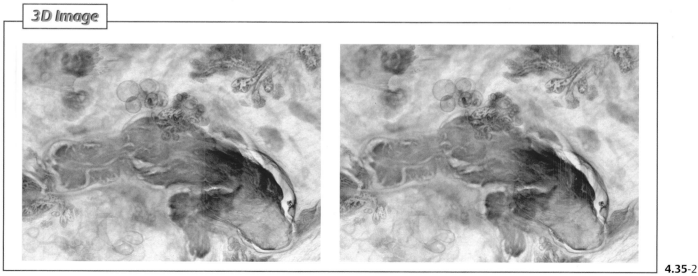

4.35-1   4.35-2

Fig. **4.35**-1 & 2   Thick-section (3D) image pair of an extremely dilated duct almost completely filled by a large benign papilloma. There are several adjacent foci of micropapillary in situ carcinoma in the upper half of the image.

Example 4.22

This 85-year-old woman with a history of right-sided mastectomy for breast cancer presented with serous discharge from the left nipple. There is no palpable tumor at clinical breast examination.

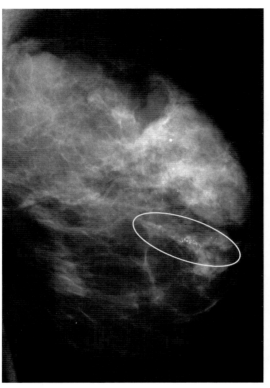
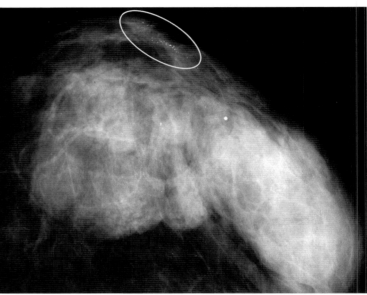

Ex. **4.22**-1

Ex. **4.22**

Ex. **4.22**-1 & 2   Left breast, MLO and CC projections. Dense fibrosis is seen over most of the breast. There is a large group of calcifications in the retroareolar region (ovals).

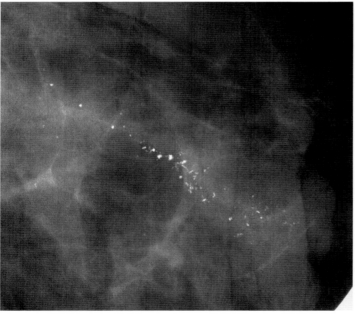
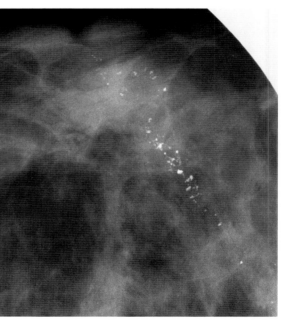

Ex. **4.22**-3

Ex. **4.22**

Ex. **4.22**-3 & 4   Spot compression with microfocus magnification, MLO and CC projections. The very irregular, discernible calcifications show a linear arrangement instead of being clustered. The analysis of their shape and density leads to the inevitable conclusion that they may be associated with a malignant process. However, there is discordance between the linear distribution and the crushed stone–like appearance, because malignant type crushed stone–like calcifications are located within TDLUs and appear as multiple clusters on the mammogram.

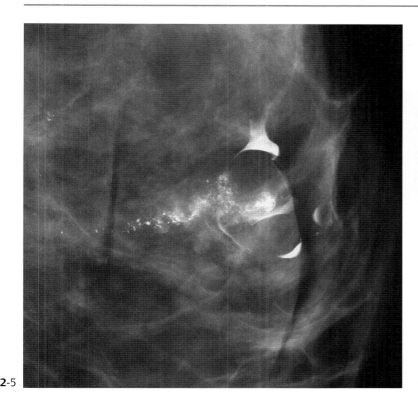

22-5

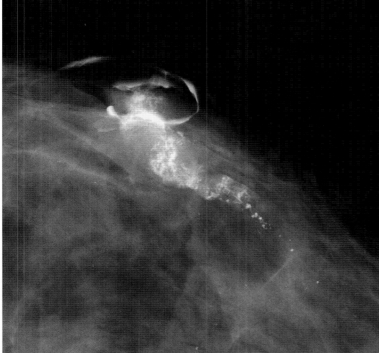

22-6

Ex. **4.22**-5 & 6   Galactography confirms that the crushed stone–like calcifications are localized within a distended duct and not within TDLUs. This indicates that the calcifications most likely represent a benign intraductal process (papilloma), rather than an in situ ductal carcinoma, since an intraductal malignant process should be associated with casting type calcifications instead of crushed stone–like calcification particles. Histological examination of the vacuum-assisted needle biopsy specimen leads to a reliable diagnosis.

Follow-up: At the most recent follow-up examination, 3 years after the biopsy, there was no evidence of malignancy in the left breast.

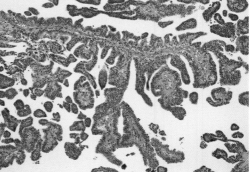

Ex.
4.22-7

Ex. **4.22**-7   Radiographs of the vacuum-assisted needle biopsy specimen containing calcifications.

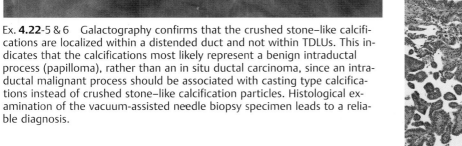

Ex.
4.22-8

Ex.
4.22-9

Ex.
4.22-10

Ex. **4.22**-8 to 10   **Histological diagnosis:** partially calcified benign papillomas. There are no signs of malignancy.

Example 4.23

A 51-year-old woman participated in mammographic screening. She was called back for further work-up of the bilateral calcifications detected on her screening mammograms.

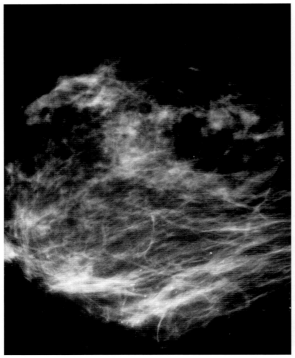

Ex. **4.23**-1

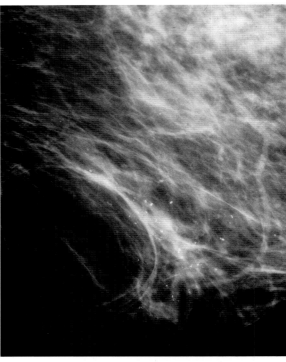

Ex. **4.23**-2

Ex. **4.23**-1 & 2   Detailed images of the right and left breasts, MLO projections. There are numerous calcifications in the lower regions of both breasts. There is no demonstrable tumor mass.

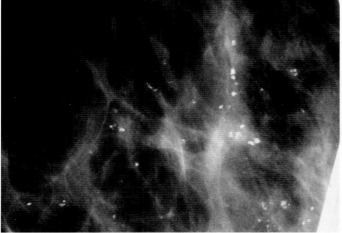

Ex.
4.23-3

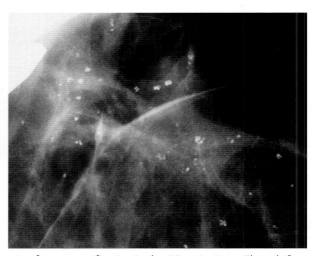

Ex.
4.23

Ex. **4.23**-3 & 4   Right and left breasts, spot compression combined with microfocus magnification in the CC projections. The calcifications are distributed in multiple clusters; their shapes and densities are variable.

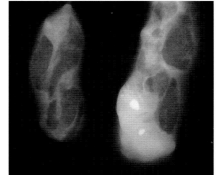

Ex. **4.23**-5   Radiograph of the vacuum-assisted specimen samples, one containing calcifications.

Ex. **4.23**-5

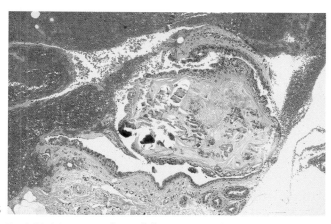

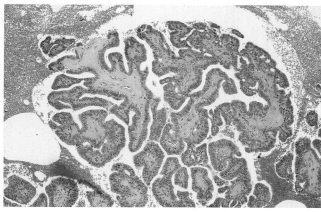

Ex. **4.23**-6

Ex. **4.23**-7

Ex. **4.23**-6 & 7 **Histological diagnosis:** multiple, partially calcified benign papillomas. There are no signs of malignancy.

The patient returned to routine mammography screening, where a gradual increase in the calcifications was observed.

Their appearance 6 years after the biopsy prompted a repeat vacuum-assisted biopsy.

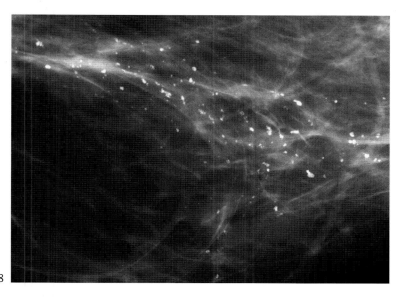

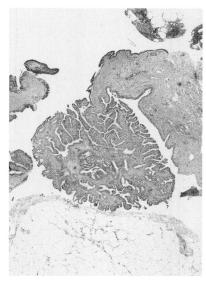

Ex. **4.23**-8

Ex. **4.23**-10

Ex. **4.23**-8 to 10   The most recent mammogram (8) and microfocus magnification (9) of the region with the increasing calcifications, 6 years after the first vacuum-assisted needle biopsy. Histological examination of the repeat vacuum-assisted biopsy specimen (10) once again shows a partially hyalinized papilloma without signs of malignancy.

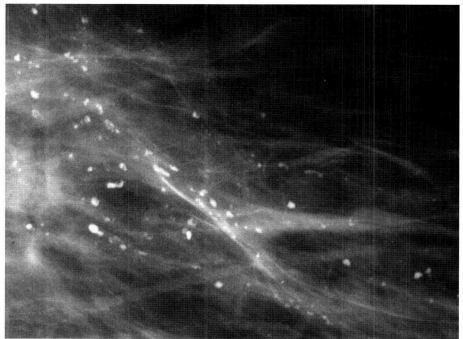

Ex. **4.23**-9

Example 4.24

A 79-year-old woman, referred to mammographic examination because of a palpable, hard lump in the lateral portion of her right breast.

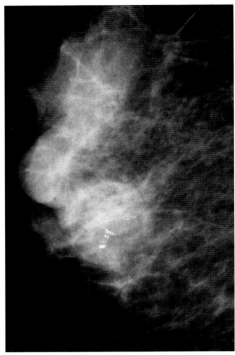

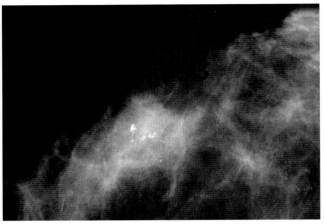

Ex. **4.24**-2

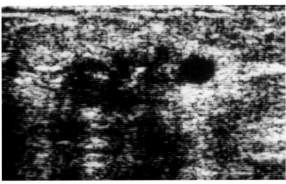

Ex. **4.24**-1

Ex. **4.24**-1 & 2   Right breast, detail of the MLO (1) and CC (2) projections. There is a 15 mm × 13 mm circular, ill-defined lesion containing irregular calcifications. The lesion corresponds to the palpable, hard lump.

Ex. **4.24**-3

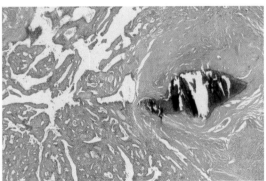

Ex. **4.24**-4

Ex. **4.24**-3 & 4   Ultrasound examination shows a lobulated lesion containing calcifications. 14-gauge core biopsy: a papillary lesion with cell proliferation. Final histology (4): partially calcified and hyalinized papilloma with no signs of malignancy.

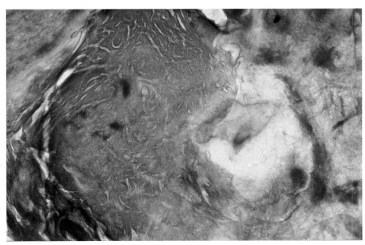

Ex. **4.24**-5   Subgross, thick-section (3D) histology of this partially calcified, benign papilloma.

Ex.
4.24-

Example 4.25

A 28-year-old woman, referred for mammographic evaluation of the multiple, "rosary bead–like" chain of nodules palpable in the lateral portion of the left breast.

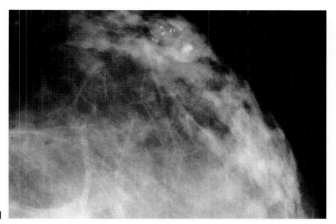 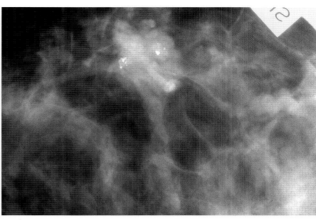

Ex. **4.25**-1

Ex. **4.25**-2

Ex. **4.25**-1 & 2 Left breast, detail of the CC projection (1) and microfocus magnification with spot compression (2). There are numerous low-density circular lesions in the lateral portion of the breast, apparently occupying a lobe. Some of them contain irregular, discernible calcifications. The palpatory finding (rosary bead–like nodules in a lobe) and the low-density multiple circular/oval masses are characteristic of juvenile papillomatosis/Swiss cheese disease, especially when calcifications are present.

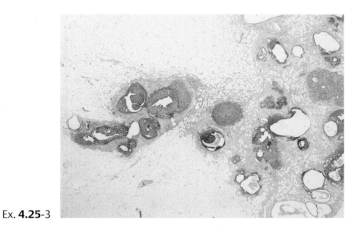 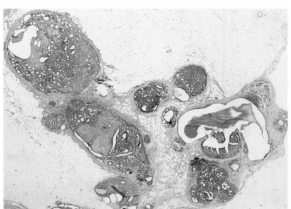

Ex. **4.25**-3

Ex. **4.25**-4

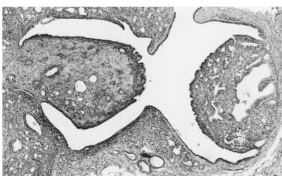 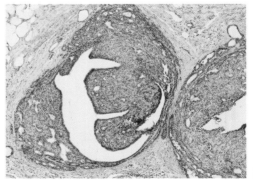

Ex. **4.25**-5

Ex. **4.25**-6

Ex. **4.25**-3 to 6 Histological examination confirms the diagnosis of juvenile papillomatosis / Swiss cheese disease. There was no sign of malignancy. The multiple cystic dilatations associated with papillomatosis explain the mammographic and clinical findings.

Comment

Juvenile papillomatosis, with a secondary name "Swiss cheese disease," was first described by Rosen and colleagues in 1980.[7, 8] This disease consists of numerous cysts of varying sizes, sclerosing adenosis, and papillomatosis with or without severe atypia.

Treatment and follow-up: The patient has attended regular mammographic follow-up for the past 26 years. There has been no evidence of malignancy.

Example 4.26

A 59-year-old asymptomatic woman, screening mammogram. She was called back for evaluation of the tiny, partially calcified mass in the central portion of her right breast.

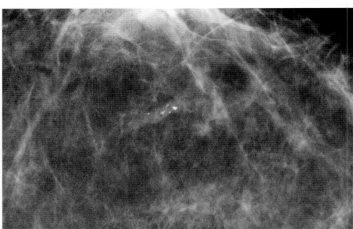

Ex. 4.26-

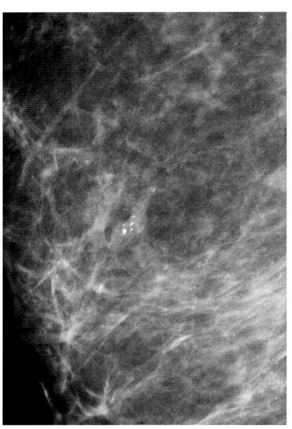

Ex. 4.26-1

Ex. **4.26**-1 & 2   Detail images of the right breast in the MLO (1) and CC (2) projections. There is a < 10 mm, ill-defined, low-density, solitary lesion containing a few irregular calcifications.

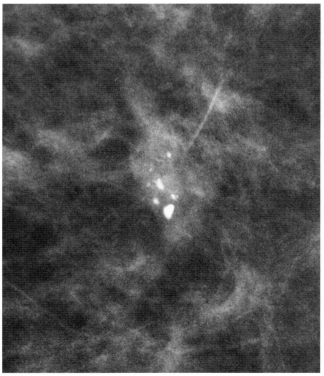

Ex. 4.26-3

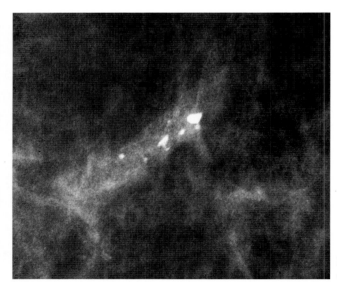

Ex. 4.26-

Ex. **4.26**-3 & 4   Detail images of the right breast, microfocus magnification in the MLO (3) and CC (4) projections. The low-density lesion has indistinct borders and is associated with high-density, irregular calcifications, suggesting malignancy.

This case predates vacuum-assisted biopsy, which is the current procedure of choice. Histological examination of the entire lesion or representative samples is necessary for correct diagnosis.

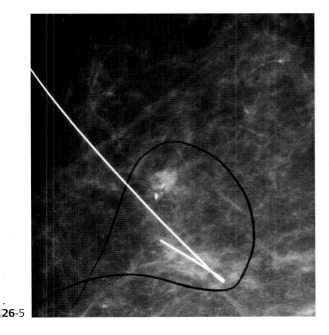

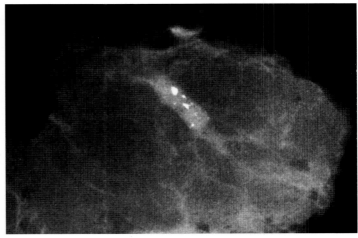

Ex. **4.26**-5

Ex. **4.26**-6

Ex. **4.26**-5 & 6 Preoperative localization mammography (5) and specimen radiography (6).

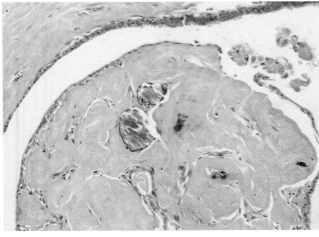

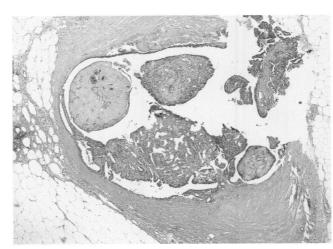

Ex. **4.26**-7

Ex. **4.26**-8

Ex. **4.26**-7 & 8 **Histology** (H&E): involuting, partly hyalinized papilloma with calcifications. There was no evidence of malignancy.

Ex. **4.26**-9 Left breast, CC projection, 10 years after surgery, showing the region with postoperative scar. No abnormality is demonstrable.

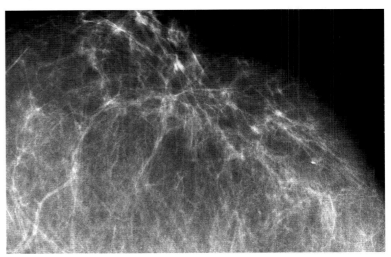

Follow-up: The patient attended regular screening during the next 10 years with no evidence of malignancy (Ex. **4.26**-9).

Ex. **4.26**-9

Chapter 5   The Prognostic Importance of Mammographic Tumor Features

We have classified 871 consecutive cases of 1–14 mm invasive breast cancers into five subgroups according to their mammographic appearance: cases having a stellate or circular tumor without associated calcifications on the mammogram and cases having either casting type, crushed stone–like or powdery calcifications with or without an associated 1–14 mm tumor demonstrable on the mammogram. We have also correlated these mammographic tumor features with long-term outcome. A striking difference has been documented between the surprisingly poor outcome of the subgroup with casting type calcifications and the excellent long-term survival of cases in the four other groups.[1–10]

Our previous volume *Casting Type Calcifications: Sign of a Subtype with Deceptive Features*[3] described in detail the well-defined subgroup having a surprisingly poor prognosis despite its being currently classified as belonging to the size range of small, 1–14 mm tumors. In reality its long-term outcome is comparable to the outcome of much larger and more advanced cancers (ref. 3, p. 226). The survival curves in advanced cancer cases and also in 1–14 mm cancers associated with casting type calcifications show a poor outcome during the first 10 years of follow-up. A strikingly different case fatality rate pattern is seen with 1–14 mm cancers associated with the remaining four mammographic tumor features.

The current volume deals with the subgroup characterized by the presence of **crushed stone–like calcifications on the mammogram**. The long-term outcome of women with 1–14 mm invasive breast cancers associated with crushed stone–like calcifications can be considered excellent. Comparison of the long-term survival curves of cases with casting type calcifications (Fig. **5.1**-1) versus crushed stone–like calcifications (Fig **5.1**-2) shows important differences:

- Size for size, there is a striking difference in outcome.
- Breast cancer-related deaths occurred predominantly during the first 10 years in cases with casting type calcifications (98%, 78%, and 51% survival at 10-year follow-up).
- In the groups with crushed stone–like calcifications, the survival rates were still 100%, 99% and 98% at 15-year follow-up.
- The few deaths that occurred among the in situ cancer cases (3/162) characterized by the presence of crushed stone–like calcifications showed the histological features of neoductgenesis. In these rare cases the tumors had features of in situ cancer but behaved as advanced invasive cancers. The most striking difference can be observed when comparing the fatality rate of 1–14 mm invasive cancers associated with casting type calcifications (22/84) versus crushed stone–like calcifications (2/93).

Since 1–14 mm invasive breast cancers without casting type calcifications have excellent long-term survival, we conclude that neoductgenesis is the single factor that best explains poor outcome in 1–14 mm invasive breast cancers. Once these cases are identified by their characteristic mammographic appearance, the remainder of all 1–14 mm screen-detected invasive breast cancers (> 90% of the total) will have excellent long-term survival. Not only does this emphasize the importance of screening in terms of a significantly better long-term survival of the individual breast cancer patient and in terms of significantly decreased breast cancer mortality in a population, but it also stresses the need for less radical treatment.

An important cause of overtreatment of early-stage breast cancers is the use of inconsistent terminology. Careful comparison of the imaging findings with modern large-section and, most importantly, subgross, thick-section, 3D histology can more accurately describe the precise location of the accumulated cancer cells, which appears to be a decisive factor in determining the final outcome of the mammographically detected, nonpalpable breast cancers. Many examples in this series of books illustrate entirely different disease entities that are unfortunately lumped together under the common term "ductal carcinoma in situ" (DCIS). As Figs. **5.1**-1 & 2 demonstrate, the outcomes of equally small, 1–9 mm and 10–14 mm invasive tumors associated with two different types of "DCIS" may be significantly different. Mammographic analysis confirmed by examination of the large, subgross, thick-section histology specimen can make a distinction between the malignant process that is confined to the TDLUs (cases with excellent outcome) and cases localized in the duct system and in neoducts (cases with a strikingly poor outcome).

Giving the name "ductal" to a malignant process that is localized to the TDLUs is confusing. The use of expressions such as "extensive intraductal component" (EIC) of an invasive cancer further exacerbates the confusion since it fails to make the important distinction between the in situ component localized in the TDLUs and that localized in the ducts. The long-term outcome curves based upon the mammographic tumor features in combination with careful analysis of the large thin- and thick-section, modern histology specimens clearly show that this distinction has profound clinical relevance. In the new era, when the majority of breast cancers are detected mammographically, it is important to make full use of the mammographic tumor features when planning the management of breast cancer patients.

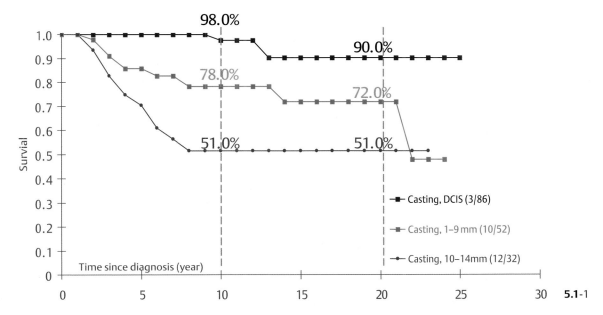

Fig. **5.1**-1   Cumulative long-term survival of 40–69-year-old women with breast cancer associated with casting type calcifications.

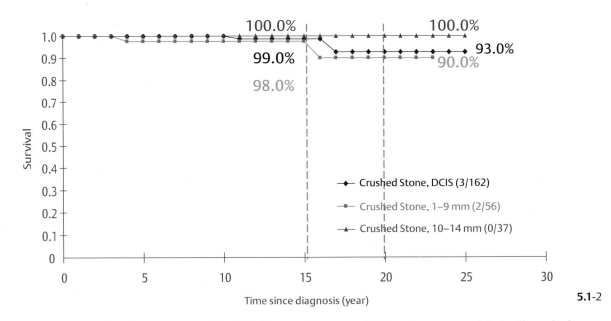

Fig. **5.1**-2   Cumulative long-term survival of 40–69-year-old women with breast cancer associated with crushed stone–like type calcifications.

References

■ Chapter 1

1 Tabár L, Tot T, Dean PB. *Breast Cancer: Early Detection with Mammography. Casting Type Calcifications: Sign of a Subtype with Deceptive Features.* Stuttgart: Georg Thieme Verlag; 2007.
2 Lagios MD. Classification of duct carcinoma in situ (DCIS) with a characterization of high grade lesions: defining cohorts for chemoprevention trials. *J Cell Biochem Suppl.* 1996;25:108–11. [Review].
3 Tot T. The limited prognostic value of measuring and grading small invasive breast carcinomas: the whole sick lobe versus the details within it. *Med Sci Monit.* 2006 Aug;12(8):RA170–5. [Review].
4 American College of Radiology (ACR). *Breast Imaging Reporting and Data System Atlas* (BI-RADS® Atlas). Reston, VA: American College of Radiology; 2003.
5 Hughes LE, Mansel RE, Webster DJ. Aberrations of normal development and involution (ANDI): a new perspective on pathogenesis and nomenclature of benign breast disorders. *Lancet.* 1987 Dec 5;2(8571):1316–9.

■ Chapter 2

1 Jensen HM, Rice JR, Wellings SR. Preneoplastic Lesions in the Human Breast. *Science.* 1976;191:295–7.
2 Tabár L, Tot T, Dean PB. *Breast Cancer: The Art and Science of Early Detection with Mammography. Perception, Interpretation, Histopathologic Correlation.* Stuttgart: Georg Thieme Verlag; 2005.
3 Tabár L, Tot T, Dean PB. *Breast Cancer: Early Detection with Mammography. Casting Type Calcifications: Sign of a Subtype with Deceptive Features.* Stuttgart: Georg Thieme Verlag; 2007.

■ Chapter 3

1 Sapino A, Frigerio A, Peterse JL, Arisio R, Coluccia C, Bussolati G. Mammographically detected in situ lobular carcinomas of the breast. *Virchows Arch.* 2000 May;436(5):421–30.
2 Georgian-Smith D, Lawton TJ. Calcifications of lobular carcinoma in situ of the breast: radiological-pathological correlation. *AJR Am J Roentgenol.* 2001 May;176(5):1255–9.
3 Fadare O, Dadmanesh F, Alvarado-Cabrero I, et al. Lobular intraepithelial neoplasia [lobular carcinoma in situ] with comedo-type necrosis: A clinicopathological study of 18 cases. *Am J Surg Pathol.* 2006 Nov;30(11): 1445–53.

■ Chapter 4

1 Hughes LE, Mansel RE, Webster DJ. Aberrations of normal development and involution (ANDI): a new perspective on pathogenesis and nomenclature of benign breast disorders. *Lancet.* 1987 Dec 5;2(8571):1316–9.
2 Lanyi M. [Differential diagnosis of the microcalcifications. The calcified mastopathic microcyst (author's translation; in German)]. *Radiologe.* 1977 May;17(5):217–8.
3 Sickles EA, Abele JS. Milk of calcium within tiny benign breast cysts. *Radiology.* 1981 Dec;141(3):655–8.

4 Bannister FA, Hey MH. Report on some crystalline components of the Weddell Sea deposits. *Discovery Repts.* 1936;13:60–9.
5 Frappart L, Boudeulle M, Boumendil J, et al. Structure and composition of microcalcifications in benign and malignant lesions of the breast: study by light microscopy, transmission and scanning electron microscopy, microprobe analysis, and X-ray diffraction. *Hum Pathol.* 1984 Sep;15(9): 880–9.
6 Frouge C, Meunier M, Guinebretiere JM, et al. Polyhedral microcalcifications at mammography: histological correlation with calcium oxalate. *Radiology.* 1993 Mar;186(3):681–4.
7 Rosen PP, Cantrell B, Mullen DL, DePalo A. Juvenile papillomatosis (Swiss cheese disease) of the breast. *Am J Surg Pathol.*1980 Feb;4(1):3–12.
8 Rosen PP, Kimmel M. Juvenile papillomatosis of the breast. A follow-up study of 41 patients having biopsies before 1979. *Am J Clin Pathol.* 1990 May;93(5):599–603.

■ Chapter 5

1 Tabár L, Chen HH, Duffy SW, et al. A novel method for prediction of long-term outcome of women with T1a, T1b, and 10–14 mm invasive breast cancers: a prospective study. *Lancet.* 2000;355(9202): 429–33.
2 Tabár L, Chen Tony HH, Yen Amy MF, et al. Mammographic tumor features can predict long-term outcomes reliably in women with 1–14-mm invasive breast carcinoma. *Cancer.* 2004;101(8): 1745–59.
3 Tabár L, Tot T, Dean PB. *Breast Cancer: Early Detection with Mammography. Casting Type Calcifications: Sign of a Subtype with Deceptive Features.* Stuttgart: Georg Thieme Verlag; 2007.
4 Eusebi V, Feudale E, Foschini MP, et al. Long-term follow-up of in situ carcinoma of the breast. *Semin Diagn Pathol.* 1994;11(3):223–35.
5 Malik HZ, Wilkinson L, George WD, Purushotham AD. Preoperative mammographic features predict clinicopathological risk factors for the development of local recurrence in breast cancer. *Breast.* 2000;9(6):329–33.
6 Thurfjell E, Thurfjell MG, Lindgren A. Mammographic finding as a predictor of survival in 1–9 mm invasive breast cancers, worse prognosis for cases presenting as calcifications alone. *Breast Cancer Res Treat.* 2001;67(2):177–80.
7 Zunzunegui RG, Chung MA, Oruwari J, Golding D, Marchant DJ, Cady B. Casting-type calcifications with invasion and high-grade ductal carcinoma in situ: a more aggressive disease? *Arch Surg.* 2003;138(5):537–40.
8 Yagata H, Harigaya K, Suzuki M, et al. Comedonecrosis is an unfavorable marker in node-negative invasive breast carcinoma. *Pathol Int.* 2003;53(8):501–6.
9 Peacock C, Given-Wilson RM, Duffy SW. Mammographic casting-type calcification associated with small screen-detected invasive breast cancers: is this a reliable prognostic indicator? *Clin Radiol.* 2004;59(2):165–70.
10 Pálka I, Ormándi K, Gaál S, Boda K, Kahán Z. Casting-type calcifications on the mammogram suggest a higher probability of early relapse and death among high-risk breast cancer patients. *Acta Oncol.* 2007;46(8):1178–1183.

Subject Index

Notes
The abbreviation TDLUs in sub entries refers to terminal ductal lobar units.
Page numbers in **bold** refer to tables.
Page numbers in *italics* refer to figures including those used in the examples.

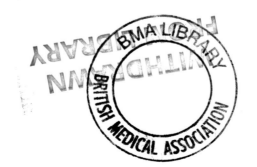